Obstetrics ar
Gynaecology

AN ILLUSTRATED COLOUR TEXT

Commissioning Editor: Ellen Green
Project Development Manager: Jim Killgore/Helen Leng
Project Manager: Nancy Arnott
Designer: Sarah Russell

Obstetrics and Gynaecology

AN ILLUSTRATED COLOUR TEXT

Joan Pitkin BSc FRCS FRCOG
Consultant Obstetrician and Gynaecologist
Northwick Park & St Mark's Hospital
NW London Hospitals NHS Trust
Harrow
Honorary Senior Lecturer, Faculty of Medicine
Imperial College
London
UK

Alison B. Peattie FRCOG
Consultant Obstetrician and Gynaecologist
The Countess of Chester Hospital
Chester
UK

Brian A. Magowan MRCOG
Consultant Obstetrician and Gynaecologist
Borders General Hospital
Melrose
UK

Illustrated by Ian Ramsden

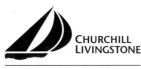
CHURCHILL
LIVINGSTONE

EDINBURGH   LONDON   NEW YORK   OXFORD   PHILADELPHIA   ST LOUIS   SYDNEY   TORONTO   2003

CHURCHILL LIVINGSTONE
An imprint of Elsevier Science Limited

First published 2003

ISBN 044305035X

British Library Cataloguing in Publication Data
A catalogue record for this book is available from the British Library

Library of Congress Cataloging in Publication Data
A catalog record for this book is available from the Library of Congress

> **Note**
> Medical knowledge is constantly changing. Standard safety precautions must be followed, but as new research and clinical experience broaden our knowledge, changes in treatment and drug therapy may become necessary or appropriate. Readers are advised to check the most current product information provided by the manufacturer of each drug to be administered to verify the recommended dose, the method and duration of administration, and contraindications. It is the responsibility of the practitioner, relying on experience and knowledge of the patient, to determine dosages and the best treatment for each individual patient. Neither the publisher nor the authors assumes any liability for any injury and/or damage to persons or property arising from this publication.

ELSEVIER SCIENCE
your source for books, journals and multimedia in the health sciences
www.elsevierhealth.com

Cover image
Infertility: false-colour hysterosalpingogram of the abdomen of a woman suffering from blocked fallopian tubes.

Credit
Science Photo Library

The publisher's policy is to use **paper manufactured from sustainable forests**

Printed in China

Preface

Obstetrics and gynaecology is a dynamic and rapidly changing speciality. Great advances have been made in prenatal diagnosis, the management of infertility and contraceptive techniques. The introduction of minimally invasive surgical procedures has reduced bed occupancy and analgesic requirements allowing women to return home more rapidly. Service delivery development, required to meet improving NHS standards, has seen the introduction of a new multidisciplinary approach, new roles for midwives and the emergence of the gynaecological nurse practitioner.

Obstetrics and gynaecology is both rewarding and demanding. Maternity care challenges all of us to be more women-centred and to provide similar standards of care worldwide. Nowhere else in medicine are we faced with the exhilaration of the arrival of new life; equally, our speciality remains the highest area for litigation – an added burden for clinicians – so that audit, clinical governance and an evidence-based approach are especially pertinent.

There continues to be areas of great controversy surrounding the speciality, especially assisted conception, termination of pregnancy and hormone replacement therapy. In no other branch of medicine are such private and intimate details discussed regarding dysparunia, vaginal discharge and psychosexual problems. The trust placed in the clinician by the woman is a privilege to be valued and respected.

This book aims to encompass the breadth and depth of our speciality in a vivid, easy-to-use fashion. Based on a double-spread format for each topic, the subject comes alive through the generous use of illustrations but retains considerable up-to-date detail and covers some topics overlooked in other texts. The use of tables and 'key-point' boxes facilitates easy reference. We hope it will be instructive and enjoyable to read.

London
2003

Joan Pitkin
Alison Peattie
Brian Magowan

Acknowledgements

We would like to acknowledge all those who have lent material, the secretarial support received and the patience of the publishers and our long-suffering partners.

London   Joan Pitkin
2003   Alison Peattie
              Brian Magowan

Contents

Obstetrics

Gynaecology

Normal pregnancy – physiological signs and symptoms

Changes to the maternal physiology in pregnancy (Fig. 1) allow maximum efficiency of fetal growth and metabolism. As this is very different from the normal maternal physiology it cannot be equally advantageous. Normally homeostatic mechanisms, after detecting a change, return the organism to the resting state, but manipulation of the mother's homeostatic mechanisms is done by the fetus in anticipation of its needs as it grows. So, many changes are noted by the mother in early pregnancy when the actual needs of the fetus are minimal.

Changes to the energy balance and respiratory control occur via the hypothalamus and are typically mediated by progesterone, while changes to the more peripheral functions such as blood volume, blood constituents and coagulation, and total body water are mediated by oestrogen.

Table 1 **Changes in the cardiovascular system**	
Change	**Results/requirements**
Increased blood volume 2600 to 3800 ml	Raised from early in pregnancy (8-9 weeks)
Increased red cell mass 1400 to 1650-1800 ml	Needs ready iron supply for optimal rise (see p. 3)
Decreased haemoglobin (Hb) and haematocrit	Proportional to the above two factors- termed the physiological anaemia of pregnancy
Increased resting cardiac output 4.5 to 6 l/min	Early rise maintained through pregnancy and labour. Declines in puerperium
Raised heart rate 80 to 90 bpm	Needs increased stroke volume
Increased oxygen consumption by 30-50 ml/min	Increased cardiac output needed to distribute this
Decrease in total peripheral resistance (TPR) to parallel rise in cardiac output (CO)	Vasodilatation - also allows dissipation of heat produced by the fetus
Mid trimester fall in blood pressure due to greater drop in TPR than rise in CO	Need to know blood pressure (BP) in first trimester when assessing a raised BP in pregnancy (see p. 20)
Increased incidence of heart murmurs due to increased flow across valves	Need to distinguish pathology from functional murmurs – consider antibiotics in labour for structural heart disease

Cardiovascular system

The main changes seen in the cardiovascular system are shown in Table 1. At term the distribution of the raised cardiac output is:

- Uterus 400 ml/min extra
- Kidneys 300 ml/min extra
- Skin 500 ml/min extra
- Elsewhere 300 ml/min extra.

Urinary tract

The anatomy of the renal tract changes in pregnancy. Cellular hypertrophy causes a 1 cm increase in renal length. The diameter of the ureters is increased due to the relaxant effect of progesterone on the smooth muscle and in later pregnancy there may be ureteric obstruction due to uterine enlargement. Increased filtration of glucose may lead to glycosuria as the proximal tubular ability to reabsorb glucose is overloaded. The patient is aware of urinary frequency due to increased renal blood flow and the pressure of the pregnant uterus on her bladder in early pregnancy. There is a diuresis immediately following delivery of the placenta as the vascular bed is contracted down by nearly 500 ml. Table 2 lists the changes in values seen during pregnancy.

Gastrointestinal tract

Progesterone causes smooth muscle relaxation and thus decreased gut motility with adverse effects for the mother. The resultant constipation can be very uncomfortable and may be exacerbated by treatment with oral iron therapy. Straining at stool may

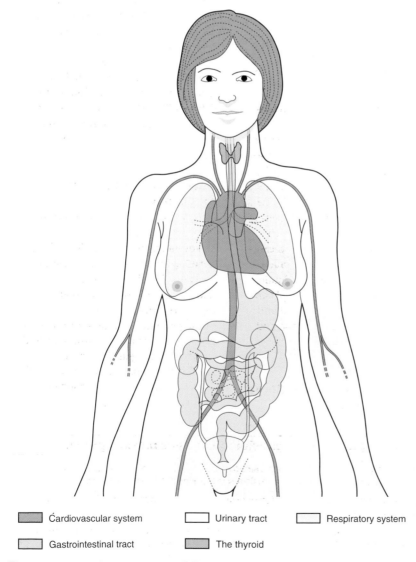

Cardiovascular system   Urinary tract   Respiratory system

Gastrointestinal tract   The thyroid

Fig. 1 **Maternal systems changed by pregnancy.**

Table 2 Changes in values	
Renal blood flow increases	From 1.2 l/min to 1.5 l/min
Glomerular filtration rate rises due to raised blood flow	140 ml/min up to 170 ml/min
Serum urea falls due to increased filtration	4.3 mmol/l down to 3.1 mmol/l
Serum creatinine falls due to greater filtration	73 mmol/l falls to 47 mmol/l

increase the pain of haemorrhoids caused by raised pressure in the venous system with blockage to venous drainage due to the enlarged gravid uterus.

Heartburn due to reflux of acid stomach contents is common in pregnancy. It is caused by relaxation of the gastro-oesophageal sphincter combined with delayed gastric emptying. Diagnosis of acute surgical problems such as appendicitis can prove difficult due to the altered site of intra-abdominal contents with the enlarged uterus displacing organs upwards and outwards.

The thyroid

Many patients may have enlargement of their thyroid during pregnancy as a result of changes in the renal handling of plasma inorganic iodide. Raised filtration of this causes a fall in plasma levels and the thyroid hypertrophies in an attempt to maintain normal iodide concentrations. Development of a goitre in pregnancy may indicate mild relative iodine deficiency.

Body water

Total body water increases by 8.5 l : 6 l distributed to placenta, amniotic fluid, blood volume, uterus and breasts – 2.5 l as extracellular water causing oedema. It is normal in pregnancy to experience dependent oedema (legs). The ground substance of the connective tissues stores much of the increase making ligaments softer, which can result in backache due to lumbar lordosis putting abnormal strain on the lower back and separation of the symphysis pubis causing pain during walking.

Tingling of the fingers supplied by the median nerve may be due to extra fluid causing compression as the nerve passes under the flexor retinaculum. A beneficial effect is the increased stretchability of the cervix noted during labour.

Respiratory system

The respiratory centre is reset to less than 4 kPa pCO_2 (from 6 kPa) under the influence of progesterone, enabling the fetus to offload its waste gas. Ventilation is increased by 40% in the first trimester due to increased tidal

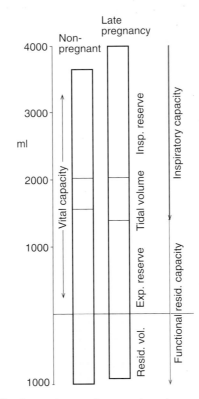

Fig. 2 **Respiratory changes of pregnancy.**

volume but as pregnancy progresses there is a decrease in total lung capacity by 200 ml due to uterine size. There is no change noted in expiratory peak flow rate during pregnancy (Fig. 2)

Dyspnoea noted in early pregnancy may be due to the lowered pCO_2 which the mother is unused to. Mild exercise may reduce pCO_2 to a level which reduces cerebral blood flow and causes dizziness. The low pCO_2 is paralleled by low plasma bicarbonate to maintain normal pH. The resulting low plasma osmolality remains uncorrected and may be responsible for polyuria and thirst in early pregnancy.

Energy balance

The average weight gain in pregnancy is 12 kg in the second half of

pregnancy. This is distributed between the fetus, uterus, breasts, increased blood volume and body fat. The body fat is distributed centripetally and is increased due to both extra intake and decreased utilization due to the more sedentary lifestyle dictated by pregnancy.

Glucose

The handling of a glucose load is altered during pregnancy with the rise higher than in non-pregnant females and elevated for longer. However, insulin levels are also raised above the usual – pregnancy is a time of insulin resistance most marked in the third trimester. Fasting plasma glucose is lowered in early pregnancy but rises in weeks 16–32. These facts mean that gestational diabetes is most likely to be detected in the third trimester.

Iron

As the red cell mass increases (18%) by less than the blood volume there is a fall in haemoglobin as pregnancy progresses. A lowered mean cell volume (MCV) is the most sensitive indicator of iron deficiency – serum iron is low and total iron-binding capacity raised. Routine iron supplementation is associated with an increased red cell mass of 30% and debate still exists as to whether to offer routine iron to all pregnant women or to treat those found to be iron deficient.

Coagulation changes in pregnancy

A hypercoagulable state exists from early in the first trimester, thought to be advantageous to meet the sudden haemostatic demand as the placenta separates. The increased ability to neutralize heparin in late pregnancy rapidly returns to normal on delivery of the placenta – important to note in patients on heparin therapy. Increased levels of fibrinogen, factors VII, VIII, and X are found, with decreased levels of factors XI, XIII and fibrinolytic activity.

Normal pregnancy – physiological signs and symptoms

- Changes to maternal physiology *anticipate* the needs of the fetus rather than the usual mechanism where change returns physiology to the normal state once disturbed.
- Progesterone causes relaxation of smooth muscle, so changes are seen in the urinary and gastrointestinal tracts.
- Many symptoms the mother experiences due to these physiological alterations are normally signs of disease. Therefore, interpret symptoms in pregnancy with caution.

Antenatal care

Aims of antenatal care

The main aim of antenatal care is to have a healthy mother and a healthy baby at the end of the pregnancy. Antenatal care thus becomes risk assessment – trying to identify from the patient's history and from examination whether there are any factors which may have an adverse effect on the patient or her fetus during the pregnancy and the correction of these problems.

Pattern of antenatal care

The traditional pattern for antenatal care was laid out in the early 20th century with monthly visits until 28 weeks' gestation, visits every 2 weeks until 36 weeks and weekly visits until delivery. This entails 12 to 14 visits per pregnancy and is probably more than is necessary to enable detection of the major complications of pregnancy such as hypertension and fetal growth restriction. The usual aim is to hold the booking visit early in the pregnancy – if possible in the first trimester – to enable advice to be given on diet, smoking, alcohol, and medication, much of which might be more appropriately dealt with under pre-conceptual counselling (see p. 6). A detailed history is usually taken at this visit enabling identification of factors which would place the patient at higher risk of perinatal mortality:

Epidemiological factors
- teenager – at risk of hypertension, intrauterine growth restriction (IUGR)
- elderly primigravida (over 35 years) – increases in fetal chromosomal abnormalities, perinatal mortality, and obstetric intervention.

Past obstetric history
- previous stillbirth or neonatal death (NND)
- previous fetal abnormality
- preterm labour or precipitate labour
- caesarean section
- pregnancy complication likely to be repeated – pre-eclampsia, IUGR, abruption, postpartum haemorrhage (PPH).

Maternal medical history
- cardiac disease, diabetes, thyroid disorder, drug misuse, renal problem, thromboembolic disorder, hypertension, epilepsy (see p. 25)
- factors on examination: cardiac

murmur, hypertension, size of mother (large with risk of gestational diabetes, small with risk of IUGR), pelvic mass, uterine size not in keeping with dates.

Clinical examination

Few women have had any medical examination since starting school and routine examination to exclude disease should cover cardiovascular, respiratory, renal and locomotor systems. Clinical examination to exclude breast disease is supplemented in pregnancy by an examination of the nipples so that the woman who wishes to breast feed may be prepared, with treatment for inverted nipples as appropriate (nipple shields or massage). The presence of varicose veins should be managed by adequate support hosiery during pregnancy to prevent worsening varicosities with the possibility of thrombophlebitis.

Palpation of the pregnant abdomen

This skill is developed with much practice but a structured approach will ensure maximum information is obtained.

- **Inspection** – look for the degree of distension; the presence of umbilical eversion suggests excessive distension (consider twins or polyhydramnios). Watch for fetal movements (presence confirms this is distension due to pregnancy and not an ovarian cyst). The linea alba may become pigmented during pregnancy – called a linea nigra.
- **Fundus** – determination of the position of the fundus (uppermost part of the uterus) is with the ulnar border of the left hand palpating gradually down from the xiphisternum.
- **Symphysis fundal height** (SFH) – measured with a tape measure from the fundus through the umbilicus to the upper border of the symphysis pubis. The measurement in centimetres in the third trimester corresponds approximately to the number of weeks' gestation (± 3 weeks).
- **Lateral palpation** – to determine the lie (longitudinal axis of the fetus with respect to the longitudinal axis of the uterus) both hands are placed

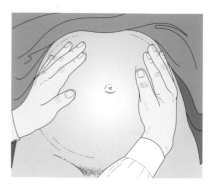

Fig. 1 **Lateral palpation of the pregnant abdomen.**

flat, one on either side of the maternal abdomen (Fig. 1). The fetus is then gently ballotted between the hands to ascertain the fetal parts. The lie may be longitudinal (most commonly), oblique or transverse (see p. 53). The volume of amniotic fluid is described as clinically normal when fetal parts can be felt through a fluid cushion, increased (clinical polyhydramnios) when fluid prevents determination of the fetal parts, or decreased (clinical oligohydramnios) when fetal parts can easily be felt through the abdominal wall.

- **Presenting part** – both hands are used to palpate the lower pole of the uterus and determine what fetal part lies there (Fig. 2). It is usual to decide whether the presenting part is engaged (widest presenting diameter has passed through the pelvic inlet) or not engaged. Alternatively with a cephalic presentation you may say how many fifths of the head you can feel (Fig. 2).
- **Fetal health** – auscultation for the fetal heart with a Pinard's stethoscope or Doppler hand-held device completes the examination. Maternal reporting on fetal movements may replace listening for the fetal heart.

Presentation of the findings

It is usual to start with a one-line summary of your history details – for example: Mrs X is a 30-year-old, para 2+0 at 36 weeks with raised blood pressure. On examination the abdomen is distended compatible with pregnancy and old striae are noted.

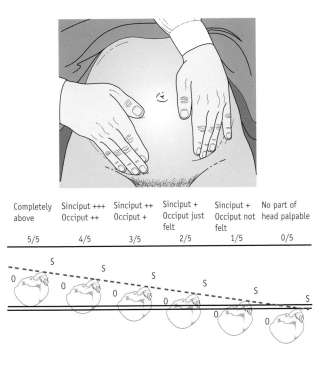

Completely above	Sinciput +++ Occiput ++	Sinciput ++ Occiput +	Sinciput + Occiput just felt	Sinciput + Occiput not felt	No part of head palpable
5/5	4/5	3/5	2/5	1/5	0/5

Fig. 2 **The relationship between abdominal palpation of the presenting part and degree of engagement.**

The SFH is 35 cm (1), with a longitudinal lie (2) of a singleton infant (3). There is a cephalic presentation (4), 3/5 head palpable (5), fetal heart sounds heard (6) and an adequate liquor volume (7). (Remember – 7 points to relate regarding your examination.)

The antenatal visit

Enquiry as to the mother's well-being and whether fetal movements have been satisfactory often opens the discussion at an antenatal visit. Some units will ask mothers to keep a fetal movement chart after 28 weeks. This is based on the finding that the movements diminish or disappear up to 24 hours before fetal demise. A 'count to ten' chart is kept with recording of 10 movements from 09.00 – if fewer than 10 movements are noted by 21.00 the mother is asked to contact her local hospital and attend for fetal assessment (usually a CTG).

Blood pressure is measured and urine tested for proteinuria. The development of hypertension in later pregnancy may have profound effects on fetal well-being and maternal health (see p. 20). Oedema is common in later pregnancy but is usually peripheral.

All recent tests (Table 1) should be reviewed and treated as required. Anaemia may develop, needing iron therapy. Rhesus negative patients need antibody checks at 28 and 34 weeks. Examination of the abdomen to check for normal growth of the fetus and to determine its position is then carried out. A growth scan may be requested if the fetus is smaller than expected. This can be repeated at 2-weekly intervals to ensure a reasonable growth rate. A larger than expected uterus may be due to polyhydramnios.

In the primigravid patient the presenting part should be engaged by 37 weeks, so check to exclude placenta praevia or fetal abnormality if the head is high. As the mother comes closer to labour she may have worries she wishes to discuss. Some draw up a birth plan which needs careful discussion of

Table 1	**Blood and urine tests in pregnancy**
Tests	**Interpretation**
Haemoglobin	Anaemia should be corrected before labour
Sickle cell screen	For Afro-Caribbeans ± prenatal diagnosis
Haemoglobin electrophoresis	For thalassaemia (see p. 34)
Rhesus status and antibody titres	Rhesus negative will need monitoring
Rubella titres	Most will be immune as vaccinated in school
Hepatitis B	Routine testing: if positive check HIV status
HIV antibodies	Only tested after counselling
FTA and TPHA	Allows treatment to prevent congenital syphilis
Urine for protein	Treatment needed for infection or bacteriuria
Urine for sugar	Renal threshold decreased therefore frequently positive even if serum glucose normal

any points where the mother's wishes diverge from accepted principles.

Mothercare and parentcraft classes are offered in developed countries, though in the developing world facilities are more variable, to prepare the mother for labour by ensuring understanding of the process. Fear of the unknown enhances perceived pain (see p. 70). Teaching on breathing techniques to help the sense of control during contractions is set alongside teaching on posture when lifting and how to lessen backache. A visit to the delivery ward may be reassuring. Baby handling is taught to both parents and feeding covers the benefits of breast feeding.

Much of the above will be impossible to achieve in developing countries where blood sampling may be limited to only haemoglobin assessment and a test for HIV status. There may be no ultrasound facility. Care personnel will therefore have different aims in delivering antenatal care. All women should receive iron orally (see p. 32) and folic acid. Regular antimalarial prophylaxis in endemic areas has been shown to reduce the incidence of anaemia and increase birthweight. As hypertension is a major cause of maternal mortality, blood pressure screening may save lives. Female circumcision is common in some countries and necessitates discussion about how to avoid damage at delivery, perhaps with elective incision before labour starts.

Delivery itself may not have any formally qualified person present, the traditional birth attendant having trained by observing a more experienced birth attendant in action. In many countries training programmes for traditional birth attendants have been developed as a means of increasing the quality of care available for women and children, under the guidance of the World Health Organization.

Antenatal care

- Antenatal care is risk assessment.
- The quality of antenatal care delivered correlates with the perinatal mortality.
- Antenatal care covers all aspects of the mother's life whilst pregnant.
- There are seven key findings on palpation of a pregnant abdomen.

Pre-conceptual counselling

Pre-conceptual counselling is helpful in a wide variety of circumstances. There is potential for general advice, an opportunity to plan care in those with background medical disease, a chance to review those with previous obstetric complications and a discussion with those at increased risk of fetal anomaly. In reality, what should ideally be pre-conceptual counselling is often carried out in the first trimester of the pregnancy.

General

Mothers at extremes of reproductive age are at increased risk of obstetric complications, particularly hypertensive disorders, and they carry an increased perinatal mortality. Smoking also increases the perinatal mortality and should ideally be stopped. Alcohol may reduce fertility and is also a potential teratogen. Poor nutrition is rare in the UK, but significant maternal malnutrition is associated with intrauterine growth restriction (IUGR) and subsequent risks to the offspring of coronary heart disease, non-insulin-dependent diabetes and stroke (Fetal Origins Hypothesis).

Daily folic acid taken from before conception reduces the recurrence risk of neural tube defects in those who have had a previously affected child (Fig. 1). A pre-conceptual prophylactic dose for all pregnant women probably also offers some protection. There are, at present, no known teratogenic effects from folate.

Medical

Chronic maternal disease may have a deleterious effect on fertility that may lessen as the disease process itself improves. Maternal disease can affect the fetus, and the pregnancy itself may affect the disease. See particularly SLE (p. 24), Diabetes (p. 28), HIV(p. 16), Renal disorders (p. 26), Thromboembolic disease (p. 42) and Thyroid disorders (p. 27).

It is rare to advise against pregnancy in those with cardiac disease, although those with fixed pulmonary output may be advised that the risks to their own health are too great (e.g. in those with pulmonary hypertension). Active SLE nephritis is associated with significant maternal and perinatal mortality, and in particular with a risk of pre-eclampsia.

Those on warfarin for valvular problems or venous thromboembolic disease are at increased risk of teratogenic problems (particularly midfacial hypoplasia). Consideration should be given to timing of pregnancy and whether a change to heparin, at least in very early pregnancy, is appropriate. As anticonvulsants for epilepsy may also be teratogenic (Fig. 2), seizure control with a single drug regime is ideal or, if seizure-free for 2–3 years, drug withdrawal may be considered (this may have implications for the patient's work and/or driving licence). Pre-conceptual folate supplements should be given because anticonvulsants lead to a reduction in serum folate.

Obstetric

Women who have experienced obstetrical difficulties in a previous pregnancy are often anxious to talk these through and consider the likelihood of recurrence. This is frequently a listening exercise so that anxieties and occasionally anger can be expressed, especially in cases of previous fetal or neonatal loss. An explanation followed by discussion of

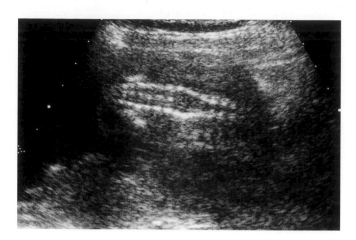

Fig. 1 **Spina bifida – large lumbosacral myelomeningocele.** Folic acid should ideally be started pre-conceptually.

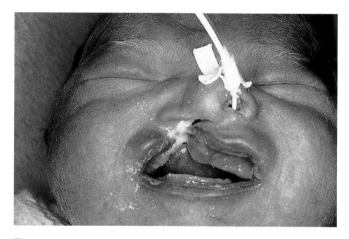

Fig. 2 **Anticonvulsants are associated with neural tube defects, cardiac and craniofacial defect.** The figure shows a unilateral cleft lip.

possible recurrence risks and a plan for the next pregnancy are useful. It is also an opportunity to identify those with abnormal grief reactions who might benefit from further counselling before considering another pregnancy.

Pre-eclampsia tends to improve with subsequent pregnancies, with the possible exception of severe pre-term disease. The incidence of proteinuric pre-eclampsia in a second pregnancy is 10–15 times greater if there was pre-eclampsia in the first pregnancy compared to those with a normal first pregnancy. It has been suggested that low-dose aspirin taken from early pregnancy (< 17 weeks and probably from the first trimester) may reduce the incidence of IUGR or perinatal mortality in those with previous severe disease. Studies in this area have provided conflicting evidence.

Those who have had a previous difficult instrumental delivery usually have a much more straightforward delivery next time around, but may occasionally request an elective caesarean section. This is controversial, and careful consideration of the advantages and disadvantages is required (see p. 56). In general, those with a previous caesarean section for a non-recurrent indication, e.g. breech, fetal distress or relative cephalopelvic disproportion secondary to fetal malposition, should be offered a trial of labour, but repeat elective caesarean section may be considered in certain circumstances.

In situations where there has been previous IUGR or an intrauterine death, subsequent management depends on the cause and the estimated likelihood of recurrence. More intensive antenatal monitoring is usually offered and the outcome is usually good, particularly when the loss was 'unexplained'.

Risk of fetal anomaly

Those who have had a previous baby with a fetal anomaly are often anxious to know the risk of this happening again and whether any prenatal testing can be carried out. This discussion has usually taken place after the problem pregnancy, but further discussion is sometimes welcomed.

A couple who have had a previous Down's syndrome baby, or fetal loss from Down's syndrome, carry a risk of 0.75% above their baseline age-related risk (p. 11). Down's, however, may rarely also be inherited from a parental translocation (e.g. 14 : 21) or mosaicism, which increases this recurrence risk significantly. The complexities of these issues often require specialist advice from a clinical geneticist (Fig. 3). This also applies to many other abnormalities, for example congenital heart disease: while in general the recurrence risk of this is ≈ 5%, it is dependent on the family history, drug history and whether the anomaly was isolated or part of some other syndrome. Other structural abnormalities, for example Potter's syndrome or diaphragmatic herniae, usually carry a low recurrence risk.

There may be a family history of certain conditions, and others have a racial predisposition, e.g. Tay–Sachs disease in Ashkenazi Jews or haemoglobinopathies in those of Mediterranean origin. Invasive fetal testing may be appropriate after parental gene testing if both partners are homozygous for a recessive condition. It is possible to test for some of the trinucleotide repeat disorders (e.g. myotonic dystrophy, Huntington's chorea or fragile X syndrome) but the ethics of such testing is complex and it is not necessarily desirable in every couple. Other autosomal recessive conditions are also amenable to testing, e.g. the screening of saliva for the commoner mutant alleles of cystic fibrosis (the

commonest being Δ F508), and again subsequent invasive fetal testing if both parents are carriers.

Lifestyle education

Smoking is associated with low- birthweight babies, probably related to fetal hypoxaemia and ischaemia from both carbon monoxide and nicotine. Although there is no evidence to support association with fetal abnormality, long-term follow-up has demonstrated intellectual and emotional impairment. Smoking is also associated with an increased risk of abruption, preterm labour, intrauterine fetal demise and sudden infant death syndrome. Alcohol and drug misuse also carry significant fetal risks and, in the ideal world, all of these substances should be avoided in pregnancy.

Those whose work environment exposes them to radiation, hazardous gases or specific chemicals should be appropriately counselled. There is no evidence that VDUs are harmful, or indeed that work itself is harmful to the mother or fetus. The mother should be advised that she may continue working providing she is not unduly tired. Moderate exercise is likely to be of benefit and should be encouraged, but should probably be avoided if there are complications, e.g. hypertension, multiple pregnancy, cardiorespiratory compromise, antepartum haemorrhage or preterm labour.

Drug treatment in pregnancy

It is never possible to confirm the safety of any drug in pregnancy; one can only report on problems that seem to have arisen. As a general principle, all drugs should be avoided in pregnancy unless clinical benefits are likely to outweigh the risks to the fetus. A useful treatment, however, should not be stopped without good reason.

The major body structures are formed in the first 12 weeks (organogenesis) and drug treatment before this time may cause a teratogenic effect. If a drug is given after this time it will not produce a major anatomical defect, but may affect the growth and development of the baby.

Drug-related teratogenic problems were highlighted by the drug thalidomide introduced in West Germany in 1956 to combat morning sickness. By the end of 1961, thalidomide, sold under 51 brand names in at least 46 countries, was identified as a human teratogen and removed from the market. More than 10 000 infants worldwide were born with malformations attributed to the use of thalidomide in pregnancy.

Other drugs known to cause fetal abnormality include anticonvulsants, warfarin and isotretinoin, a vitamin A derivative, which is highly teratogenic and can produce almost any type of malformation in small doses. Ionising radiation kills rapidly dividing cells and can produce virtually any type of birth defect depending on the dose.

Alcohol is able to cross from the maternal circulation through the placenta into the fetal circulation and is potentially teratogenic. Fetal alcohol syndrome is discussed on page 44.

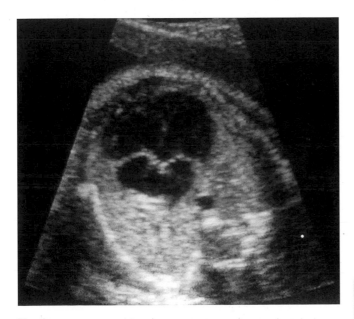

Fig. 3 **Atrioventricular canal defect in a baby with Down's syndrome.** There is a large ventricular septal defect (VSD) and no identifiable atrial septum.

Pre-conceptual counselling

- Folic acid reduces the incidence of neural tube defects.
- Certain medical disorders, particularly structural cardiac disease and renal failure, may have major implications for mother and baby.
- Screening for structural or genetic fetal abnormality may be possible.

Fetal chromosomal abnormality

About 2–3% of couples are at high risk of producing offspring with genetic disorders and 5% of the population will have displayed some form of genetic disorder by the age of 25 years. Particular risk factors are:

- Advanced maternal age (e.g. Down's syndrome)
- Family history of inherited diseases (e.g. fragile X syndrome, Huntington's chorea)
- Previous child with genetic disorder (e.g. Tay–Sachs disease, congenital adrenal hyperplasia).

The techniques for prenatal diagnosis that can be used and the appropriate timings are given in Table 1.

Here we will focus on screening for Down's syndrome which is characterized by an extra chromosome 21. The overall incidence is 1 : 600 live births, but depends on maternal age, being 1 : 2000 at age 20 and 1 : 100 at age 40. In affected individuals, although walking, language and self-care skills are usually attained, independence is rare. There is mental retardation (with a mean IQ of around 50) and an association with congenital heart disease, particularly atrioventricular canal defects, ventriculoseptal defect, atrioseptal defect and Fallot's tetralogy. Gastrointestinal atresias are common and there is early dementia with similarities to Alzheimer's disease. Twenty per cent die before age 1 but 45% reach age 60.

Serum screening

Antenatal screening for Down's syndrome is possible by measuring levels of serum markers at 15+ weeks – low levels of α-fetoprotein (AFP) ± high levels of unconjugated oestriol and human chorionic gonadotrophin (hCG) are corrected for maternal weight and age. This allows ~ 60% of cases of Down's syndrome to be picked up, with amniocentesis required on ~ 4% of the screened population. The pick-up rate is higher in older women, but the chance of being recalled with an elevated risk is also higher. It is therefore *not* essential to advise women over the age of 35 years to have an amniocentesis as serum screening is more sensitive in this age group. Fluorescent in situ hybridization (FISH) techniques may be used to exclude the commoner aneuploidies within 72 hours. Routine karyotyping does take up to 3 weeks because of the need to culture cells first.

Screening for open neural tube defects is also carried out by measuring the maternal serum AFP at 16 weeks.

Nuchal translucency

Screening for aneuploidy is also possible by measuring the fetal nuchal thickness on first trimester ultrasound. Sensitivities of 70–90% have been quoted for detecting Down's syndrome, particularly when combined with first trimester serum levels of specific fetal proteins. Increased nuchal translucency is also a marker for structural defects (4% of those > 3 mm) particularly cardiac, diaphragmatic hernia, renal, abdominal wall and other more rare abnormalities. The overall survival for

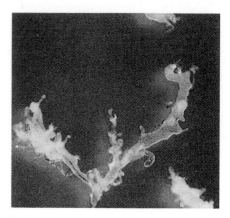

Fig. 1 **Low-power view of chorionic villi.**

those with nuchal translucency > 5 mm is ~ 53%.

Both these tests are screening tests for chromosomal problems. This allows selection of a group of mothers who can then be considered for an invasive diagnostic test.

Methods of obtaining tissue

Chorionic villus sampling (CVS)

Samples of mesenchymal cells of the chorionic villi are obtained for chromosomal and DNA analysis. The transabdominal technique is now more favoured, as the transcervical technique may give a higher infection and fetal loss rate.

Chorionic villus sampling is performed at 11–14 weeks' gestation. A needle is introduced through the maternal abdomen under ultrasound guidance, into the placenta and along the chorionic plate. A sample of the villi (Fig. 1) is aspirated. Cells from the direct preparation allow preliminary karyotype and DNA analysis within 24 hours, but this is usually confirmed with a cultured preparation as well.

Chorionic villus sampling only rarely leads to erroneous results, due to placental mosaicism (placental tissue of different cell lines can be identified from one placenta, e.g. XO, XX) but errors from this can be virtually eliminated providing decisions are deferred until both the direct and culture results are available. Karyotypic discrepancy between fetus and placenta increases with increasing gestation and if rapid results are required over 20 weeks fetal blood sampling or amniocentesis with FISH is preferable (see below).

Table 1 **Techniques for prenatal diagnosis**		
Technique	**Tests employed**	**Indications**
Chorionic villus sampling (11–14 weeks)	Chromosomal analysis DNA analysis Enzymology	Chromosomal abnormalities, fetal sexing in X-linked conditions Inborn errors of metabolism Haemoglobinopathies, Duchenne muscular dystrophy
Amniocentesis (15+ weeks)	Chromosomal analysis	As above As above As above
Maternal venous blood sample	AFP, Triple test screening for Down's syndrome	High incidence of neural tube defects
Ultrasound (10–20 weeks)	USS	Spina bifida, anencephaly, hydrocephaly, cystic renal disease, renal tract dilatation, exomphalos, gastroschisis, duodenal atresia, limb abnormalities, cardiac abnormalities
Cordocentesis (>18 weeks)	Enzymology Chromosomal analysis Blood testing	As above As above Heamoglobin studies, fetal viral infection, rhesus disease, unexplained hydrops and fetal anaemia pH

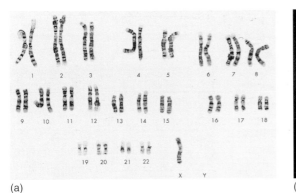

(a)

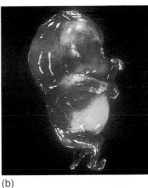

(b)

Fig. 3 **Karyotyping for Turner's syndrome. (a)** 45, XO karyotype. **(b)** Fetus with Turner's syndrome.

Fig. 4 **FISH analysed cell showing trisomy 21 (Down's syndrome).**

The advantage of chorionic villus sampling is that there is no breach of the amniotic cavity and that it allows an early diagnosis with the option of a suction termination of pregnancy. There is, however, good evidence to suggest that psychological parental morbidity is independent of whether a diagnosis is made in the first or second trimester and indeed medical termination of pregnancy may carry less psychological morbidity than surgical (even if medical complications are higher).

Amniocentesis

Amniocentesis involves withdrawing a sample of amniotic fluid containing fetal cells by passing a needle (using direct ultrasound control) through the maternal abdomen (Fig. 2). A karyotype of the fetal cells is obtained (see above). In approximately 98% of cases cell culture will be successful, enabling karyotypic analysis. This is performed from 15 weeks' gestation so that sufficient viable fetal cells can be obtained but at a fetal loss rate of about 1%. Amniocentesis performed in the presence of a raised maternal AFP level appears to be associated with a significant increase in miscarriage rates.

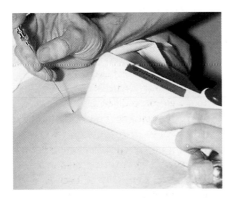

Fig. 2 **Insertion of needle under ultrasound guidance**

Cordocentesis

This technique may be used later in pregnancy when a rapid result is required. Often this will be at a later gestation after an ultrasound scan has shown an anomaly that is strongly associated with a genetic defect.

A needle is introduced transabdominally into the umbilical artery or vein. The most stable portion of the cord suitable for this is at the point of insertion. The blood sample obtained can be used for karyotyping and for the diagnosis of other conditions such as haemoglobinopathies, viral infections and metabolic disorders. The disadvantage of cordocentesis is that it requires a highly skilled operator. Complications include fetal haemorrhage, cord haematoma and fetal bradycardia.

Diagnostic tests for chromosome abnormality

Karyotyping

Human chromosomes can be examined directly in rapidly dividing tissue. However it is more usual to culture cells and then use colchicine to inhibit the formation of the spindle and arrest cell division at metaphase which allows the preparations that we are familiar with (Fig. 3). Chromosomes can then be paired according to their size, position of the centromere, and the Giemsa stain (this shows a characteristic banding pattern for each chromosome allowing individual identification).

DNA analysis

In an increasing number of inherited diseases it is now possible to identify a single gene defect or omission that is responsible. Fetal cells obtained by the various sampling techniques are cultured and their chromosomal DNA separated. This DNA is digested with restriction enzymes. The resulting fragments are separated by Southern blotting. A radioisotope-labelled DNA probe is then added and autoradiography allows identification of any hybridization. Specific probes are available for sickle cell disease, thalassaemia, and cystic fibrosis.

Fluorescent in situ hybridization (FISH)

In situ hybridization permits the analysis of genetic material of a single nucleus, by incubating a fixed dried cell with a specific probe, which binds to the gene of interest (Fig. 4). The use of a fluorescent marker tagged to the gene probe leads to the acronym FISH. This technique is sensitive enough to demonstrate each allele on individual chromatids but is not yet reliable enough for single cell analysis so is applied to larger samples. It provides a rapid diagnosis of trisomy, triploidy or sex chromosome problems if appropriate markers are used.

Fetal chromosomal abnormality

- Screening tests for genetic abnormality include nuchal translucency measurement, maternal serum screening and ultrasound examination of the fetus.

- Screening tests will *not* detect all abnormalities.

- Diagnostic tests are usually used after an abnormal screening test and include chorionic villus sampling, amniocentesis and cordocentesis. Amniocentesis is associated with the lowest fetal loss rate.

Fetal abnormality

The finding of some 'abnormality' in pregnancy transforms what was previously an exciting and joyous event into an extremely worrying and distressing time. This remains true even when the potential risks are small; for example being recalled with an abnormal level of α-fetoprotein (AFP), or with the finding of a choroid plexus cyst on routine ultrasound scan. The very greatest of care should be taken in explaining any findings to parents. Tact, understanding and reassurance (if appropriate) are paramount. The advice given to parents is of such importance that it will frequently be necessary to involve senior members of the obstetrics team as well as members of other specialties, particularly paediatricians, clinical geneticists and radiologists.

The aims of prenatal diagnosis are fourfold:

- the identification at an early gestation of abnormalities incompatible with survival, or likely to result in severe handicap, in order to prepare parents and offer the option of termination of pregnancy
- the identification of conditions which may influence the timing, site or mode of delivery
- the identification of fetuses who would benefit from early paediatric intervention
- the identification of fetuses who may benefit from in utero treatment (rare).

It should not be assumed that all parents are going to request termination of pregnancy even in the presence of lethal abnormality. Many couples have opted to continue pregnancies in the face of severe defects that have resulted in either intrauterine or early neonatal death, and have expressed the view that they found it easier to cope with grief having held their child. Others say that they were glad of the opportunity to terminate the pregnancy at an early stage and that they could not have coped with going on. More controversial still are the problems of chronic diseases with long-term handicap and long-term suffering for both the child and its parents. The parents themselves must decide what action they wish to take – it is they who will have to live with the consequences. It is our role to advise, guide and respect their final wishes, irrespective of our own personal views.

Screening for fetal abnormalities

Structural anomalies are best seen on ultrasound scan and many clinicians advocate that all mothers should be offered at least one detailed ultrasound at around 18–20 weeks or earlier. This has the advantage that previously unsuspected major or lethal anomalies (e.g. spina bifida, renal agenesis) can be offered termination, and it also allows planned deliveries of those conditions which may require early neonatal intervention (e.g. gastroschisis, transposition of the great arteries). It has the disadvantage, however, that many defects are not identified (it is likely that < 50% of cardiac defects are recognized) and the false reassurance provided by this scan may become a source of parental resentment. Furthermore, problems may be uncovered; for example one of the 'soft markers' (see below), the natural history of which is uncertain. This may generate unnecessary anxiety and increase the number of invasive diagnostic procedures (and thereby the loss rate) in otherwise healthy pregnancies.

Chromosomal abnormalities are much more difficult to identify on scan. While around two-thirds of fetuses with Down's syndrome will look normal at 18 weeks, most with Edwards' or Patau's syndrome do show some abnormality, even though these are often not specific or diagnostic.

In the absence of routine ultrasound scans, it is possible to screen for open neural tube defects by measuring the maternal serum AFP at 16 weeks. AFP is an alpha-globulin of similar molecular weight to albumin, which is synthesized by the fetal liver. Any break in the integrity of the fetus allows the AFP to escape into the maternal circulation and therefore be elevated on serum testing. Those with levels greater than 2.0–2.5 multiples of the median should be recalled for an ultrasound scan, giving a sensitivity for picking up neural tube defects of around 85%. Raised levels are also found following first trimester bleeding, or with intrauterine death (fetal autolysis), abdominal wall defects, or multiple pregnancy

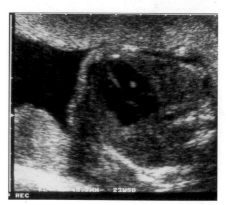

Fig. 1 **Echogenic focus in the left ventricle of a four-chamber cardiac view.**

(increased synthesis). Even if the scan is normal, raised AFP is still a marker for later pre-eclampsia or intrauterine growth restriction.

Increased nuchal translucency (NT) is also a marker for structural defects (4% of those > 3 mm), particularly cardiac, diaphragmatic hernia, renal, abdominal wall and other more rare abnormalities. The overall survival for those with NT > 5 mm is ≈ 53%.

Aneuploidy — soft markers

These are structural features found on ultrasound scan which in themselves are not a problem, but which may be pointers to chromosomal problems. Examples include choroid plexus cysts, mild renal pelvic dilatation, an echogenic focus (Fig. 1) in the heart ('golf-ball'), or mild cerebral ventricle dilatation. They are found in approximately 5% of all pregnancies in the second trimester and are the cause of a lot of parental anxiety. If isolated, the risk of chromosomal problems is low, but if more than one is found, or if there are any other structural defects, the risk is very much higher.

Congenital heart disease

This is the commonest congenital malformation in children and affects about 5–8:1000 live births. Of defects diagnosed antenatally, about 15% are associated with aneuploidy, most commonly trisomies 18 and 21.

The four-chamber view of the heart can be used as a screening test (Fig. 1) and will identify 25–40% of all major abnormalities, particularly ventricular septal defect, ventricular hypoplasia, valvular incompetence and arrhythmias. In addition, viewing the aorta and pulmonary artery increases

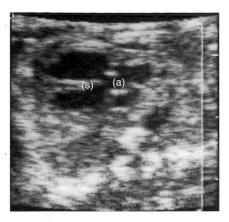

Fig. 2 **Fallot's tetralogy.** The aorta (a) overrides the interventricular septum (s).

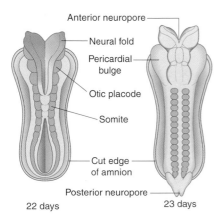

Fig. 3 **Dorsal view of embryo on days 22 and 23, demonstrating neural tube closure**

Anterior neuropore
Neural fold
Pericardial bulge
Otic placode
Somite
Cut edge of amnion
Posterior neuropore
22 days   23 days

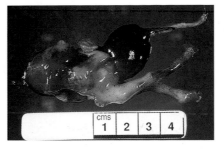

Fig. 4 **Spina bifida in association with large exomphalos.**

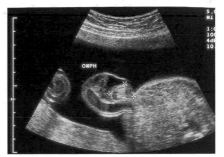

Fig. 5 **Small exomphalos.**

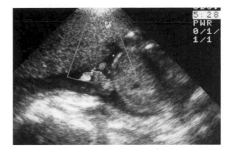

Fig. 6 **Gastroschisis, with Doppler flow to highlight the cord.**

the sensitivity to 60+% by screening for Fallot's tetralogy (Fig. 2) and transposition of the great arteries. At 18 weeks most of the major connections can be seen, but high-risk pregnancies (e.g. those with diabetes, or taking anticonvulsants, or who have a personal or family history of congenital heart disease) should be re-scanned at 22–26 weeks for more minor defects.

Neural tube defects

The neural tube is formed from the closing of the neural folds, with both anterior and posterior neuropores closed by 6 weeks' gestation (Fig. 3). Failure of closure of the anterior neuropore results in anencephaly or an encephalocele, and failure of posterior closure in spina bifida.

Anencephaly. The skull vault and cerebral cortex are absent. The infant is either stillborn or, if liveborn, will usually die shortly after birth (although some may survive for several days).

Encephalocele. There is a bony defect in the cranial vault through which a

dura mater sac (± brain tissue) protrudes. This may be occipital or frontal. Isolated meningoceles carry a good prognosis, whereas those with microcephaly secondary to brain herniation carry a very poor prognosis.

Spina bifida (Fig. 4). In a meningocele, dura and arachnoid mater bulge through the defect, whereas in a myelomeningocele, the central canal of the cord is exposed. Those with spinal meningoceles usually have normal lower limb neurology and 20% have hydrocephalus. Those with myelomeningoceles usually have abnormal lower limb neurology and many have hydrocephalus. In addition to immobility and mental retardation, there may be problems with urinary tract infection (UTI), bladder dysfunction, bowel dysfunction, and social and sexual isolation.

Spina bifida and anencephaly make up more than 95% of neural tube defects. There is wide geographical variation in births with a higher incidence in Scotland and Ireland 3 : 1000), and a lower incidence in England (2 : 1000), USA, Canada, Japan and Africa (< 1 : 1000). There is good evidence that the overall incidence has fallen over the past 15 years (independently of any screening programmes). Daily folic acid taken from before conception reduces the recurrence risk of neural tube defects in those who have had a previously affected child. A pre-conceptual prophylactic dose for all pregnant women probably also offers some protection. There are, at present, no known teratogenic effects from folate. There is an increased incidence of recurrence in subsequent pregnancies.

Abdominal wall defects

Exomphalos (Fig. 5)
This occurs following failure of the gut to return to the abdominal cavity at 8

weeks' gestation and results in a defect through which the peritoneal sac protrudes. This may contain both intestines and liver. There are chromosomal abnormalities in 30% (especially trisomy 18) and 10–50% have other lesions, particularly cardiac and renal. There is also an association with ectopia vesicae and ectopia cardia (midline bladder and cardiac hernias). If the exomphalos is isolated (i.e. no other structural abnormalities), the chromosomes are normal and there is no bowel atresia or infarction, the prognosis is good (> 80% long-term survival). The sac rarely ruptures at vaginal delivery.

Gastroschisis (Fig. 6)
There is an abdominal wall defect, usually to the right and below the insertion of the umbilical cord. Small bowel (without a peritoneal covering) protrudes and floats free in the peritoneal fluid. Gut atresias and cardiac lesions occur in 20% but the association with chromosomal abnormality is very small (probably < 1%). The prognosis is good if the bowel is viable, although 10% end in stillbirth despite apparently normal growth. Gut dilatation may be associated with bowel obstruction or ischaemia but is not directly linked to prognosis. These babies are usually small for dates and require very close surveillance. The recurrence risk is < 1%.

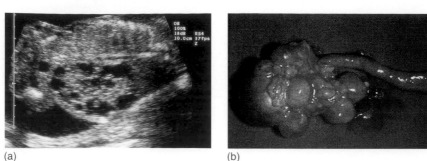

(a)   (b)

Fig. 7 **Dysplastic renal scan.** Note the enlarged kidney containing fluid-like cysts. **(a)** Ultrasound. **(b)** Postmortem specimen.

Genitourinary abnormalities

Renal dysplasia (Fig. 7)

Multicystic dysplastic kidneys (sporadic inheritance). The kidneys have large, discrete, non-communicating cysts with a central, more solid core and are thought to follow early developmental failure (Fig. 7a). If the cysts affect only one kidney, the other is normal, and there is adequate liquor, the prognosis is good. If the cysts are bilateral and the liquor is reduced, the prognosis is poor.

Polycystic kidney disease

Adult polycystic kidney disease (AD). The corticomedullary junction is accentuated and the condition is relatively benign, often not producing symptoms until the fifth decade of life. Many individuals have ultrasonically normal kidneys at birth. There are at least two genes on different chromosomes, however, so that DNA studies are only possible in families with multiple affected members.

Infantile polycystic kidney disease (AR). There is a wide range of expression with the size of cysts ranging from microscopic to several millimetres across. Both kidneys are affected, and there may also be cysts present in the liver and pancreas. Ultrasound features of oligohydramnios, empty bladder and large symmetrical bright kidneys (Fig. 8) may not develop until later in

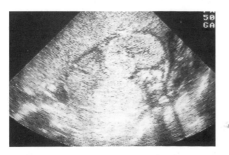

Fig. 8 **Infantile renal cystic scan.** Note anhydramnios and bright real echoes from the microscopically small cysts.

pregnancy. If there is survival beyond the neonatal period, there may be later problems with raised blood pressure and progressive renal failure. Long-term survival is rare.

Pyelectasis

Renal pelvic dilatation may be unilateral (79–90%) or bilateral. It is probably caused by a neuromuscular defect at the junction of the ureter and the renal pelvis, and presents with increasing pelvic dilatation in the presence of a normal ureter. As there is an association with postnatal UTIs and reflux nephropathy, it is reasonable to start all neonates on prophylactic antibiotics and arrange postnatal radiological follow-up. Even in those with mild dilatation (≥ 5 mm and < 10 mm) there is vesicoureteric reflux in 10–20%, although only a small proportion require surgery.

Posterior urethral valves

Folds of mucosa at the bladder neck prevent urine leaving the bladder. The fetus is usually male, there is often oligohydramnios and on ultrasound there are varying degrees of renal dysplasia. There is a chromosomal abnormality in 7% of isolated defects, and in one-third of those with other abnormalities. It may be possible to insert a pigtail shunt between the bladder and amniotic cavity to relieve the obstruction, but the long-term prognosis is still poor as the renal damage may not be reversible.

Potter's syndrome

There is bilateral renal agenesis which is associated with extreme oligohydramnios and leads to the Potter's sequence of pulmonary hypoplasia (see below) and limb deformity (due to fetal compression). The condition is lethal. The recurrence risk is approximately 3% although AD forms with variable penetrance have been described.

Lung disorders

Pulmonary hypoplasia

Liquor is important for alveolar maturation, particularly in the second trimester when the alveoli are forming. Without liquor there will be pulmonary hypoplasia. Severe oligohydramnios occurs with very preterm pre-labour membrane rupture or Potter's syndrome (see above). Pulmonary hypoplasia also occurs with diaphragmatic herniae as there is no room for lung expansion.

Diaphragmatic hernia

Stomach, colon and even spleen can enter the chest through a defect in the diaphragm, usually on the left. The heart is pushed to the right and the lungs become hypoplastic. The incidence of aneuploidy is 15–30% and there is an association with neural tube defects, congenital heart disease and renal and skeletal abnormalities. The overall survival of those diagnosed antenatally is ~20% with a better prognosis for isolated left-sided herniae. Polyhydramnios, mediastinal shift and left ventricular compression are poor antenatal prognostic factors. Postnatally, those that survive undergo surgery to reduce the hernia and close the diaphragmatic defect.

Cystic fibrosis

The UK gene frequency is 1 : 25 (i.e. heterozygote frequency), giving an estimated overall couple risk for a live birth around 1 : 2500. Clinically there is respiratory, gastrointestinal, liver and pancreatic dysfunction and azoospermia is the rule. The prognosis is very variable and although death in the 20–30 age group still occurs, the prognosis is improving and many now live considerably longer. The health of an affected sib is not a prognostic guide to the health of other sibs. Four mutant alleles account for 85% of the gene defects in the UK (the commonest being ΔF508) and antenatal screening for these is possible using saliva specimens, with chorionic villus sampling (CVS) being performed if both parents are gene carriers.

Other disorders

Cystic hygroma (Fig. 9)

Cystic hygromas are fluid-filled swellings at the back of the fetal neck and probably develop from a defect in the formation of lymphatic vessels – it

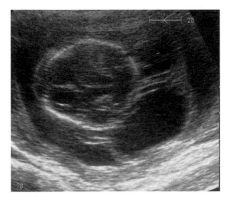

Fig. 9 **Cystic hygroma.**

Table 1 Polyhydramnios: causes and pathology	
Cause of polyhydramnios	Pathology
Increased production from high urine output	Macrosomia, diabetes, recipient of twin–twin transfusion, hydrops fetalis
Gastrointestinal obstruction	Oesophageal atresia, duodenal atresia, small intestine or colonic obstruction, Hirschsprung's disease
Poor swallowing because of neuromuscular problems or mechanical obstruction	Anencephaly, myotonic dystrophy, maternal myasthenia, facial tumour, macroglossia or micrognathia

is likely that the lymphatic system and venous system fail to connect and lymph fluid accumulates in the jugular lymph sacs. Larger hygromas are frequently divided by septae and may be associated with skin oedema, ascites, pleural and pericardial effusions, and cardiac and renal abnormalities. There is also an association with aneuploidy (particularly Turner's, Down's, Edwards') and it is appropriate to offer karyotyping. If generalized hydrops is present the prognosis is bleak. Isolated hygromas may be surgically corrected postnatally and have a good prognosis. Only rarely are they so large as to result in problems with labour.

Fragile X syndrome
This is the commonest cause of moderate mental retardation after Down's syndrome and the commonest form of inherited mental handicap. It is X-linked. Males are usually more severely affected than females. Speech delay is common and there is an associated behavioural phenotype with gaze aversion. The condition is caused by the expansion of a CGG triplet repeat on the X chromosome. Normal individuals have an average of 29 repeats but for an unexplained reason this may increase to a pre-mutation of 50–200 repeats. Those with a pre-mutation are phenotypically normal but the pre-mutation is unstable during female meiosis and

can expand to a full mutation of more than 200 repeats. There is an approximately 10% chance of this occurring (in the absence of a full mutation in that generation already). This causes the fragile X phenotype in 99% of males and around 30–50% of females. Parental screening is possible and CVS may be used to identify the degree of amplification of the CGG repeats in potential offspring.

Huntington's chorea
The onset of this autosomal dominant condition is usually after the age of 30, although it may present as early as 10–15 years of age. There is dementia, mood change (usually depression) and choreoathetosis, progressing to death in approximately 15 years. There is a CAG trinucleotide expansion on chromosome 4p allowing accurate carrier and prenatal testing.

Tay–Sachs disease
The gene frequency is 1:30 in Ashkenazi Jews, but is rare in other groups. There is a build-up of gangliosides within the CNS leading to retardation, paralysis and blindness. By the age of 4 years, the child is usually dead or in a vegetative state. Carriers may be screened by measuring the level of hexosaminidase A in leucocytes.

Polyhydramnios
Liquor is produced by fetal kidneys and is swallowed by the fetus. Excess liquor, polyhydramnios, may be defined as more than 2–3 litres of amniotic fluid, but for practical clinical purposes may be considered as:

- a single pool > 8 cm
- amniotic fluid index > 90th centile.

This is a measurement of the maximum depth of liquor in the four quadrants of the uterus.

Polyhydramnios occurs in 0.5–2% of all pregnancies and is associated with maternal diabetes (~20%) and congenital fetal anomaly (~5%). Its causes are listed in Table 1.

Even in the absence of an identifiable cause (>60%), polyhydramnios is associated with an increased rate of:

- placental abruption
- malpresentation
- cord prolapse
- requiring a caesarean section
- perinatal death
- carrying a large for gestation age infant.

It is important to arrange a growth and detailed ultrasound scan, glucose tolerance test (GTT), and fetal well-being assessment. The rhesus status should also be checked to exclude immune hydrops fetalis. Only rarely is it necessary to aspirate fluid for maternal comfort or decrease the chance of preterm labour. Increased antenatal fetal surveillance is important, and an increased awareness of the risks of intrapartum complications. A paediatrician should be present for delivery.

Investigations may suggest that the baby is large for dates. It should be remembered that clinical examination and ultrasound measurements are relatively poor predictors of birthweight and it is rarely justifiable to use these assessments alone to plan an elective caesarean section.

Fetal abnormality
- Not everybody wishes prenatal diagnosis, and not everybody wishes the option of termination if there is a severely abnormal fetus.
- Ultrasound scanning is the best screening tool for structural abnormalities but will still miss many problems, particularly cardiac defects.

Infections in pregnancy

Infections in pregnancy are important because of potential risks to the fetus. A number of agents are known to be teratogenic, particularly in the first and early second trimesters. Others carry the risk of miscarriage, premature labour, severe neonatal sepsis or long-term carrier states.

Infection risks
Occupation
Farm workers

A chlamydia (which causes miscarriage in sheep), toxoplasma (which causes abortion in cows and sheep) and listeria can all cause miscarriage in humans.

Working with farm animals should therefore be avoided when pregnant, particularly in the lambing and calving seasons. At these times, basic hygiene precautions should be observed by everyone else on the farm to prevent transmission.

Nurses

Nurses may be concerned about cytomegalovirus (CMV), particularly

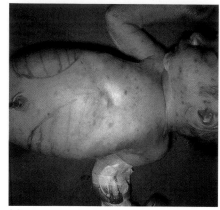

(a)

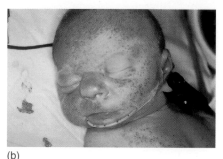

(b)

Fig. 1 **Hepatosplenomegaly (a) and thrombocytopenia (b) occur with congenital CMV infection.**

those in contact with small children (Fig. 1). Serology is of little benefit as the presence of antibodies does not necessarily denote immunity (see Table 1). If hands are washed well and often, the risk of transmission is very small.

Food

The following foods carry potential infection risks in pregnancy:

- *Soft cheeses.* Unpasteurized milk and its products may contain listeria. Those made from pasteurized milk are safe.
- *Raw eggs.* These must be avoided as there is a risk of salmonella (remember puddings).
- *Meat or pâté.* Undercooked meat may transmit toxoplasma or rarely listeria.
- *Fruit.* This should always be washed before eating as it may be contaminated with salmonella, toxoplasma or one of several intestinal parasites.

Table 1 **Infections in pregnancy**

Agent	Epidemiology	Maternal features	Fetal features	Risk	Treatment
Rubella	Person to person UK immunity now 97% and congenital infection is rare	Asymptomatic or mild maculopapular rash	IUGR, ↓ platelets, hepatosplenomegaly, jaundice, deafness, CHD, mental retardation, cataracts, microphthalmia, abortion, microcephaly and cerebral palsy (Fig. 2)	Risk of affected fetus: < 4 weeks 50% 5–8 weeks 25% 9–12 weeks 10% > 13 weeks 1%	Consider TOP if < 12 weeks Postnatal vaccination if not immune
Toxoplasmosis (protozoan – *Toxoplasma gondii*)	From cats, uncooked meats and unwashed fruits	May have fever, rash and lymphadenopathy, but most are asymptomatic	Hydrocephalus, chorioretinitis, intracranial calcification, ↓ platelets	< 12 weeks transmission is 10–25%, of which 75% will be severely affected 12–28 weeks transmission is 54%, of which 25% will be severely affected > 28 weeks transmission is 65–90%, of which < 10% will be severely affected	Consider TOP only if primary infection < 20 weeks
CMV (herpes virus)	Person to person	Nearly always asymptomatic	Hepatosplenomegaly, ↓ platelets, IUGR, microcephaly, sensorineural deafness, CP, chorioretinitis, hydrops fetalis, exomphalos	40% of fetuses infected. Risk is unaffected by gestation Of these, 90% are normal at birth, although 20% develop late sequelae Of the 10% who are symptomatic, 33% die and the rest have long-term problems	Even primary infection carries only a 10–25% risk of severe abnormality
Parvovirus B19	Respiratory transmission Seroprevalence 50%	Erythema infectiosum (slapped cheek disease) May be asymptomatic	Aplastic anaemia, hydrops fetalis and myocarditis ± fetal loss (if < 20 weeks) Transmission < 20 weeks ≈ 10% of which ≈ 10% are lost If > 20 weeks, transmission 60%, but no adverse effects have been demonstrated	If less than 20 weeks and fetus survives the infection (≈ 90%), it is likely to result in a healthy live birth	Intrauterine transfusion may be possible
Chickenpox (varicella zoster virus)	Person to person	Papules and pustules	Limb hypoplasia, skin scarring, IUGR, neurological abnormalities and hydrops fetalis	25% transmission. Probably < 1–2% have problems if < 20 weeks. No structural problems > 20 weeks See 'Chickenpox at term'	Treat with ZIG (zoster immunoglobulin) if < 10 days from contact or < 4 days from onset of rash, although the benefits are not proven

Key: CHD, congenital heart disease; CMV, cytomegalovirus; CP, cerebral palsy; IUGR, intrauterine growth restriction; TOP, termination of pregnancy

Specific infections
General principles
The fetus does not make IgM until beyond 20 weeks' gestation. Absence of fetal IgM at birth does not mean that infection has not occurred and IgG is usually passive (i.e. transplacental from the mother) unless the baby is older than 1 year. Evidence of infection does not imply damage.

Chickenpox
Chickenpox at term (see Table 1 for early pregnancy). Severe and even fatal cases of chickenpox can occur in neonates whose mothers develop chickenpox from 7 days before to 1 month after delivery (usually 2 days before to 2 days after). This is because the baby is born before maternal IgG production has increased sufficiently to allow passive transplacental protection. The baby should be given varicella zoster immunoglobulin (VZIG) as soon as possible if maternal symptoms develop.

Hepatitis
Hepatitis A has not been associated with significant complications in pregnancy. All mothers should be screened antenatally for hepatitis B virus as vertical transmission can occur. The initial serological response is with HBsAg, followed by HBeAg, a marker of high infectivity.

Transmission is most likely to occur with acute infection (especially third trimester), or in the presence of HBeAg. The risk of maternofetal transmission for mothers who are HBeAg +ve is 90%, falling to 10% in those with antibodies to the HBeAg. The baby should be given hepatitis B immunoglobulin i.m. at birth as well as active hepatitis B immunization, the latter repeated at 1 month and at 6 months.

With hepatitis C, vertical transmission is related to viral load but is unlikely in the absence of detectable RNA. There is no evidence that treatment during pregnancy reduces the chance of transmission and ribavirin is probably teratogenic. Caesarean section or breast feeding is unlikely to alter the incidence of neonatal infection. Hepatitis E infection in pregnancy, whilst uncommon, carries a 30% maternal mortality rate and possible risk of fetal loss.

Herpes simplex virus
An acute attack of primary herpes shortly before delivery may lead to a neonatal infection (≈ 40%) and this may be localized or systemic, occasionally including encephalitis. The risk of infection is greatest with a primary infection, but can occur with recurrence, although this risk decreases with time from the first attack. Antenatal screening at 36 weeks does not predict transmission, and indeed, 70% of neonatal infections occur to mothers with no overt signs of infection. Membrane rupture in the presence of a primary infection (i.e. within 6 weeks of delivery) is considered by many to be the only indication for caesarean section, providing the operation is carried out within the first 4 hours. It is possible, however, that caesarean section is appropriate in recurrent herpes if active lesions are present. The very small risk of fetal infection in this situation must be weighed against the risk to the mother of caesarean section.

Rubella
Rubella infection is discussed in Table 1 but its importance lies in its potential for prevention through vaccination. Immunity from natural infection is lifelong. Seroconversion and lifelong immunity occur in about 95% of vaccinated individuals, and as the benefits of herd immunity have been clearly demonstrated, many countries now immunize all preschool children. Rubella antibodies are commonly checked at booking, and postnatal vaccination is offered to those with low titres.

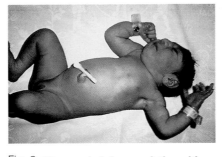

Fig. 2 Microcephaly in association with congenital rubella infection. Now rare in countries with childhood vaccination programmes.

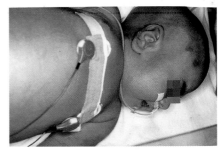

Fig. 3 Jaundice and sepsis with perinatal group B β-haemolytic streptococcal infection.

Listeria monocytogenes
This is a rare bacterial infection transmitted in food (usually soft ripe cheeses, pâté, cooked–chilled meals and ready-to-eat foods that have not been thoroughly cooked). Following an initial gastroenteritis, which may be fleeting, bacteraemia results in bacilli crossing the placenta leading to amnionitis, preterm labour (which may result in stillbirth) or spontaneous miscarriage. There may be meconium, neonatal jaundice, conjunctivitis or meningoencephalitis. Diagnosis is made by blood culture or by culture of liquor or placenta. Treatment is with high-dose amoxicillin or erythromycin.

β-haemolytic streptococci – group B
Between 5% and 20% of women carry this organism in the vagina. It is associated with preterm rupture of the membranes. About 50% of babies become colonized at delivery but only about 1% of these develop infection. The mortality from infection may be up to 80%, with 50% of those surviving meningitis having subsequent neurological impairment (Fig. 3). Antenatal screening is not indicated in the UK (initial screen positives may become negative and vice versa) but those with known infection should receive intrapartum antibiotics (e.g. amoxicillin or erythromycin). There is no evidence to support antenatal treatment of asymptomatic carriers, as carriage is rapidly re-established following treatment.

Infections in pregnancy

- CMV, toxoplasmosis and rubella are teratogenic.
- Parvovirus B19 may lead to hydrops fetalis.
- Primary varicella zoster and herpes simplex infections just before the onset of labour may result in serious neonatal morbidity and mortality.

Human immunodeficiency virus (HIV)

HIV is a retroviral infection which may be transmitted sexually, via blood or blood products, or from mother to child (vertical transmission). The incidence worldwide is steadily rising (Fig. 1) with HIV-1 most widely found and HIV-2 predominantly in West Africa and Portugal.

The median interval between HIV infection and development of AIDS is 8–10 years (Fig. 2). HIV-2 has a longer incubation period and slower rate of progression. More than 70% of HIV infections worldwide have occurred in sub-Saharan Africa, the major route of transmission being heterosexual, but there is a markedly expanding epidemic affecting South East Asia.

Over five million people worldwide acquired HIV infection in 1999 and it is estimated that 34.3 million adults and children were living with HIV/AIDS at the end of 1999, 24.5 million of them in sub-Saharan Africa. Publicity campaigns are essential to keep the risks of HIV infection in the public mind.

Clinical features

Pneumocystis carinii pneumonia (PCP) presenting with dyspnoea on exertion and a non-productive cough, Kaposi's sarcoma (which is rare in women) and cervical carcinoma are agreed AIDS-defining illnesses when present in HIV-positive individuals. Viral load (monitored by HIV-1 plasma RNA) is the most important prognostic marker of risk of progression. Those with a low ($< 500 \times 10^6/l$) CD4 count (a T-cell subset) need antiretroviral therapy (Fig. 3).

Early symptoms and signs of progression include malaise, weight loss, fevers and night sweats. Persistent generalized lymphadenopathy is common throughout the course of the disease and has no prognostic significance, but asymmetrical or atypical lymphadenopathy needs further evaluation as it

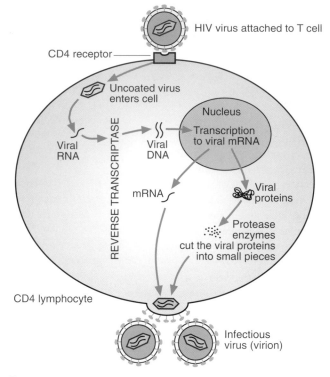

Fig. 2 **HIV entry into a CD4 lymphocyte.**

may represent a neoplastic process such as a lymphoma.

Obstetrics

The vertical transmission rate is somewhere between 13 and 30% before treatment, with 90% of all infants infected

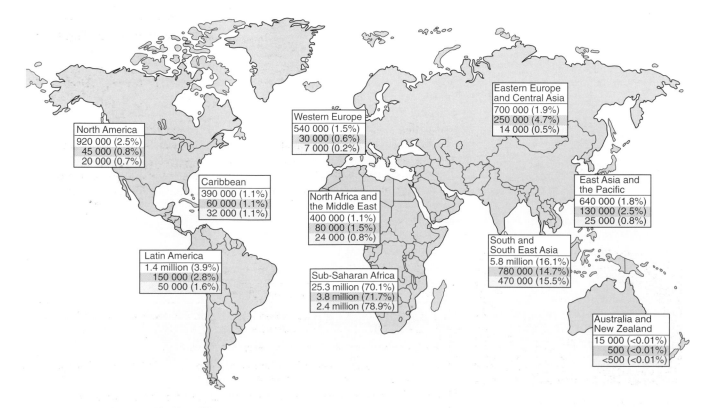

Fig. 1 **Numbers of people living with HIV/AIDS, numbers of new infections and numbers of deaths due to HIV/AIDS in 2000.**

perinatally being born in sub-Saharan Africa. There are obvious advantages to the mother in knowing her HIV status during pregnancy (Fig. 4).

A very small minority of women may wish to terminate their pregnancy but knowledge of HIV status allows an informed decision about future pregnancies. Antenatal testing thus has advantages and should be on offer to all patients, though uptake of testing is low in the UK compared to France and Sweden. A 1997 survey of children born in the UK and developing AIDS found that 53% of the maternal infections were diagnosed only once the child developed AIDS. Only 4.5% were diagnosed during pregnancy. Most women who know they are HIV-positive act to reduce the risk of vertical transmission (Fig. 4), so uptake of testing antenatally must be more universally encouraged.

There are also advances in the treatment of HIV in adults, including combination drug therapies, leading to increased benefits to the woman herself in knowing that she is HIV-infected. The use of triple therapy (generally consisting of two nucleoside analogues and a protease inhibitor) hopes to prevent emergence of drug-resistant strains due to incomplete suppression of replication (note: protease inhibitors are teratogenic).

Gynaecology

There are three areas where HIV-positive status impacts on gynaecology:

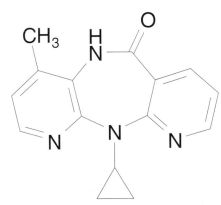

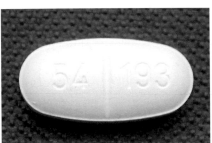

Fig. 3 **AZT (zidovudine), an antiretroviral drug.**

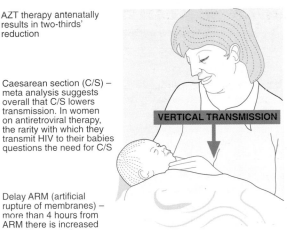

AZT therapy antenatally results in two-thirds' reduction

Caesarean section (C/S) – meta analysis suggests overall that C/S lowers transmission. In women on antiretroviral therapy, the rarity with which they transmit HIV to their babies questions the need for C/S

Delay ARM (artificial rupture of membranes) – more than 4 hours from ARM there is increased rate of transmission

VERTICAL TRANSMISSION

Avoid use of fetal scalp electrode and fetal blood sampling in labour – these interventions bring maternal and fetal blood into contact

Douches to the birth canal may limit spread – under investigation

Avoid breast feeding – halves the rate of transmission. Where there is high infant mortality associated with malnutrition and infectious disease, WHO/UNICEF support breast feeding by the baby's own mother, regardless of her HIV status

Fig. 4 **Reducing vertical transmission from mother to baby.**

gynaecological manifestations of HIV, termination of pregnancy and infection control.

Gynaecological manifestations of HIV

Immunosuppressed HIV-positive patients are at increased risk of genital tract malignancy and an annual cervical smear is probably appropriate. Cervical carcinoma is an AIDS-defining diagnosis but the malignancy may be multifocal with lesions of the cervix, vagina, vulva and perianal area. Human papilloma virus (HPV) types 16 and 18 have oncogenic effects which may be enhanced in the HIV-positive patient who also has a higher prevalence of such infection.

The risk of developing neoplasia is directly related to the degree of HIV-induced immunosuppression as measured by decreasing CD4 lymphocyte number and advancing clinical disease.

There is a strong association between HIV and other sexually transmitted diseases (STDs), particularly those involving genital tract ulceration, such as chancroid, syphilis and genital herpes. These disrupted mucous membranes allow organisms to bypass normal defences but are also a potent source of virus in those who are seropositive. Vigorous treatment of STDs would help to reduce the worldwide progression of HIV infection.

Pelvic inflammatory disease has not been found to occur more often in the HIV-positive patient but may be more severe and ideally requires inpatient therapy to prevent peritonitis and abscess formation.

Termination of pregnancy

Once pregnancy is confirmed a full discussion of the risks to mother and baby should be available. Though some patients who are HIV-positive may wish termination, others will proceed successfully with their pregnancy. Proper disposal of the products of conception, handling them as high risk and sending for incineration in line with all contaminated hospital waste, is important.

Infection control

Gynaecological and obstetric practice exposes practitioners to bodily fluids infected by HIV so universal use of safe handling techniques is logical.

Human immunodeficiency virus

- HIV is important in obstetrics and gynaecology because of the contact with bodily fluids and the impact of AIDS on gynaecological diseases.
- Knowledge of HIV status can have a large impact on pregnancy management.
- Reduction of vertical transmission can be achieved by two-thirds with the use of AZT therapy and by half with avoidance of breast feeding.
- Low rates of diagnosis of HIV antenatally limit the ability to reduce vertical transmission.

Preterm labour and preterm premature rupture of the membranes (PPROM)

Preterm labour

Preterm labour is defined as labour occurring before 37 completed weeks. It affects 5–10% of all pregnancies but it accounts for approximately 75% of perinatal mortality.

Diagnosis

Diagnosis is made with difficulty as uterine activity is not always associated with cervical dilatation and may settle down with no untoward effect on the pregnancy, hence the apparent spontaneous cessation of the labour in 50% of cases. Causes of preterm labour include:

- preterm rupture of the membranes
- polyhydramnios
- multiple pregnancy
- cervical incompetence
- uterine abnormalities
- antepartum haemorrhage
- fetal death
- maternal pyrexia, particularly associated with urinary infection
- idiopathic – the majority of cases.

Management

The benefits of in utero existence are weighed against the risks of threatened preterm delivery and in each case a decision is reached about the best treatment options. Maternal infection should be sought and treated appropriately – mid-stream urine sample (MSU), full blood count (FBC) and high vaginal swab (HVS) should be obtained on admission, as should a clean-catch liquor sample in cases with ruptured membranes.

A cardiotocograph (CTG) will determine the status of the fetus but interpretation of the CTG in the extremely preterm infant (24–26 weeks) is complicated by lack of knowledge about normal parameters (see p. 50). Assessment of cervical dilatation over the first few hours after admission will show if there is progressive cervical dilatation and the need for uterine suppression.

Uterine suppression (tocolysis)

Various medications are used to try to suppress uterine contractions including intravenous betamimetic drugs, calcium channel blockers, oxytocin receptor antagonists and antiprostaglandins. Side effects which limit use of the betamimetics are palpitations, tremor, headache, restlessness, nausea and vomiting, and hypotension. If chest discomfort or breathlessness develops this may indicate pulmonary congestion – one of the more serious side effects of therapy.

There are no studies which show any decrease in perinatal mortality with the use of betamimetics, though there is a reduction in the proportion of deliveries occurring within the next 24–48 hours. This allows time to administer steroid therapy and transfer the patient to a centre with neonatal intensive care facilities.

Intravenous ritodrine has been studied extensively but salbutamol and fenoterol are also used. All will have an effect on carbohydrate metabolism and should be used with caution in the diabetic patient. Maintaining uterine suppression after the acute event by use of oral therapy has not been shown to reduce the incidence of preterm delivery.

As there is good evidence that prostaglandins are involved in the initiation of labour, suppressing prostaglandin synthesis is logical. Indomethacin, p.r. or orally, has been shown to suppress uterine contractility, reducing delivery within 48 hours and reducing preterm birth. It too has side effects – gastrointestinal tract irritation even amounting to peptic ulceration, nausea and vomiting, diarrhoea and headache. For the fetus, the theoretical adverse effects include impaired renal function and prolonged bleeding time but the major worry is constriction of the ductus arteriosus which may result in persistent pulmonary hypertension in the new-born.

Nifedipine (a calcium channel blocker) and glyceryl trinitrate have also been used, with possible success. Magnesium sulphate is the preferred treatment in the US. As infection may be an aetiological feature, there may be a role for empirical treatment with broad-spectrum antibiotics, particularly following preterm premature rupture of the membranes (PPROM).

When should tocolysis be used?

- Where prolongation of the pregnancy will have beneficial effects for the fetus, to allow time to administer steroids to ensure fetal lung maturation; tocolysis works only in early labour (less than 4 cm cervical dilatation)
- Not in the presence of an antepartum haemorrhage as the vasodilatation caused may potentiate the bleed
- With caution in the diabetic patient as betamimetics cause gluconeogenesis and may precipitate diabetic ketoacidosis
- Not with evidence of chorioamnionitis – maternal pyrexia, uterine tenderness, raised white blood count (WBC) (steroids used for fetal lung maturation cause a rise in WBC, so use of C-reactive protein may be more accurate), fetal tachycardia
- Not with evidence of fetal compromise when conditions ex utero may be more favourable.

Cervical cerclage

There are two main ways this technique is employed:

1. In the acute situation when the cervix is found to be dilated on admission – usually in a patient with suspected preterm labour. If the cervix does not continue to dilate whilst the patient rests in bed then a suture may be placed (rescue cerclage) to prevent further passive dilatation. This may be unsuccessful with membrane rupture during suture placement. The suture may cut through the thinned cervical tissue or intrauterine infection may follow.

2. In patients with a history of previous cervical incompetence, or history of gynaecological procedures which may leave the cervix incompetent, cerclage may be considered. The suture is placed circumferentially at the level of the internal os taking four large bites into the substance of the cervix.

A large, multi-centre study assessing cervical cerclage failed to show benefit in prolonging pregnancy. Practice is to assess cervical length ultrasonically in the high-risk patient and use cerclage if there is evidence of shortening of the cervix.

The cerclage suture is usually removed at around 37 weeks and onset of spontaneous labour is awaited. This may occur some days later.

Benefits and risks of in utero existence

The survival rates for infants between 24 and 28 weeks' gestation vary from 25% early to 80% later and determine whether intervention will offer benefits over the in utero state. From 28 weeks onwards the survival rates climb gradually from 80% to 98% and give greater confidence in delivering a preterm infant. Extremely preterm infants have better survival prospects if delivered in a neonatal intensive care unit and should be transferred in utero if possible.

Delivery

If labour ensues, a controlled delivery with intact membranes and a short second stage offers the best outcome for the infant. The preterm breech presentation risks delivery of the small trunk through an incompletely dilated cervix resulting in fetal head entrapment. In these circumstances it may be best to deliver by caesarean section, between 26 and 34 weeks' gestation – though the evidence for this is limited. The lower uterine segment will be poorly formed in these circumstances, so a longitudinal incision in the lower uterine segment may be needed (de Lee incision).

PPROM

Premature rupture of the membranes (PROM) is when the membranes rupture before the onset of labour. In 80% of patients labour ensues within 24 hours. Once the membranes are ruptured the barrier to ascending infection is gone and if labour does not follow within 24–48 hours, induction of labour to prevent chorioamnionitis in the mother and systemic neonatal infection is usual.

Preterm PROM (PPROM) is when the membrane rupture occurs before 37 weeks and induction of labour may not be the optimal management. It occurs in 2–3% of pregnancies and accounts for about one-third of preterm deliveries. A more conservative approach may be used dependent on the gestation (see Fig. 1). In uncomplicated cases:

< 34 weeks – benefits of in utero development outweigh the risks of ascending infection and a conservative approach is appropriate. Pulmonary hypoplasia and skeletal deformities may be seen due to oligohydramnios following spontaneous rupture of the membranes (SRM) in extreme prematurity. Pulmonary hypoplasia after SRM occurs in 50% of cases less than 20 weeks but in only 3% over 24 weeks. Two doses of corticosteroid given 12 hours apart are associated with increased fetal surfactant production so long as there are 24 hours after the completion of the dose before delivery. The use of antibiotics prophylactically is of unproven benefit for the fetus.

34–37 weeks – no suppression of uterine activity and if no evidence of infection conservative management. The risk of respiratory distress syndrome (RDS) in the infant is about 5% and this dictates conservative management. Antibiotic therapy may be given to reduce maternal infection but it may be preferable to treat infection if detected rather than subject all patients to therapy. Induction of labour at 36 weeks avoids the continued risk of ascending infection, whilst the chance of RDS is small.

> 37 weeks – if no labour ensues within 24–48 hours of membrane rupture then induction of labour avoids the development of infection with the associated morbidity.

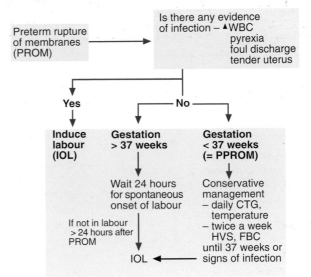

Fig. 1 **Management plan.**

Complications include:

- infection
- antepartum haemorrhage
- fetal compromise.

The presence of complications makes a more active approach to delivery appropriate. If there are no complications it is acceptable to wait up to 96 hours for labour.

Making the diagnosis

After palpation of the abdomen to confirm the fetal lie, presentation and size, a *sterile* speculum examination is performed to observe the cervix for amniotic fluid leakage – unless there is obvious liquor at the vulva or on a pad. Amniotic fluid has a characteristic odour and presence of vernix caseosa is diagnostic. A high vaginal swab should be taken to check for infection or amniotic fluid aspirated and sent for microscopy and culture. If doubt exists the patient may be asked to wear a pad whilst ambulant and check the pad for presence of liquor. If there is still doubt, then an ultrasound scan to measure the amniotic fluid index and a check for the presence of fluid below the presenting part will refute the diagnosis.

Management of chorioamnionitis

Labour should be induced with Syntocinon and a continuous CTG is needed. Caesarean section is only performed if clinically indicated as there will be an increased risk of postoperative pelvic sepsis and subsequent tubal blockage. Intravenous antibiotics should be broad spectrum.

Preterm labour and PPROM

- Preterm labour accounts for 75% of perinatal mortality.
- Most preterm labour is due to unknown reasons.
- Rupture of the membranes is associated with ascending infection.

Hypertension

Hypertension in pregnancy may be coincidental (usually background essential hypertension) or related to pregnancy (gestational hypertension, pre-eclampsia or in association with eclampsia).

- Hypertension in pregnancy is defined as a diastolic blood pressure (BP) > 110 mmHg on any one occasion or > 90 mmHg on two occasions ≥ 4 hours apart.
- Severe hypertension is a single diastolic BP > 120 mmHg on any one occasion or > 110 mmHg on two occasions ≥ 4 hours apart.

In normal pregnancy the BP will fall during the first trimester, reaching a nadir in the second trimester and rising slightly again during the third trimester. It should be measured in the sitting position with an appropriate size of cuff (Fig. 1a). Although controversial, it is suggested that the phase IV Korotkoff sound (i.e. 'muffling' rather than 'disappearance') should be taken when reading the diastolic pressure.

Raised BP at booking (e.g. before 16 weeks) is usually due to chronic hypertension (usually essential hypertension, only rarely renal disease

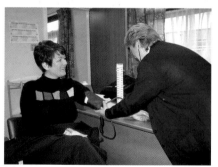

(a)

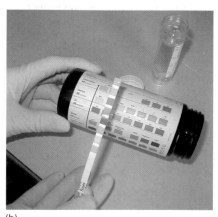

(b)

Fig. 1 **Early detection of pre-eclampsia is paramount.**

or phaeochromocytoma). Gestational hypertension and pre-eclampsia (hypertension and proteinuria) only very rarely occur before 20 weeks (unless associated with trophoblastic disease).

Essential hypertension

This is commoner in older women and the prognosis overall for pregnancy is good. The main risk is from superimposed pre-eclampsia (which is more common with pre-existing essential hypertension). The hypertension itself is rarely of significance, although there might be a slightly increased risk of placental abruption. Those women who are already taking antihypertensive drugs, and who have mild to moderate hypertension (140/90–170/110), may be able to discontinue the medication in pregnancy. Those with more severe hypertension should continue. Appropriate preparations include methyldopa, β blockers (e.g. labetalol) or nifedipine. Diuretics and ACE inhibitors may cause fetal compromise and are contraindicated.

Gestational hypertension and pre-eclampsia (gestational hypertension and proteinuria)

- Gestational hypertension: see definitions above, but note that some authorities also consider an incremental diastolic rise of > 25 mmHg above the level recorded at booking to be significant.
- Gestational proteinuria: ≥ 300 mg/ 24 hours (≈ '+' or more on Dipstix testing).

Pre-eclampsia is a multisystem disorder of unknown aetiology specific to pregnancy characterized by hypertension, proteinuria and often fluid retention. Those with bilateral

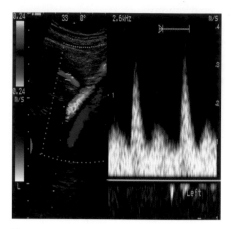

Fig. 2 **Uterine artery Doppler notching at 24 weeks is predictive of pre-eclampsia and IUGR in high-risk mothers.**

uterine artery Doppler notching (Fig. 2) at 24 weeks are at increased risk of developing pre-eclampsia.

Primary placental pathology

There is a lack of trophoblast infiltration of placental arterial walls leading to failure of arterial dilatation, and acute atherosis with aggregates of fibrin and platelets blocking the arteries.

Secondary effects

These are summarized in Table 1.

It is an extremely variable and unpredictable condition, and progression is often more rapid the earlier in pregnancy it occurs. Some have minimal symptoms and then have fits, others look worryingly unwell and are fine. The purpose of antenatal screening is to prevent both the maternal complications (cerebral injury, multisystem failure) and fetal complications (intrauterine growth restriction (IUGR), intrauterine death and abruption) of severe disease by timely delivery of the baby. Treatment of the mother with antihypertensives masks the sign of hypertension but

Table 1 **Secondary effects of primary placental pathology**	
System	**Effects**
Cardiovascular system	Increased peripheral resistance leading to hypertension Reduced maternal plasma volume and increased vascular permeability
Renal	Glomerular damage leading to proteinuria, hypoproteinaemia, reduced oncotic pressure, which further exacerbates the hypovolaemia. May develop acute renal failure ± cortical necrosis
Clotting	Hypercoagulable, with increased fibrin formation and fibrinolysis
Liver	Fibrin deposition in the hepatic sinusoids. HELLP syndrome
Central nervous system	Thrombosis and fibrinoid necrosis of the cerebral arterioles Eclampsia (convulsions), cerebral haemorrhage and cerebral oedema
Fetus	Impaired uteroplacental circulation leading to IUGR and increased perinatal mortality

does not alter the course of the disease, although it may allow prolongation of the pregnancy and thereby improve fetal outcome. The only true 'cure' is delivery of the placenta.

Management of gestational hypertension

The following may be used as guidelines:

- If the BP is found to be elevated at an antenatal clinic, it should be rechecked after 10–20 minutes. If it has settled, no further action is required.
- If the BP is elevated on two or more occasions ≥ 4 hours apart, fetal size should be appraised clinically and enquiry made about maternal well-being. Serum urate (rises with pre-eclampsia). U & Es, and platelets (which fall with pre-eclampsia) should be checked twice weekly along with BP recording and urine Dipstix measurement (Fig. 1b). Advice should be given to present if unwell, or if there is frontal headache or epigastric pain.
- If there are abnormal blood results, the diastolic is > 100 mmHg or has risen from booking by > 25 mmHg, or there is clinical suspicion of IUGR, poor fetal well-being or maternal compromise, arrangements should be made for a cardiotocograph (CTG) and ultrasound assessment of fetal size and liquor volume. Also arrange BP recording and Dipstix three times per week, with at least weekly measurement of serum urate, U & Es, full blood count, and platelets.

It is important to consider the overall picture rather than make decisions on the basis of a single parameter. It is appropriate to admit the mother for more intensive monitoring if there are symptoms or if she has significant proteinuria or severe hypertension. Oral antihypertensives may be considered and plans can be made for delivery.

The decision to deliver and the method of delivery are dependent on many of the above factors. There are advantages to conservative management up to 34 weeks if BP, laboratory values and fetal parameters are stable.

It has been suggested that low-dose aspirin taken from early pregnancy (< 17 weeks and probably from the first trimester) may reduce the incidence of IUGR or perinatal mortality in those with previous disease. Studies in this area have provided conflicting evidence.

Severe disease

The aim is to:

- Reduce diastolic BP to < 100 mmHg with labetalol, hydralazine or nifedipine.
- Consider delivery, the timing of which depends on maternal well-being, and fetal gestation and well-being. Delivery is the only thing that will improve the course of the disease.
- Assess fluid balance. There is increased vascular permeability and a reduced intravascular compartment – giving too little fluid risks renal failure and giving too much risks pulmonary oedema. Urine output should be measured hourly, and SaO_2 also monitored. U & Es, liver function tests (LFTs), albumin, urate, haemoglobin (Hb), haematocrit, platelets and clotting should be monitored. Central monitoring with a central venous pressure (CVP) or Swan–Ganz line is often helpful in oliguria to differentiate intravascular depletion from renal impairment.
- There is very good evidence supporting the use of anticonvulsants in established eclampsia, and magnesium sulphate is known to be significantly more effective than phenytoin or diazepam in preventing further convulsions. Although the use of magnesium sulphate in severe pre-eclampsia has been shown to be effective in preventing eclampsia, treatment is not without risk.

Eclampsia is said to have occurred when there has been a convulsion. The UK national incidence is 4.9/10 000 maternities with 38% antepartum, 18% intrapartum and 44% postnatal. Of these, 38% occur before proteinuria and hypertension have been documented. The maternal mortality is 1.8% with a neonatal death rate of 34/1000. In the developing world, incidences of 20–80/10 000 maternities have been quoted, with a maternal mortality around 10%.

- The patient should be turned onto her side to avoid aortocaval compression. An airway and high-flow O_2 should be given.
- $MgSO_4$ should be given immediately by intravenous injection to terminate the convulsion and then by intravenous infusion to reduce the chance of further convulsions. $MgSO_4$ can depress neuromuscular transmission, so the respiratory rate and patellar reflexes should be monitored.
- Consideration should be given to urgent delivery if the fit has occurred antenatally.
- Consideration should also be given to paralysis and ventilation if the fits are prolonged or recurrent.

HELLP syndrome

HELLP is an acronym from **h**aemolysis, **e**levated **l**iver enzymes (particularly transaminases) and **l**ow **p**latelets. It is a variant of pre-eclampsia, affecting 4–12% of those with pre-eclampsia/eclampsia and is commoner in multigravidae. There may be epigastric pain, nausea, vomiting, and right upper quadrant tenderness. There may be acute renal failure and disseminated intravascular coagulation (DIC), and there is an increased incidence of placental abruption. There is also an increased incidence (although still rare) of hepatic haematoma and hepatic rupture leading to profuse intraperitoneal bleeding. Management is to stabilize coagulation, assess fetal well-being and consider the need for delivery. It is generally considered that delivery is appropriate for moderate to severe cases, but management may be more conservative (with close monitoring) if mild. Postpartum vigilance is required for at least 48 hours. The incidence of recurrence in subsequent pregnancies is about 20%.

Hypertension

- Pre-eclampsia is a multisystem disorder, and a major cause of fetal and maternal morbidity and mortality.
- Medication, including antihypertensive agents, does not alter the progress of the condition; the only cure is delivery.
- HELLP syndrome is a variant of pre-eclampsia and is an acronym from **h**aemolysis, **e**levated **l**iver enzymes (particularly transaminases) and **l**ow **p**latelets.

Small for dates fetus

The detection of poor fetal growth is one of the aims of antenatal care. Perinatal mortality rises from 12 in 1000 in those over 5th centile for growth to 190 in 1000 in those less than 10th centile. Although there is little that can be done to promote growth in utero, the option exists for delivery of the fetus when it is decided that the environment outside the uterus is healthier than that inside. There is increased risk of intrauterine death, intrapartum hypoxia, neonatal hypoglycaemia and possible long-term neurological impairment for the small fetus.

Categories of small infants

Born too soon

These babies are a normal size for their gestation. Perinatal mortality is more strongly associated with low gestation than with birth weight.

Low birth weight

These infants are by definition < 10th centile for gestation.

Intrauterine growth restriction (IUGR)

Infants in this category may show two different patterns of growth.
Asymmetric IUGR. In this case uteroplacental insufficiency means the fetus fails to achieve its growth potential. There is an association with pre-eclampsia, abruptio placentae, maternal disease and maternal smoking. The asymmetry arises from the 'brain-sparing' effect with blood preferentially diverted to the fetal brain, maintaining its growth at the expense of the liver. Thus the head circumference follows the same centile for growth while the abdominal circumference falls to a lower centile. These infants are born with a wasted appearance – being long and thin.
Symmetric IUGR. The fetus is noted to be growing in proportion but is small. Some of these infants will just be at the lower end of the normal range for size (e.g. babies of Asian parents) but others will be small due to an insult such as viral infection or chromosomal abnormality.

In practice all infants where growth is on a lower centile than predicted are monitored, looking for other signs of a problem (decreased liquor volume or Doppler abnormality).

Assessment of the fetus

Fetal movement charts

Asking the mother to record the time at which 10 fetal movements have been noted is based on the recognition that a reduction or cessation in fetal movements may precede fetal death by 24 hours or more. This is not true in all cases and thus action to prevent fetal loss is not always possible. Trials assessing movement counting do not show a reduction in the incidence of intrauterine fetal death in late pregnancy but in the high-risk pregnancy this method does allow daily monitoring and is sometimes used.

Symphysis–fundal height (SFH)

Assessment of fetal size is undertaken by all involved in antenatal care, with palpation of the maternal abdomen performed at each antenatal visit. This is notoriously unreliable at predicting either large or small infants but use of a tape measure to record the symphysis–fundal height may give a useful guide for an individual observer. This may then be plotted against a chart of expected measurements and any change from the expected size noted (Fig. 1). The inter-observer error

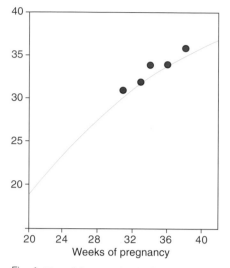

Fig. 1 **Plot of the symphysis–fundal height.**

with this measurement is large but studies of the ability of SFH measurement to predict low birth weight have shown quite good sensitivity.

Ultrasound

Ultrasound measurements of the fetus can give an idea of the growth pattern by plotting the measurements serially against standardized charts (Fig. 2).

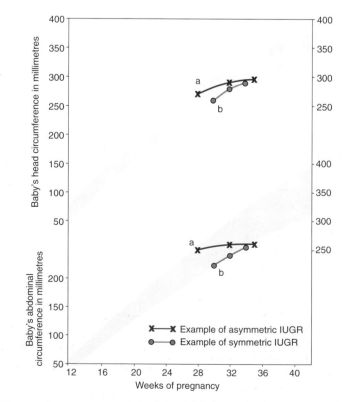

Fig. 2 **Ultrasound measurement of the fetus. (a)** Asymmetric IUGR. **(b)** Small for dates (symmetric IUGR).

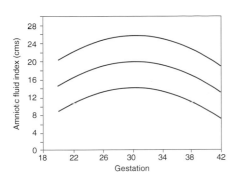

Fig. 3 **The amniotic fluid index plotted against gestation showing normal range (mean ± 2 standard deviations).**

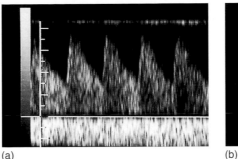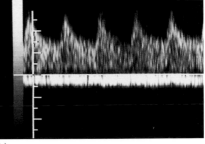

(a)   (b)

Fig. 4 **Doppler ultrasound of the umbilical artery. (a) Normal. (b) Absent end diastolic blood flow.**

The fetal head circumference is measured to try to get around the problem of variations in the biparietal diameter (BPD) due to different head shape depending on fetal position (e.g. dolicocephaly or the more oval head shape in the breech infant). This is plotted against the abdominal circumference on the charts and the pattern of growth noted. Curve a depicts asymmetric IUGR and curve b shows a small for dates fetus.

Ultrasound is also used to measure the amount of liquor around the fetus. This varies with the gestation but also changes with IUGR when, due to poor perfusion of the fetal kidneys, there is less liquor than usual at that gestation. The volume is assessed by measuring the pools of liquor without limbs or cord in them. Pools between 3 and 8 cm are normal but are not thought to give a very representative overall picture of the volume, so an amniotic fluid index measuring the greatest pool in each quadrant of the uterus may be preferred (Fig. 3). The amniotic fluid index has been plotted against gestation to give a normal range.

Alterations in fetal umbilical blood flow may occur as an early event in conditions of placental insufficiency. Doppler ultrasound (Fig. 4) of the umbilical artery is used as an assessment of downstream vascular resistance (i.e. placental resistance) and may help to identify placental insufficiency in high-risk pregnancies (e.g. IUGR, PET). The Doppler probe is directed at the umbilical cord and detects velocity (the Doppler shift – the effect noted as an ambulance with its siren on passes and you note a change in the tone).

Figure 4a shows the normal pattern obtained with flow during systole and diastole indicated and below the line the continuous venous flow. Reduction of end diastolic blood flow may

identify those at risk of hypoxia (Fig. 4b). It is likely that the hypoxia precedes the Doppler changes. This can give further information to aid a decision on whether to deliver a small fetus early to achieve a better outcome.

Biophysical profile
This looks at five variables (fetal movement, tone, reactivity, breathing and amniotic fluid volume) considered to be of prognostic significance in assessment of the high-risk pregnancy. Comparison of this profile with antenatal CTG for care of high-risk pregnancies does not result in improved outcome for the baby so the test is not universally used, though it often produces useful information.

Monitoring
Once the small infant has been identified there is usually a period of monitoring to try to assess the optimal time to deliver the baby. Twice weekly measurement of amniotic fluid volume (plotted against the chart – see above) and CTG may be supplemented by Doppler studies. Abnormalities in any of these tests may make the obstetrician feel that the extrauterine environment may be safer for the baby. The decision is based on the likely

survival rates of infants at the gestation the pregnancy has reached once tests become abnormal.

Management
Delivery of the baby removes the infant from a hostile intrauterine environment but the mode of delivery has to be decided upon. A caesarean section offers immediate extrauterine conditions but there is a higher risk of respiratory distress syndrome in babies born by caesarean section compared with babies born vaginally at the same gestational age. Vaginal delivery, however, is recognized to be stressful for the infant and if there are already signs of fetal compromise, it is not reasonable to induce labour. There are no scientific studies to give an answer, and each case is assessed individually in the light of all the facts to try to decide on the best method of delivery.

Antenatal corticosteroid therapy has been shown to reduce the incidence of respiratory distress syndrome. Maximum benefit is achieved for babies delivered more than 24 hours and less than 7 days after commencement of the medication. In elective preterm deliveries it is usual to give corticosteroid therapy between 24 and 34 weeks' gestation.

Small for dates fetus

- Asymmetrical growth restriction is associated with low amniotic fluid index and raised perinatal mortality, and may necessitate early delivery.

- Ultrasound measurements of the fetal abdominal and head circumference plotted on growth charts allow detection of the fetus whose growth pattern deviates from the normal.

- Symphysis–fundal height is better than abdominal palpation alone in detecting low birth weight for gestation.

- Doppler ultrasound gives additional information when monitoring the high-risk pregnancy.

Medical disorders in pregnancy

(See also Diabetes mellitus, p. 28; Hypertension, p. 20; Venous thromboembolic disease, p. 42; Infections in pregnancy, p. 14.)

Cardiac disease

Heart disease of varying types complicates less than 1% of all pregnancies but accounts for 9% of UK maternal deaths. While rheumatic heart disease remains a significant problem in the developing world, there are increasing numbers of fertile women in western countries who have had surgery for congenital heart disease (CHD) as children. Maternal mortality is highest in those conditions where pulmonary blood flow cannot be increased to compensate for the increased demand during pregnancy, e.g. in those with pulmonary hypertension (particularly Eisenmenger syndrome, where maternal mortalities of 40–50% have been reported).

Unfortunately, many of the symptoms and signs usually considered indicative of heart disease occur commonly in normal pregnancy, making clinical diagnosis difficult: breathlessness and syncopal episodes are present in 90% of normal pregnancies, atrial ectopic beats are common and up to 96% of women may have an audible ejection systolic murmur. Further investigation should be considered if the murmur is > 3/6, a thrill is present, or if there are any other suspicious features.

If significant problems are discovered, a cardiologist should be involved. If there is no haemodynamic compromise (e.g. as with congenital mitral valve prolapse), then the prognosis is good and, after initial assessment, there is no need for cardiac follow-up, although antibiotic prophylaxis may be required. If there are significant potential haemodynamic problems, then consideration of pregnancy termination is an option (e.g. with Eisenmenger syndrome, primary pulmonary hypertension and pulmonary veno-occlusive disease). If the maternal pO_2 is decreased, the fetus is at risk from asphyxia and intrauterine growth restriction (IUGR) and should be monitored with regular ultrasound scans (USS) for growth, Doppler studies, cardiotocographs

(CTGs) and biophysical profiles.

Severe cardiac disease can cause problems at delivery, particularly in those with prosthetic valves, aortic stenosis, severe mitral stenosis and those with pulmonary hypertension. Important aspects of the management of delivery in cases of severe cardiac disease are listed in Table 1.

Puerperal cardiomyopathy is rare (< 1 : 5000), carries a 25–50% mortality, and is associated with hypertension in pregnancy, multiple pregnancy, high multiparity and increased maternal age. It presents with sudden onset of heart failure and there is a grossly dilated heart on echocardiography.

Connective tissue disease

Although these diseases are rare, they occur most commonly in women during their child-bearing years and it is therefore relatively common to find them in association with pregnancy.

Systemic lupus erythematosus (SLE)

There is no effect of pregnancy on the long-term prognosis of SLE. There is probably an increased chance of flare-ups occurring in pregnancy (Fig. 1). Women should be discouraged from becoming pregnant during disease flare-ups to minimize fetal problems. Active SLE nephritis during pregnancy is associated with a significant maternal and perinatal mortality and in particular with a risk of pre-eclampsia.

SLE is associated with increased fetal loss rates from an increase in spontaneous miscarriages and preterm delivery. This is particularly so in those with raised anticardiolipin antibodies (p. 93). There is an increased incidence of pre-eclampsia and this may be difficult to differentiate from a disease

Table 1 **Cardiac disease and delivery**
■ Labour should be conducted in a high-dependency or intensive care unit setting, aiming for a vaginal delivery, and avoiding ↓ BP, hypoxia or fluid overload
■ Epidural analgesia may be used, and is probably preferable to spinal or general anaesthesia
■ Endocarditis prophylaxis should be given if required
■ The second stage should be kept short
■ Particular care is required in the immediate postpartum period as there is an increased circulating volume following uterine retraction, which may lead to fluid overload and congestive failure

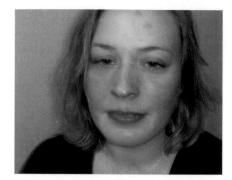

Fig. 1 **There is a characteristic butterfly rash.** This patient's SLE flared up at 22 weeks, with marked hypertension and renal impairment.

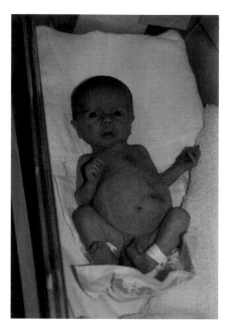

Fig. 2 **Pacemaker in baby with congenitaling heart block in association with anti-Ro antibodies.**

flare-up, as both are associated with hypertension and proteinuria. There is no increase in the rate of fetal abnormalities, although there is a risk of fetal congenital heart block in association with the presence of anti-Ro and anti-La antibodies (Fig. 2). Neonatal lupus may rarely occur and is characterized by haemolytic anaemia, leucopenia, thrombocytopenia, discoid skin lesions, pericarditis and congenital heart block.

If lupus anticoagulant or anticardiolipin antibodies are present, low-dose aspirin should be given, and, in those with a previous history of thromboembolic disease, low-dose heparin may also be required. Careful monitoring of renal function is also appropriate. Flare-ups should be managed where possible with oral prednisolone (if not already on oral prednisolone) and there should be regular growth scans looking for IUGR as well as regular fetal monitoring with CTGs and biophysical profiles in the third trimester.

Epilepsy

Around a third of those with epilepsy have an increase in seizure frequency independent of the effects of medication, particularly those with secondary generalized or complex partial seizures. The fall in anticonvulsant levels owing to dilution, reduced absorption, reduced compliance and increased drug metabolism is partially compensated for by reduced protein binding (and therefore an increase in the level of free drug). There is an increased incidence of fetal anomaly in those with epilepsy irrespective of the effects of drugs (3–4% vs 2% in the general population), possibly owing to a combination of hypoxic and genetic factors (Fig. 3). For those on anticonvulsants, the incidence of anomaly is ≈ 6%. Single-drug regimens are less teratogenic than multidrug therapy.

The management of epilepsy in pregnancy is summarized in Table 2.

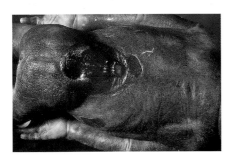

Fig. 3 **Anticonvulsants are associated with neural tube defects, cardiac and craniofacial defects.**

Hepatic disorders

A history of a prodromal illness, overseas travel or high-risk group for blood-borne illness may suggest viral hepatitis. Itch is suggestive of cholestasis. Abdominal pain is associated with gallstones, HELLP syndrome and acute fatty liver. Clinical signs are often unhelpful in diagnosis. U & Es, urate, liver function tests (LFTs), blood glucose, platelets and coagulation screen should be checked and blood sent for hepatitis serology. An abdominal ultrasound scan of the liver may show obstruction or fat infiltration.

Liver disorders specific to pregnancy

Hyperemesis gravidarum

This may be associated with abnormal LFTs.

Intrahepatic cholestasis of pregnancy

Jaundice is mild, usually presenting after 30 weeks' gestation, possibly because of a genetic predisposition to the cholestatic effect of oestrogens. Pruritus is generally severe, affecting limbs and trunk. There is a positive family history in up to 50% of cases.

Transaminases are increased (less than threefold), and alkaline phosphatase levels are raised (above normal pregnancy values). Bilirubin is usually < 100 µmol/l, and there may be pale stools and dark urine. Serum total bile acid concentration is increased early in the disease and may be the optimum marker.

There are no serious long-term maternal risks but there is a risk of preterm labour, fetal distress and intrauterine fetal death. The fetus must be monitored closely and there is growing evidence that delivery at 37–38 weeks is appropriate. The combined oral contraceptive pill is contraindicated.

HELLP syndrome
See page 21.

Acute fatty liver of pregnancy

This is very rare, but carries a high maternal and fetal mortality and may progress rapidly to hepatic failure. It usually presents with vomiting in the third trimester associated with malaise and abdominal pain followed by jaundice, thirst and alteration in consciousness level. LFTs are elevated, urate is very high and there is often profound hypoglycaemia.

Liver disorders coincidental to pregnancy

Viral hepatitis

This is the commonest cause of abnormal LFTs in pregnancy. Titres for hepatitis A, B and C as well as for cytomegalovirus (CMV) and toxoplasmosis should be checked.

Gallstones

Asymptomatic gallstones do not require treatment. Cholecystitis should be managed conservatively.

Cirrhosis

In severe cirrhosis there is usually amenorrhoea. If pregnancy occurs, and the disease is well compensated, there is usually no long-term effect on hepatic function. The main risk is from bleeding oesophageal varices.

Chronic active hepatitis

This is usually associated with amenorrhoea. Pregnancy does not usually have any long-term effect on liver function. Obstetric complications are common and fetal loss rate is high. Immunosuppressant therapy with prednisolone and azathioprine should be continued in those with autoimmune disease.

Table 2 **Management of epilepsy in pregnancy**	
Consider	**Discussion**
Pre-pregnancy counselling	Monotherapy ideal. Folate supplementation should be continued until at least 12 weeks
Anticonvulsant dosage	Anticonvulsant doses adjusted on clinical grounds. There are fetal risks from the anticonvulsant medication as well as from not taking the drugs (from increased fit frequency)
Detailed ultrasound scan at 18–22 weeks	Neural tube, cardiac and craniofacial abnormalities as well as diaphragmatic herniae are more common
Vitamin K for women on enzyme-inducing anticonvulsants	Vitamin K p.o. daily from 36 weeks (anticonvulsants are vitamin K antagonists and increase the risk of haemorrhagic disease of the newborn). The baby should be given vitamin K i.m. stat. at birth and the paediatrician alerted to the possibilities of anticonvulsant drug withdrawal
Fits	Most fits in pregnancy will be self-limiting but if prolonged give diazepam p.r./i.v. ± ventilation
Postnatal	Postnatally, the mother may breast feed safely (drugs pass into the milk but are of little clinical significance). Advice should be given about safe and suitable settings for feeding, bathing, etc. Carbamazepine, phenytoin, primidone and phenobarbital induce liver enzymes, reducing the effectiveness of standard dose combined oral contraceptives, therefore a higher-dose oestrogen preparation is required

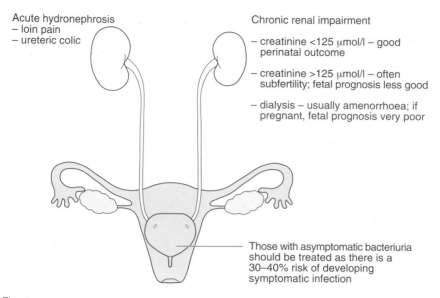

Acute hydronephrosis
– loin pain
– ureteric colic

Chronic renal impairment

– creatinine <125 μmol/l – good
  perinatal outcome

– creatinine >125 μmol/l – often
  subfertility; fetal prognosis less good

– dialysis – usually amenorrhoea; if
  pregnant, fetal prognosis very poor

Those with asymptomatic bacteriuria
should be treated as there is a
30–40% risk of developing
symptomatic infection

Fig. 4 **The genitourinary system in pregnancy.**

Primary biliary cirrhosis

This is variable in severity. The prognosis for mother and fetus is good in mild disease. It may present during pregnancy for the first time in a similar way to intrahepatic cholestasis of pregnancy.

Renal disorders (Fig. 4)

In pregnancy, there is an increase in the size of both kidneys and dilatation of the ureter and renal pelvis. This is greater on the right than on the left because of the dextrorotation of the uterus. There is also an increase in creatinine clearance because of the increased glomerular filtration rate (GFR) (maximal in the second trimester). Urea should be < 4.5 mmol/l and creatinine < 75 μmol/l.

Infection

Urinary tract infections (UTIs) occur in 3–7% of pregnancies and if untreated may lead to septicaemia and premature labour. Asymptomatic bacteriuria should be treated in all pregnant women, as there is a 30–40% risk of developing a symptomatic UTI. Pyelonephritis should be treated aggressively.

Obstruction

Acute hydronephrosis is characterized by loin pain, ureteric colic, sterile urine and a renal USS showing dilatation of the renal tract greater than normal in pregnancy (Fig. 5). If the symptoms are not settling and the USS does not demonstrate the cause of the obstruction, a limited intravenous urogram (IVU) should be considered.

Chronic renal impairment

The fetal prognosis with chronic renal disease in pregnancy is best if maternal renal function and BP are optimized. If the plasma creatinine is < 125 μmol/l, the maternal and perinatal outcome is usually good. If it is > 250 μmol/l, there is usually amenorrhoea and if pregnancy occurs there may be a risk of renal deterioration (therefore consider termination of pregnancy). Between these levels, women should be advised that pregnancy may cause their renal function to deteriorate and that there are also risks to the fetus (mainly IUGR). Pre-existing hypertension, proteinuria and a pre-pregnancy GFR < 70ml/minute are also associated with a poorer maternal and fetal outcome. Some renal diseases carry a worse prognosis than others (specialist advice is required).

Close fetal monitoring is important in the third trimester. It is difficult to distinguish pre-eclampsia from increasing renal compromise as both may present with hypertension and proteinuria.

Pregnancy should be discouraged in patients on dialysis as the fetal prognosis is poor. Pregnancy in patients with renal transplant is possible.

Respiratory disorders

Breathlessness due to the physiological increase in ventilation is a common symptom in pregnancy. This is due partly to low pCO_2, the effect of progesterone, and partly to a raised diaphragm, which occurs even before the uterus causes direct physical pressure. A normal chest X-ray and physical examination virtually excludes a pathological problem in the absence of other symptoms.

Asthma is common. In most, the disease is unchanged, but it may improve, or less commonly, deteriorate. Treatment is similar to that in the non-pregnant patient. Inhaled β-sympathomimetics and inhaled steroids are safe. Oral steroids may be indicated.

Thrombocytopenia

Maternal thrombocytopenia in pregnancy

In the second half of 8% of normal pregnancies there is a mild thrombocytopenia (platelet count $100–150 \times 10^9/l$) which is not associated with any risk to the mother or fetus. Pre-eclampsia (see p. 20) should be excluded.

Autoimmune thrombocytopenic purpura is the commonest cause of thrombocytopenia in early pregnancy (but can also arise in later pregnancy) and may be acute or chronic.

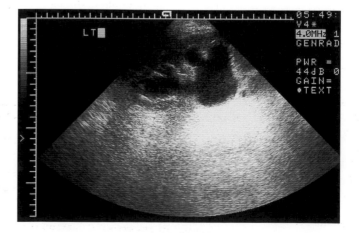

Fig. 5 **Ultrasound of left kidney with ureteric obstruction and calyceal clubbing.** There was a calculus in the lower third of the ureter.

Antiplatelet antibodies may be detected. These may cross the placenta and cause fetal thrombocytopenia, although this is rarely associated with long-term morbidity (cf. alloimmune thrombocytopenia). No treatment is required in the absence of bleeding, providing the platelet count remains above $50 \times 10^9/l$. If the platelet count falls below this level, steroids and immunoglobulin can be given.

Fetal (alloimmune) thrombocytopenia

This is a rare disorder in which there are maternal antibodies to fetal platelets (similar to Rhesus disease except for platelets rather than red blood cells). The maternal platelet level is normal, but there may be profound fetal thrombocytopenia and antenatal or intrapartum intracranial bleeds. The diagnosis should be suspected when a previous child has had neonatal thrombocytopenia and maternal antiplatelet antibodies have been identified (often to the HPA-1a antigen). Treatment is usually with antenatal immunoglobulin and elective caesarean section.

Thyroid disorders

1% of pregnant women in the western world are affected by thyroid disease, with hypothyroidism being commoner than hyperthyroidism. The fetal thyroid gland is active and secretes thyroid hormones from the 12th week. It is independent of maternal control, although maternal thyroid hormones do cross the placenta.

Hypothyroidism

This may present with fatigue, hair loss, dry skin, abnormal weight gain, poor appetite, cold intolerance, bradycardia and delayed tendon reflexes. If untreated, there is double the rate of spontaneous miscarriages and stillbirths compared to the normal population, as well as a risk of fetal neurological impairment. There is minimal fetal risk if the mother is treated and euthyroid. Thyroid function should be regularly monitored, aiming to keep thyroid-stimulating hormone within the normal range and free thyroxine (T4) at the upper end of the normal range. Fetal hypothyroidism may occur when the mother carries antithyroid antibodies or is receiving antithyroid drugs.

Hyperthyroidism

Thyrotoxicosis presents with weight loss, exophthalmos, tachycardia and restlessness. It is usually due to Graves' disease but may occur secondary to toxic thyroid adenoma or multinodular goitre. Untreated thyrotoxicosis is associated with approximately 50% fetal mortality and a risk of maternal thyroid crisis at delivery. Well-controlled hyperthyroidism is not associated with an increase in fetal anomalies but there is a tendency for babies to be small for gestational age. Graves' disease usually improves during pregnancy. Carbimazole and propylthiouracil cross the placenta and can potentially cause fetal thyroid suppression. In low doses, however, this is rarely significant. Radioactive iodine is absolutely contraindicated, and surgery is indicated only for those with a very large goitre or poor oral compliance.

Postpartum thyroiditis

This occurs following 5–10% of all pregnancies, with initial hyperthyroidism followed by hypothyroidism (at around 1–3 months, which therefore may be confused with depression) and then recovery. Symptoms of hyperthyroidism may be treated with propranolol (antithyroid drugs accelerate the appearance of hypothyroidism). Hypothyroidism may be treated with thyroxine as above, withdrawing it around 6 months postnatally. A small proportion may require long-term treatment or may develop hypothyroidism later in life.

Gastrointestinal disorders

Peptic ulceration

Ulcers are rare in pregnancy but, when present, tend to improve. If ulcer symptoms occur, first-line treatment is with simple antacid/alginate compounds. If not resolving then ranitidine, an H2 antagonist, should be started. Those with problematic recurrent ulcers should also take ranitidine. Endoscopy is the investigation of choice, if necessary.

Inflammatory bowel disease

Fetal loss rate is similar to that of the normal population providing that the disease is not active at the start of the pregnancy. Flare-ups of the disease occur most commonly in the first trimester. There is no evidence of fetal problems with prednisolone or sulfasalazine and these should be continued at the minimum dose necessary. Constipation should be avoided and the mother should receive folic acid supplementation.

Acute episodes of inflammatory bowel disease present with abdominal pain, diarrhoea and passage of blood and mucus p.r. Patients should be admitted and fluid and electrolyte balance checked. Stool samples should be sent for culture to exclude gastroenteritis. Treatment is with topical steroid enemas, oral sulfasalazine and prednisolone daily. If the patient deteriorates, the possibility of intestinal perforation or toxic megacolon should be considered.

Colostomies and ileostomies may become temporarily obstructed during pregnancy. Vaginal deliveries are preferable to caesarean section (as there is a risk of adhesions from previous surgery), although care is needed with operative vaginal deliveries if the disease involves the perineum. Although sulfasalazine crosses into breast milk, there is no evidence of any neonatal problems.

Coeliac disease

Presentation may occur in pregnancy with non-specific gastrointestinal symptoms, anaemia and weight loss. Diagnosis is by duodenal biopsy via endoscopy. Treatment is with gluten-free diet and vitamin supplementation. Patients with known coeliac disease should be encouraged to comply with a strict gluten-free diet in pregnancy. Iron and folate supplements are recommended. The prognosis for the mother and fetus is good.

Medical disorders in pregnancy

- Structural heart disease in pregnancy has potentially serious implications for both mother and fetus.
- Abnormal liver function tests may be related to the pregnancy, but are commonly coincidental.
- Asymptomatic UTIs should be treated.
- The fewer anticonvulsants, the less the risk of fetal abnormality.
- Well-controlled thyroid disease poses little serious risk.

Diabetes in pregnancy I

Physiology

The hormonal changes of pregnancy profoundly affect carbohydrate metabolism. The levels of oestrogen, progesterone, human placental lactogen (HPL), prolactin and free cortisol rise progressively throughout pregnancy. Cortisol and HPL, especially, are insulin antagonists, so women become relatively insulin resistant in pregnancy. To overcome this trend, normal women compensate by producing increased amounts of insulin.

Definitions

When the obstetrician is faced with diabetes in pregnancy it represents either gestational diabetes or pre-existing disease.

Gestational diabetes

By definition, this is carbohydrate intolerance that develops during pregnancy and disappears after delivery. Normally in the second half of pregnancy, and particularly in the third trimester, there is a further increase in insulin resistance and a slight deterioration in glucose tolerance. Women who develop gestational diabetes are unable to meet this with a compensatory rise in insulin production and pregnancy-onset diabetes is therefore most commonly detected at this time.

The situation is often not as clear-cut as this. Some women have had pre-existing subclinical diabetes which was missed and therefore they appear to present as 'gestational' diabetes, since the diabetes was first detected in pregnancy. Some women with true pregnancy-related diabetes will continue to be diabetic post-delivery (about 15%). These are often missed, as postnatal glucose tolerance tests (GTTs) are not widely performed. Some will develop diabetes in later life.

Pre-existing diabetes

The classical syndrome of diabetes is characterized by hyperglycaemia due to a deficiency or diminished effectiveness of insulin. This results in the well-known symptoms and signs of polyuria, polydipsia, weight loss and glycosuria. The effects, if untreated, are profound. Eventually, cellular damage can occur, especially to vascular endothelial cells in the eye, kidney and central nervous systems.

In general the majority of diabetics are non-insulin dependent (NIDDM), controlled by diet or oral hypoglycaemic agents. There is a hereditary element and an association with obesity. NIDDM is less common in the childbearing years.

Insulin-dependent diabetes (IDDM) occurs most often in young adults and is due to cellular and humoral autoimmunity to pancreatic beta cells.

In pregnancy, diabetic control needs to be as careful for NIDDM as IDDM to avoid adverse perinatal outcome. White's classification (Table 1) is often used to grade the severity of the disease. In general, the more severe the disease the greater the perinatal mortality and incidence of congenital malformations.

Potential diabetes

This term is often used to define a group of women who are more likely to develop diabetes at some time in their lives than normal based on family, medical or obstetric history. These risk factors are still widely used in antenatal clinics today as part of screening for gestational diabetes (Table 2).

Diagnosis and screening

Screening and diagnosis aims to identify

Table 1   White's classification of established diabetes

A	Asymptomatic diabetes diagnosed by GTT
B	Diabetes onset after age 20 years
	Diabetes duration 0–9 years
	No vascular complications
C	Diabetes onset 10–19 years
	Diabetes duration 10–19 years
	No vascular disease
D	Diabetes onset before 10 years of age
	Diabetes duration > 20 years
	Vascular disease present
F	Diabetes with nephropathy
R	Diabetes with retinopathy

Table 2   Antenatal screening risk factors for gestational diabetes

- Significant glycosuria on two occasions in antenatal clinic, or one occasion if a fasting urine sample is tested, or one if less than 16 weeks' gestation
- Family history of diabetes, particularly parents or siblings (IDDM in the father is of greater predictive value than in the mother; predictive value is greater if a sibling or both parents are diabetic; grandparents are less significant)
- Previous big babies > 90th centile for gestational age and sex
- Diabetes in a previous pregnancy
- Previous unexplained intrauterine death or stillbirth
- Polyhydramnios
- Maternal obesity (> 20% above the ideal weight)

all women who may develop gestational diabetes. Various risk factors may be assessed from the booking history (Table 2) and if a patient exhibits two or more of these, then a glucose tolerance test (GTT) can be organized for 24–28 weeks' gestation.

Impaired glucose tolerance (IGT) is present if the fasting glucose is > 6 and < 7.8 but rises to 8.0–10.9 mmol/l within 2 hours of the 75 g glucose load. These women may develop gestational diabetes as the pregnancy progresses or remain with slightly impaired metabolism as pregnancy advances, reverting to normal afterwards. The significance of IGT is controversial. There is no evidence that treatment is of benefit but commonly, if the preprandial sugar is > 6 or the postprandial value is > 8, treatment with dietary control and possibly insulin can be introduced.

Gestational diabetes is diagnosed if the fasting glucose is > 8 mmol/l and the 2-hour level is > 11 mmol/l.

Alternative screening

Although the above method is most widely used there are considerable limitations:

- 30% of gestational diabetics have *none* of the recognized risk factors
- glycosuria can be found in up to 50% of all pregnant women at some stage in their pregnancy
- not all women with gestational diabetes, or even IGT, have *persistent* glycosuria and may be clear on testing.

Thus some gestational diabetics are missed and a lot of normal women have unnecessary GTTs. Routine screening for everyone has been suggested as a more accurate approach, performing random blood glucose tests at booking, 28 weeks and 32 weeks (referring equivocal cases for a GTT). Some centres perform a modified GTT at booking.

Pre-conceptual counselling

For the patient with pre-existing diabetes pre-conceptual counselling is vital (see p. 6). There is an increased incidence of congenital malformations amongst babies born to mothers whose diabetes is poorly controlled, with a 3–4 times higher rate of abnormality than in their non-diabetic counterparts. The incidence of *all* malformations is increased, especially congenital heart disease and neural tube defects.

Multiple abnormalities are common. Caudal regression syndrome (absence of vertebrae anywhere below T10) is rare but peculiar to diabetics. The most common form is sacral agenesis (Fig. 1). Tight diabetic control is therefore very important at the time of organogenesis to reduce the incidence of congenital malformations. As organogenesis occurs during the first 7–9 weeks of fetal life, and patients rarely book for antenatal care before 10–12 weeks, pre-conceptual counselling is the only way to gain diabetic control in time. At the pre-conception clinic the patient receives:

- general advice regarding diet, smoking and lifestyle
- establishment of tight diabetic control with advice for its maintenance
- examination of optic fundi
- assessment of baseline renal function
- plans made for early antenatal referral and booking
- commencement on folic acid.

Ongoing diabetic control
Control of diabetes remains essential throughout pregnancy for pre-existing and gestational disease. The movement of glucose across the placenta is by carrier-mediated facilitated diffusion (Fig. 2). Fetal blood-glucose levels usually remain 20–30 mg/dl lower than those of the mother. There is close correlation between fetal glucose uptake and blood levels. The fetal level is normally maintained within narrow limits because maternal glucose homeostasis is well regulated. Protein hormones such as insulin, glucagon, growth hormone and HPL do not cross the placenta. Ketoacids appear to diffuse freely and serve as fetal fuel during periods of maternal starvation. Periods of maternal hyperglycaemia result in fetal hyperglycaemia.

Perinatal mortality rates (PNMRs) (see p. 78) are closely linked to the severity of the diabetes and the degree of control achieved. Good control, however, does not completely preclude the development of macrosomia (large birthweight infants > 90th centile for gestational age and sex, with polycythaemia, adiposity and organomegaly) as up to 30% incidence has been reported in well-controlled diabetics (Figs 3 and 4).

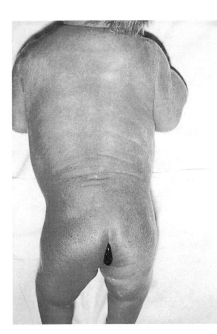

Fig. 1 **Sacral agenesis.**

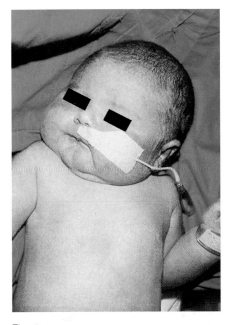

Fig. 3 **Macrosomic baby.**

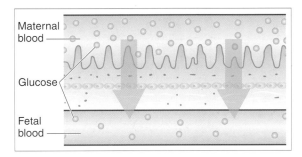

Fig. 2 **Facilitated diffusion of glucose molecules through the placenta.**

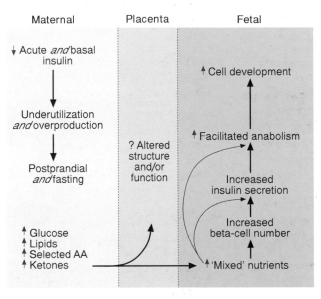

Fig. 4 **The modified Pedersen hypothesis.** Glucose and other substrates stimulate fetal insulin release resulting in macrosomia and other morbidity observed in the infant of a diabetic mother.

Diabetes in pregnancy I

- Pregnancy is a relatively insulin-resistant state.
- Gestational diabetes occurs if the increased insulin output fails to compensate.
- Antenatal screening methods are controversial; screening may be selective, based on risk factors, or offered to all.
- Existing diabetics have a higher incidence of congenital fetal malformations.
- The PNMR is closely linked to the severity of the disease and the degree of control.
- Pre-conceptual counselling and control is vital for established diabetics.

Diabetes in pregnancy II

Antenatal care

Antenatal care for both existing and gestational diabetes should take place jointly between physicians and obstetricians, preferably at a specially run clinic which involves a dietician. 'Brittle' diabetics may need to be seen weekly. The support of a diabetic Management Sister is invaluable as she can visit the patient at home, offering advice and supervision on self-monitoring of blood sugars and assessment of compliance to therapy.

Therapy

In general, gestational diabetics are treated with diet alone – unless there is evidence that this is failing to produce good control, when insulin is substituted.

Established diabetics are changed to insulin in early pregnancy if they were previously managed by diet or oral hypoglycaemics. As hypoglycaemic agents cross the placenta it is preferable to change to insulin, although in developing countries they may have an important role.

Good control can be achieved by a combination of a short-acting insulin such as Soluble or Actrapid, with a medium-acting insulin, such as Isophane or Monotard, given twice daily. Human or highly purified porcine insulins reduce the risk of developing antibodies which can cross the placenta.

Monitoring

Home-based monitoring ensures optimal control with the patient's usual diet and activity levels. Patients use a glucometer to check blood sugar profiles two or three times a week (see Fig. 1). Blood sampling by

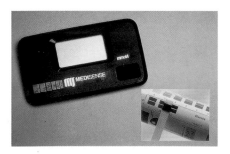

Fig. 1 **Glucometer and a Dextrostix colour indicator.** The glucometer is a more objective measurement, removing possible error when comparing the filter paper against the colour controls provided with the Dextrostix system.

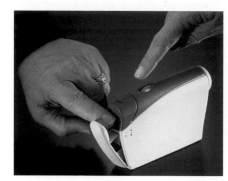

Fig. 2 **Automated finger puncturer.**

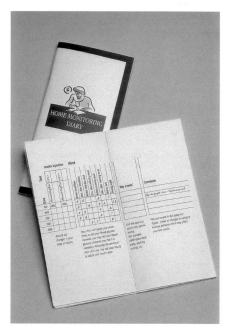

Fig. 3 **'Glucolog' log book.**

automated puncture (Fig. 2) is performed preprandially, 2-hourly postprandially and at bedtime. The results are recorded in a log book (Fig. 3) and brought to each clinic visit.

A random blood sugar is performed at each clinic visit as well as reviewing the log book results, checking the patient's weight and a urinalysis. A glycosylated haemoglobin reading is also obtained. This gives retrospective evidence of blood sugar control over the preceding few weeks rather than evidence of current control and checks the veracity of the values the patient has been reporting. Glycosylated haemoglobin is a naturally-occurring haemoglobin linked to glucose which represents a fairly constant 5–6% of the total haemoglobin mass in the non-pregnant normoglycaemic state. A level above 8% in pregnancy indicates poor sugar control.

Table 1 **Risks associated with diabetes in pregnancy**
Maternal
Adverse effects on existing retinopathy, nephropathy and neuropathy
Increased incidence of infections – urinary, monilial and other
Obstetric complications – pre-eclampsia, polyhydramnios, preterm labour
Trauma to the genital tract, e.g. haematomas and tears due to difficult delivery of large-birthweight baby (macrosomia)
Fetal
Congenital malformations
Prematurity associated with preterm labour
Intrauterine death
Fetal trauma (e.g. fractured clavicles, Erb's palsy), due to difficult deliveries
Shoulder dystocia
Neonatal metabolic problems, e.g. hypoglycaemia
Increased incidence of respiratory distress syndrome

Table 2 **Assessment of maternal and fetal well-being**
Maternal
Blood sugar control
Weight
Blood pressure
Optic fundi
Renal function
Fetal
Fetal anomalies scan at 18 weeks
Echocardiography at 20–24 weeks to detect congenital cardiac anomalies
Serial scans to assess fetal growth
Kick charts, biophysical profiles, Doppler studies and outpatient cardiotocographs in the third trimester to assess well-being
Amniotic phospholipid analysis to assess lung maturation (if preterm delivery looks likely)

Management

The aim is to maintain preprandial blood sugars at < 5 mmol/l and 1–2 hour postprandial blood sugars at < 7.5 mmol/l to reduce the potential risks to the mother and fetus (Table 1). In practice, most clinics tailor the control of blood glucose to the individual needs of the patient. Nocturnal hypoglycaemia can be treated by reducing the evening insulin or, more simply, by increasing the dietary intake just before bedtime. The disadvantage of maintaining the maternal blood sugar too low is that it may reduce the availability to the fetus of essential energy-producing substrates. Also, it may produce unpleasant and potentially damaging hypoglycaemic side effects in the mother.

The obstetric input to the clinic is to maintain a careful watch on maternal and fetal well-being as the pregnancy advances (Table 2). More intensive outpatient monitoring or admission may be indicated if:

- good glucose control cannot be achieved as an outpatient
- hypertension and/or proteinuria develop
- weight gain is excessive
- renal function deteriorates
- polyhydramnios develops
- fetal growth or well-being cause concern.

Delivery

Timing
In the past, sudden intrauterine death near term led to a policy of induction of labour between 36 and 38 weeks. This created a potential difficulty as diabetic babies have less appropriate surfactant levels for their gestational age and are more prone to respiratory distress syndrome (RDS) than neonates of non-diabetic mothers.

Improved diabetic control has encouraged many centres to allow their mothers to go into spontaneous labour if the pregnancy is uncomplicated. This has reduced the incidence of both RDS and caesarean sections for failed induction. It has not been accompanied by a rise in unexplained intrauterine deaths but it remains common practice to induce at 40 weeks.

If insulin requirements start to fall it is prudent to deliver the infant as this may indicate placental failure.

Premature labour
If the pregnancy has reached 34 weeks, no attempt should be made to stop labour. If there is genuine concern about the state of fetal lung maturity an amniocentesis can be performed or, in the case of ruptured membranes, a sample of liquor can be collected, though this is more often considered with induction, if required, preterm. The presence of phosphatadyl glycerol (a lung surfactant) indicates lung maturity and a low risk of RDS. If levels are low or absent, dexamethasone should be given to accelerate lung maturation.

Preterm labour prior to 34 weeks should generally be stopped if possible. Betasympathomimetics (e.g. salbutamol or ritodrine) should be used with caution, especially if used in conjunction with corticosteroids (see p. 18) as they cause marked hyperglycaemia. Use of tocolytics can be covered by an insulin infusion and regular blood glucose monitoring, along with potassium estimations.

Route of delivery
If there are no obstetric or other medical complications, the diabetes is well controlled and spontaneous onset of labour has been achieved, vaginal delivery is both possible and desirable. Caesarean section is indicated if there is evidence of fetal compromise or if ultrasound and clinical assessment suggest a baby so large that a vaginal delivery represents potential trauma to mother and fetus.

Intrapartum care
During labour, close control of the blood sugar is required by a continuous infusion of soluble insulin and an intravenous infusion of 10% dextrose. Blood sugars are checked hourly and kept between 5 and 8 mmol/l. Urea and electrolytes are checked 4-hourly.

Continuous fetal monitoring with cardiotocography is mandatory. An experienced obstetrician should be present at delivery because of the increased risk of shoulder dystocia (see p. 63).

Postnatal care
As insulin sensitivity increases immediately after delivery of the placenta the insulin infusion is stopped at this stage. The gestational diabetic will return to normal within 24 to 36 hours and insulin-dependent diabetics will return to their prepregnancy dose requirements.

Breast feeding is to be encouraged. An increase in the dietary allowance of carbohydrate by 50 g per day is needed to cover the extra calories required for lactation. Insulin requirements of the established diabetic do not alter during lactation.

Family planning should be carefully discussed. In the past, the combined contraceptive pill has been avoided in diabetics both because of the small but real risk of thromboembolism and because of the effect on carbohydrate metabolism. The newer low-dose pills can now be used in all but the most brittle diabetics. Progestogen-only contraception (Mirena coil, Implanon, Depo injection, progestogen-only pill) offers an alternative, especially if the woman is breast feeding, but may produce some cycle irregularities. The other forms of contraception must be considered on merit.

The neonate
The management of all infants of diabetic mothers calls for expert neonatal care. The neonate is at risk of a number of complications (Table 3).

The perinatal mortality has dropped dramatically over the past decade. In the best centres it now approaches that for other pregnancies, after mortality for congenital malformations has been excluded.

Infants of diabetic mothers have a greater than average chance of developing diabetes in later life (a risk in the order of 1% compared to 0.1% in infants of non-diabetic mothers).

Table 3 **Neonatal complications of poorly controlled diabetic pregnancy**
■ Low APGAR scores – one-third of all cases require intubation
■ Respiratory distress syndrome (RDS) (see p. 83)

■ Hypoglycaemia, secondary to pancreatic cell hyperplasia and hyperinsulinaemia
  – most commonly seen in macrosomic babies
  – usually asymptomatic, but can cause apnoea, hypertonia, excitability and fits

■ Hypocalcaemia
■ Hypomagnesaemia
■ Polycythaemia
■ Jaundice

Diabetes in pregnancy II

- Tight control of diabetes is necessary throughout pregnancy to minimize the risk of maternal and fetal complications.
- Management should be at a joint clinic run by physician and obstetrician.
- Emphasis is on home monitoring and outpatient management, minimizing hospitalization.
- Well-controlled uncomplicated pregnancies may be allowed to continue to 40 weeks to improve their chance of spontaneous labour.
- The perinatal mortality rate has been dramatically reduced and now approaches 9/100 000.

Anaemia in pregnancy

A useful guide to the acceptable lower limit of haemoglobin (Hb) for each trimester is 12.5 g/dl in the first trimester, 11.5 g/dl in the second and 10.5 g/dl in the third. The apparent fall in level throughout pregnancy is due to the relatively greater rise in maternal plasma volume compared to the rise in red cell mass. This physiological dilution of the maternal blood ensures normal circulation with less cardiac work than might be expected allowing for the increased amount of clotting factors and fibrinogen.

Anaemia may affect 10% of pregnancies in developed countries and is considerably commoner in developing countries, where it is a major source of maternal morbidity and a contributor to mortality. Up to 56% of all women living in developing countries are anaemic (Hb < 11 g/dl) due to infestations (particularly malaria – Fig. 1), frequent pregnancies or haemoglobinopathies (see p. 34). Maternal anaemia does not seem to pose substantial problems for the fetus but it is dangerous to both mother and fetus if there is superimposed haemorrhage (Fig. 2). It may also predispose the mother to thromboembolic problems and is associated with puerpural infection.

The proportion of maternal deaths due to anaemia has been reported as – India 16%, Kenya 11%, Nigeria 9% and Malawi 8%. Whether the anaemia is directly responsible for death or acts as an underlying factor in other causes is not clear. Antimalarial prophylaxis in endemic areas has been shown to decrease moderate to severe anaemia in pregnancy by over 50%. The increased incidence of low birthweight infants in affected women may be more related to the malaria than to the anaemia.

Antenatal screening

Haemoglobin is estimated at booking and during the third trimester to ensure anaemia is detected and treated. If the haemoglobin level is low, then the MCV (mean cell volume) is probably the most sensitive indicator of iron deficiency in pregnancy without measuring serum ferritin levels. Table 1 lists the indicators for anaemia. A macrocytic anaemia may suggest folate deficiency.

Iron metabolism

There is increased iron absorption during pregnancy but despite this the most common reason for anaemia is nutritional deficiency in both the developed and developing world. Iron utilization is 700–1400 mg per pregnancy with a saving of ~ 500 mg due to no menstrual blood loss. Dietary advice to eat plenty of green vegetables and high iron-containing foods may need to be supplemented with oral iron (Fig. 3).

Routine supplements are associated with a higher rise in red cell mass thus reducing the physiological haemodilution – which may have benefits in pregnancy. Conversely, maternal hypervolaemia may protect against supine hypotension and helps compensate for haemorrhage at delivery.

The question of whether to offer routine iron supplementation in pregnancy remains controversial. Iron requirements during pregnancy are increased three-fold to approximately 4 mg/day for the placenta, fetus, maternal red cells – as well as additional lactational needs. In developing countries all pregnant women should receive daily iron (60 mg) and folic acid (400 μg) and should be considered for preventive measures against malaria and hookworm.

Folate metabolism

A normal diet supplies adequate amounts of folate for pregnancy but, as

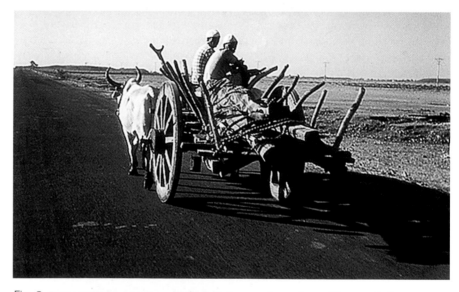

Fig. 2 **Postpartum haemorrhage is likely to be more hazardous with pre-existing anaemia, particularly if transport to hospital is a problem.**

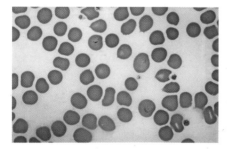

Fig. 1 **Chronic malarial infections from *Plasmodium vivax* are commonly associated with anaemia.**

Table 1	**The diagnosis of anaemia in pregnancy**
Factor	**Result indicating anaemia**
Haemoglobin	< 11 g/dl
Haematocrit	< 0.30
MCV	An MCV of < 80 fl indicates possible β-thalassaemia. If found, an estimation of haemoglobin A2 and haemoglobin electrophoresis should be made
MCH (mean cell haemoglobin)	< 28 pg
MCHC (mean cell haemoglobin concentration)	< 32 g/dl
Serum ferritin	A level of 10–50 μg/l indicates a strong possibility that anaemia will develop, whilst a level of < 10 μg/l indicates severe depletion of iron stores. In the latter case iron tablets should be prescribed, irrespective of the haemoglobin level

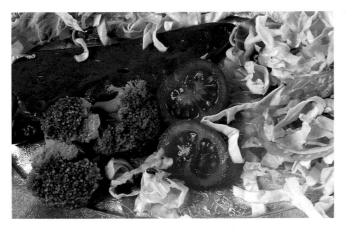

Fig. 3 **Iron-rich foods.**

Table 2 **Response to blood loss**	
Usual response in non-pregnant female	**Response in female at term post-delivery**
Fall in blood volume and compensatory vasoconstriction	Fall in blood volume (< 25% pre-delivery volume) with no vasoconstriction
Rise in plasma volume to bring blood volume to normal	Fall in plasma volume due to diuresis
Fall in haematocrit associated with rise in plasma volume	Haematocrit remains normal due to raised red cell mass of pregnancy

Table 3 **The benefits and risks of blood transfusion and parenteral iron therapy**		
	Benefits	**Risks**
Blood transfusion	Hb will rise after transfusion	Transfusion reaction
	Anaemia corrected	Transfusion of HIV
	Less risk of associated haemorrhage	CJD, hepatitis C
Parenteral iron	Malabsorption of iron avoided	Anaphylactic reaction
	Quicker response with anaemia close to term	Pain at injection site

body stores are small, any increase in demand may require supplementation. Conditions requiring folate supplementation in pregnancy are:

- anaemia responding to iron therapy
- haemolytic anaemia
- malaria
- multiple pregnancy
- antepartum haemorrhage.

Some women will have taken pre-conceptual folate as a preventive measure against neural tube defect in their infants and those on iron therapy will find most preparations are combinations of iron and folate.

Response to blood loss (Table 2)

Blood loss during delivery is inevitable and thus may be considered normal. The raised plasma volume and red cell mass return to pre-pregnancy values within 6 weeks of delivery. Vaginal delivery of a singleton infant is associated with blood loss of up to 500 ml, more loss than this being defined as a postpartum haemorrhage (see p. 60). Caesarean section or multiple delivery may be associated with greater blood loss. The average blood loss which can be tolerated without causing a significant fall in haemoglobin is around 1000 ml, dependent on a normal increase in blood volume prior to delivery.

Treatment

If iron deficiency anaemia is detected during screening, oral iron therapy is advised. This should increase the haemoglobin concentration by 1 g/dl per week of therapy after the first week (which goes to marrow stores for production). Side effects of this treatment include both constipation (already a problem in pregnancy due to the slower gut motility) and diarrhoea. Nausea may also be a problem.

Parenteral therapy is only required if there are compliance problems or prohibitive side effects with the oral route; it is contraindicated in patients with thalassaemia. It is also associated with the risk of anaphylactic reaction if given intravenously or pain at injection sites if given intramuscularly. Only if iron therapy fails should transfusion be considered. In recent years there has been much adverse publicity surrounding blood transfusion in relation to HIV, CJD and hepatitis C transmission and many patients are understandably reluctant to consider this form of therapy. A discussion of the risks of blood transfusion, versus the risks of parenteral iron, versus the risks of haemorrhage superimposed upon their anaemia should allow a reasonable treatment option to be decided in each patient (see Table 3).

On a worldwide scale, prevention of anaemia may depend on food enrichment or modification. Although genetic modification of food is controversial it is recognized that grain can be altered to reduce its phytate content and increase its content of cysteine – and so improve the absorption of iron from the intestine. This may produce a reduction in maternal mortality from anaemia in pregnancy. Food fortification would benefit both mothers and children who are at most risk of nutritional deficiencies.

Table 4 lists some valuable sources of dietary iron.

Table 4 **The iron content of some iron-rich foods** (note: absorption is 5–10%)	
Foods high in iron	**Amount per average portion (g)**
Chick pea curry	8.4
Cabbage	0.3
Spinach	1.4
Frozen peas	1.1
Frozen broccoli	0.5
Oat and wheat bran	13.5
Calves' liver	12.2
Pigs' kidney	12.7
Lamb vindaloo	10.5
Lamb chops – loin	2.9
Special K™	23.8

Anaemia in pregnancy

- The commonest worldwide cause of anaemia in pregnancy is nutritional deficiency; this could be addressed by fortification of food.
- Iron deficiency anaemia should be prevented with routine iron supplementation in developing countries.
- Routine iron supplementation should not be necessary in patients with an adequate diet.
- Anaemia at the time of delivery may compromise both mother and baby in the face of a postpartum haemorrhage.

Haemoglobinopathies in pregnancy

The haemoglobinopathies are genetic disorders of haemoglobin structure and synthesis. They are important in pregnancy because of their effect on maternal health and the possibility of transmission to the offspring, thus raising the question of prenatal diagnosis (see p. 8). Table 1 lists the various types of haemoglobinopathy. A basic résumé of haemoglobin structure and formation may aid understanding.

Formation of haemoglobin

Haemoglobin consists of four haem molecules attached to two pairs of globin chains (Fig. 1). Each globin chain has two genes which code for it, so faults in any of the genes may have effect on the structure or amount of globin produced. All types of haemoglobin have a pair of alpha chains, so a fault in alpha chain production affects all haemoglobins. The various types of haemoglobin are listed in Table 2 with their globin chain composition.

The thalassaemias

These disorders result from a reduced production of globin chains, limiting the amount of normal haemoglobin in the red cells available to transport oxygen. The clinical manifestation during pregnancy is anaemia. The beta thalassaemias have the greatest clinical impact and are found with an incidence varying from one in seven in Cyprus to one in a thousand in the UK (see Fig. 2 for affected areas). Population movement has resulted in some geographical overlap of the different haemoglobinopathies leading to double heterozygote phenotypes, e.g. HbS-beta thal.

Table 1 The haemoglobinopathies

Haemoglobinopathy	Globin gene composition	Bands on Hb electrophoresis	RBC features	Clinical
Alpha thalassaemia	α-/α α	A (i.e. normal)	Normal	Normal
	α-/α-	A	Mild anaemia	Normal
	--/α -	A, H	Severe anaemia HbH cells	Splenomegaly
	--/--	H	-	Hydrops fetalis
'Non-deletional' α-thal				
(abnormal α* gene)	α*α/α α	A, *, ± H	Variable	Variable
Beta thalassaemia				
β thal minor	normal β/reduced β	A, A₂, F	Mild anaemia	Normal
β thal intermedia	normal β/absent β	A, A₂, F	Moderate anaemia	Hepato-splenomegaly
	reduced β/reduced β	A, A₂, F		
β thal major	absent β/reduced β	(A) (A₂) F	Severe anaemia	Hepato-splenomegaly Bone deformity Delayed puberty Iron overload if transfused
	absent β/absent β	F		
Sickle cell trait	AS	A, S	Normal	Normal
Sickle cell disease	SS	S	Moderate or severe anaemia	Sickle crises Bone infarcts Asplenia Fetal loss
	SC	S, C		
	SD	S, D		

Table 2 Types of haemoglobin

	Type	Globin chains	% after 6 months old
Adult haemoglobin	HbA	$\alpha_2\beta_2$	97%
Adult haemoglobin	HbA₂	$\alpha_2\delta_2$	~ 2%
Fetal haemoglobin	HbF	$\alpha_2\gamma_2$	< 1%

Beta thalassaemias

This condition only becomes apparent after birth when the fetus moves from production of fetal haemoglobin with gamma chains to adult haemoglobin with beta chains. There are many possible abnormalities of the beta gene leading to a spectrum of clinical and laboratory abnormalities rather than to clearly defined beta thalassaemia heterozygote or homozygote appearances.

Severe disease with both beta chains affected means the disease was inherited from both parents (beta thalassaemia major with no beta chain production – see Table 1). Management is with regular transfusion but iron overload from the transfused red cells may lead to hepatic and endocrine dysfunction and myocardial damage. Cardiac failure is a major cause of death if an iron chelation programme is not used. Some patients can exist without regular blood transfusion but the expanded bone marrow leads to severe bone deformity. This group may achieve pregnancy and would require folate supplementation but iron in *any* form is contraindicated.

Beta thalassaemia minor patients may become iron deficient during pregnancy with lowered MCV, MCH and MCHC. They will need both folate and iron supplements but should *never* be given parenteral iron therapy. Unresponsive anaemia may require blood transfusion. Serum ferritin should be monitored as this is the best indicator of iron store status.

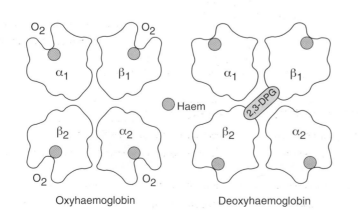

Fig. 1 **The structure of haemoglobin.**

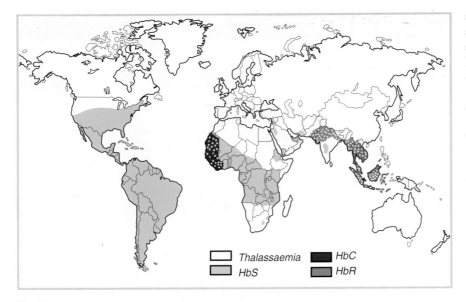

Fig. 2 **Distribution of thalassaemia.**

Table 3 Potential complications of sickle cell disease in pregnancy		
Maternal	**Fetal**	**Management plan**
Crises due to infection (UTI)	–	Check MSSU each visit
Spontaneous crises	–	Check for candidiasis
Retroplacental microthrombi	Fetal growth compromised	Serial growth scans
Anaemia	–	Iron and folate supplements
Anaesthesia risks at delivery		
– GA leads to hypoxia		O_2 and fluids
– regional block gives stasis		Fluid load
Preterm labour	Higher perinatal mortality	Need high-risk antenatal care

Alpha thalassaemias

There are four genes determining alpha chain production. The severity of the anaemia depends on the number of affected genes with production varying from reduced amount to total absence, when HbH tetramers may form. Daily oral folate supplements are needed for the chronic haemolytic anaemia, with increased supplements during pregnancy. Iron therapy is unhelpful. The unstable HbH is affected by substances known to trigger haemolysis.

Antenatal diagnosis in thalassaemias

This will be relevant in communities where the prevalence of thalassaemia is high. From the known status of the parents, prediction of the fetal thalassaemia status is possible and allows the parents to consider selective termination of an infant with a fatal variant. If an infant with severe thalassaemia is detected then the pregnancy can be associated with fulminating pre-eclampsia, a dangerous condition for the mother, and the hydropic infant is likely to die in utero.

In beta thalassaemia the diagnosis has to be made on chorionic villus sampling which allows DNA analysis. Beta chain production is negligible in the fetus and examination of fetal blood would not give a complete picture. Sampling is obtained at 9–11 weeks, so early attendance for antenatal care is essential.

Sickle cell syndromes

A variation in the beta chain structure results in sickle haemoglobin (HbS) which, although soluble in its oxygenated form, in its reduced state precipitates, distorting the cell into a sickle shape. Hypoxia, acidosis, dehydration and cold may produce sickling and the distorted cells block small blood vessels. This results in stasis, exacerbating the hypoxia and acidosis. These sickle cells may cause placental infarcts which is thought to account for the increased fetal loss rate in this disease.

Patients may be homozygous (HbSS), or heterozygous (HbS trait), or may have a combined condition with sickle cell haemoglobin C disease or sickle cell thalassaemia. Sickle trait is symptom free; HbSC and HbS-thal have the same clinical features as sickle cell disease.

Sickle cell disease and pregnancy
(Table 3)
The term sickle cell disease (SCD) includes sickle cell anaemia (SS), sickle haemoglobin C disease (SC), sickle beta thalassaemias and sickle cell anaemia with alpha thalassaemia. Pre-pregnancy counselling allows establishment of the haemoglobin status of the parents and prediction of the likelihood of an affected child. Presentation in early pregnancy is more common and discussion about prenatal diagnosis then is relevant.

Chorionic villus sampling at 9–11 weeks offers the chance of DNA analysis and establishment of the haemoglobin status of the fetus. Perinatal mortality is raised in association with higher rates of preterm labour and premature delivery.

Debate continues on whether it is necessary to offer elective exchange transfusion during pregnancy, aiming to keep the proportion of sickle cells low and keep the risk of sickle crisis to a minimum, or whether it is preferable to use exchange transfusion only if the clinical situation dictates.

Despite the theoretical risks of infection associated with intrauterine devices and the thrombotic risk of oral contraception, the risk of pregnancy is far greater and thus the most effective contraception is appropriate.

Management of sickle cell crises
Appropriate management includes:

- placing the patient in an intensive therapy unit
- oxygen therapy
- rehydration – usually with intravenous fluids
- opiate analgesia
- warmth
- appropriate antibiotics (some may already be on penicillin because of asplenia)
- exchange transfusion.

Haemoglobinopathies in pregnancy

- Haemoglobinopathy is a disorder of haemoglobin structure and synthesis.
- Thalassaemia reduces the amount of haemoglobin in the red blood cells, thus reducing the amount of oxygen carried.
- Iron overload must be avoided when treating anaemia in thalassaemic patients.
- Sickle haemoglobin causes the red blood cells to distort, producing placental infarcts and causing increased rates of fetal loss.

Antepartum haemorrhage

Antepartum haemorrhage (APH) is defined as bleeding from the genital tract after the gestation of potential viability (approximately 24 weeks). Common causes of APH include:

- placenta praevia
- placental abruption (abruptio placentae)
- local causes.

The incidence of APH is far greater than the combined incidence of placenta praevia and placental abruption and many cases remain of unknown origin.

Placenta praevia

The incidence of placenta praevia is 0.4–0.8%. It is more common in multiple pregnancy and conditions with large placental surface area, increasing maternal age and in patients with a previous caesarean section scar.

Grading (Table 1)

This grading is important as major degrees of placenta praevia are likely to require operative delivery whereas the minor grades may manage a successful vaginal delivery.

Clinical presentation

The lower uterine segment forms during the third trimester and with differential growth of the uterus antepartum haemorrhage is commoner at this stage. The classic presentation is:

- recurrent pain-free antepartum haemorrhage
- abnormal fetal lie
- non-engagement of the fetal presenting part.

Abdominal palpation will usually reveal a soft uterus with readily palpable fetal parts, an abnormal lie and a high presenting part. The fetal heart is most commonly audible except where there has been overwhelming haemorrhage. The diagnosis may be confirmed using ultrasound scanning to localize the placenta. This is still most commonly performed transabdominally where the maternal bladder delineates the upper edge of the lower uterine segment anteriorly. Without this landmark a posterior placenta praevia is more difficult to diagnose. The presenting part also obscures vision posteriorly.

Vaginal scanning enables more accurate measurement of the distance from the edge of the cervical os to the edge of the placenta – placental location greater than 2 cm from the cervical os would not be expected to cause any clinical problem. Transvaginal scanning is used with caution for fear of precipitating catastrophic haemorrhage. More clear views of the pelvis, fetus and placenta can be obtained with magnetic resonance imaging (MRI) scanning. However, this is not widely available and its fetal effects are less well known than those of ultrasound.

Management (Fig. 1)

The golden rule for APH is that no vaginal examination should be performed until placenta praevia has been excluded as this might precipitate torrential bleeding with possible maternal and fetal demise. Blood should be cross-matched, haemoglobin checked and clotting screen performed, with intravenous fluids and blood transfusion as necessary.

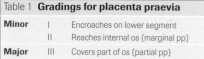

Table 1	**Gradings for placenta praevia**	
Minor	I	Encroaches on lower segment
	II	Reaches internal os (marginal pp)
Major	III	Covers part of os (partial pp)
	IV	Covers os completely (complete pp)

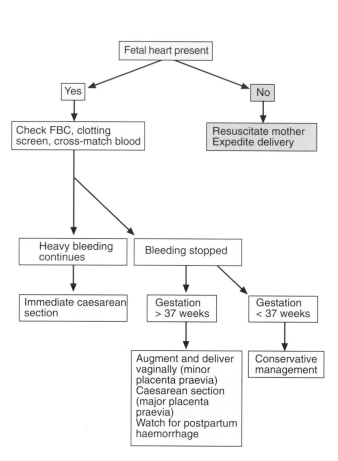

Fig. 1 **Management plan for placenta praevia.**

Abruptio placentae

Abruptio placentae (also known as accidental haemorrhage) results from retroplacental bleeding. Although it is not possible to predict, there are recognized associations:

- pregnancy-induced hypertension
- eclampsia
- renal disease ± hypertension
- rapid changes in uterine size (e.g. release of polyhydramnios or after delivery of first twin) – in reality very rare.

The classic presentation is of abdominal pain associated with an antepartum haemorrhage. There may be uterine activity. The condition is classified into whether the haemorrhage is revealed, concealed or a mixture of the two (Fig. 2).

Examination

The findings may be:

- uterus – tense or irritable
- fetus – longitudinal, if cephalic presentation head engaged.

In <u>revealed haemorrhage</u>, most of the retroplacental bleeding tracks down inside the uterus to be revealed as vaginal bleeding. The amount of uterine irritation caused by this bleeding may be less, pain not being such a great feature.

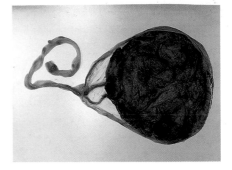

Concealed haemorrhage, however, may have only very slight vaginal bleeding with a large amount of retroplacental clot, causing a tense uterus.

In the case of <u>mixed</u> <u>haemorrhage</u> there will be some vaginal bleeding and perhaps passage of clots but also a build-up of some clot behind the placenta.

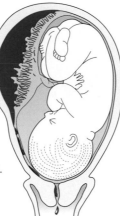

Fig. 4 Velamentous cord insertion. With rupture of the membranes a vessel may rupture and APH results. In this case the bleeding is fetal and may result in death of the baby if not delivered promptly.

Thromboplastins released from the back of the placenta into the maternal circulation may result in disseminated intravascular coagulation (DIC).

If there is a large haemorrhage, blood may be forced between the fibres of the uterine muscle. If the abdomen is opened the uterus appears bruised (Couvelaire uterus) possibly with free blood in the intraperitoneal cavity. With haemorrhage of this degree it is likely that the fetus will be dead.

Fig. 2 **Classification of abruptio placentae.**

Differential diagnosis

This should include:

- placenta praevia
- preterm labour
- other causes of acute abdomen.

Management

The management plan for abruptio placentae is shown in Figure 3.

In the case where DIC develops, delivery is best vaginally to avoid uncontrollable haemorrhage during surgery. A logical treatment for severe haemorrhage may be heparin therapy to break the clotting cascade and the consumption that is occurring of all the patient's clotting factors. In these cases the fetus is often dead, so management is not complicated by the need for urgent delivery of the fetus.

Other causes of antepartum haemorrhage

Vasa praevia

Vasa praevia may occur when the cord is inserted into the membranes and the fetal vessels run in the membranes to reach the placenta. If the vessels run over the cervix at the time of membrane rupture (vasa praevia) they themselves may rupture and lead to rapid exsanguination of the fetus (Fig. 4).

Cervical carcinoma

This is a very rare condition in pregnancy. However, it is possible for a cervical carcinoma to bleed, especially as the patient goes into labour and the cervix starts dilating.

Cervical lesions

Occasionally a cervical polyp or an infected cervix may bleed. Speculum examination of the cervix is therefore helpful in the differential diagnosis of antepartum haemorrhage.

Ruptured uterine scar

A scar on the uterus may rupture during labour, and vaginal bleeding would be associated with signs of fetal distress.

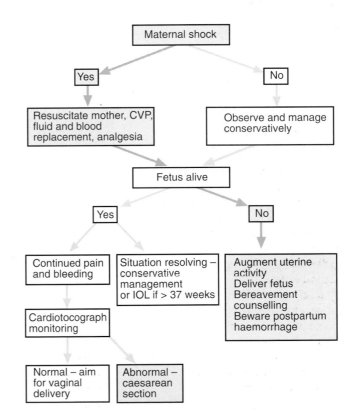

Fig. 3 **Management of abruptio placentae.**

Antepartum haemorrhage

- In APH, first exclude placenta praevia and abruptio placentae.
- In a large number of cases the cause remains unknown.
- Postpartum haemorrhage is a recognized complication of APH.
- Previous APH predisposes to APH in future pregnancies.

Multiple pregnancy

The UK incidence of twins is 12/1000 pregnancies (3/1000 of these are monozygous). Worldwide this ranges from 54/1000 in Nigeria to 4/1000 in Japan with the differences being almost entirely due to variations in dizygous rates. The incidence is higher with ovulation induction, e.g. clomifene (10%) or gonadotrophins (30%). The perinatal mortality in twin pregnancies is four or five times higher than for singleton pregnancies, largely related to preterm delivery (40% deliver before 37 weeks compared to 6% in singletons), intrauterine growth restriction (IUGR), feto-fetal transfusion sequence (FFTS), malpresentation and an increased incidence of congenital malformations.

Chorionicity (i.e. number of placentae)

Dizygous (non-identical) twins come from two eggs; monozygous twins come from one egg and are identical.

All dizygous pregnancies are dichorionic, and therefore have separate chorions and amnions. The placental tissue may appear to be continuous but there are no significant vascular communications between the fetuses. Monozygotic pregnancies may also be dichorionic, but may be monochorionic diamniotic or monochorionic monoamniotic (Figs 1–3) depending on the stage of embryonic development at which separation occurred (Table 1). Most monochorionic placentae have inter-fetal vascular connections.

Chorionicity determination is essential to allow risk stratification, and has key implications for prenatal diagnosis and antenatal monitoring (Table 2). It is most easily determined in the first or early second trimester by ultrasound:

- Widely separated first trimester sacs or separate placentae are dichorionic.
- Those with a 'lambda' or 'twin-peak' sign at the membrane insertion are dichorionic (Figs 2 and 3).
- Those with a dividing membrane > 2 mm are often dichorionic.

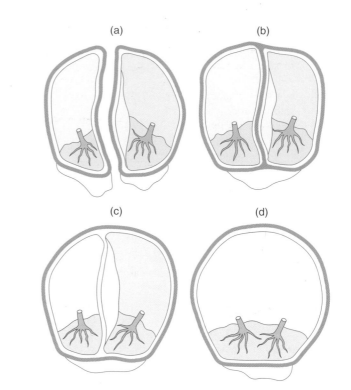

Fig. 1 **Diagram of chorionicity.** All dizygous twins are dichorionic **(a, b)**. Monozygotic pregnancies may form any of the following combinations: **(a)** dichorionic diamniotic; **(b)** dichorionic diamniotic (placentae beside each other); **(c)** monochorionic diamniotic; **(d)** monochorionic monoamniotic.

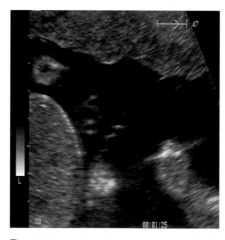

Fig. 2 **Monochorionic twins** – no lambda sign.

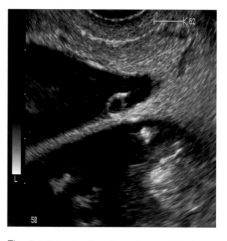

Fig. 3 **Dichorionic twins** – lambda sign.

- Different sex twin pregnancies are always dichorionic (and dizygous!).

Fetal abnormality

The incidence is not different per fetus in a dichorionic pregnancy compared to a singleton pregnancy, but the incidence is greater with monochorionicity.

Structural defects

These are usually confined to one twin (i.e. non-concordant). For example, if there is a neural tube defect in one twin, the other twin is normal in 85–90%. All multiple pregnancies should be offered a detailed mid-trimester ultrasound scan. Selective termination with

Table 1 Placentation in twin pregnancies

Number of chorions (placentae)	Number of amniotic sacs	Percentage of twins	Timing of embryonic separation post-fertilization
Dichorionic	Diamniotic	30%	Separation < 4 days
Monochorionic	Diamniotic	66%	Separation 4–7 days
Monochorionic	Monoamniotic	3%	Separation 7–14 days
Conjoined		<1%	Separation > 14 days

Table 2 Outcome of twin pregnancies

	Dichorionic	Mono-chorionic
Fetal loss before 24 weeks	1.8%	12.2%
Fetal loss after 24 weeks	1.6%	2.8%
Delivery before 32 weeks	5.5%	9.2%

intracardiac KCl is possible in dichorionic pregnancies only, and is most safely carried out before 16–20 weeks.

Chromosomal abnormalities

These are usually discordant in dizygotic twins and usually concordant in monozygotic twins. Nuchal translucency measurement is probably more appropriate than serum screening for multiple pregnancies. Two amniocenteses are required in dichorionic pregnancies (very great care must be taken to document which sample has come from which sac). Chorionic villus sampling (CVS) is less appropriate for twin pregnancies as it is difficult to be sure that both placentae have been sampled, particularly if they are lying close together.

Management of pregnancy

Initial visit

- As many as 50% of twins diagnosed in the first trimester will proceed only as singletons despite the absence of loss per vagina. Parents should be told this if twins are diagnosed in the first trimester.
- The parents are often quite shocked, so counselling should focus on the positive aspects, while also outlining that closer monitoring will be required. This can be expanded later. They should consider whether they wish antenatal screening and consider the potential problems of finding one normal and one abnormal twin.

Subsequent visits

Thereafter, scans may be arranged at:

- 18 weeks for growth discrepancy ± fetal abnormality if the patient wishes
- 24 weeks for growth (average weight for twins is 10% lighter than singletons)
- and every 2–4 weeks thereafter for growth; more frequently if there is size discordance, with or without Doppler, cardiotocograph and biophysical profile studies if appropriate.

Antenatal problems specific to multiple pregnancies

Feto-fetal transfusion sequence (FFTS) (twin-twin transfusion syndrome)

This complicates 4–35% of monochorionic multiple pregnancies. The recipient develops severe polyhydramnios with raised amniotic

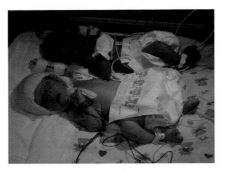

Fig. 4 **Twin-twin transfusion sequence.** These monochorionic twins were born at 37 weeks' gestation. Although their weights were almost identical, there was significant oligohydramnios around the recipient.

pressure, while the donor develops oliguria, oligohydramnios (Fig. 4) and growth restriction. Most centres support serial amnioreductions if the amniotic fluid index exceeds a certain limit, while other centres support laser division of placental vessels.

Twins with one fetal death

First trimester intrauterine death (IUD) in a twin has not been shown to have adverse consequences for the survivor. This probably also holds true for the early second trimester, but loss in the late second or third trimester commonly precipitates labour and 90% will have delivered within 3 weeks. Prognosis for a surviving dichorionic fetus is then influenced primarily by its gestation. When a monochorionic twin dies in utero, however, there are additional risks of death (approximately 20%) or cerebral damage (approximately 25%) in the co-twin.

Twin reversed arterial perfusion sequence (acardia)

If the heart of one monochorionic twin stops, the twin may continue to be partially perfused through vascular connections from the surviving twin. It is very rare, and there is a high incidence of mortality in the donor twin owing to intrauterine cardiac failure and prematurity. Cord ligation has been used in isolated cases.

Management of twin delivery

The commonest twin presentations are cephalic/cephalic (40%), cephalic/breech

(40%), breech/cephalic (10%) and others, e.g. transverse, (10%). Triplets and higher-order multiples are probably best delivered by caesarean section. In general with twins, providing the first twin is cephalic, evidence would suggest that a trial of labour is appropriate. With significant growth discordance, particularly if twin II is the smaller, it may be reasonable to consider caesarean section. It is common practice to carry out a caesarean section at 38 weeks in those not suitable for a vaginal delivery and to induce at 38–40 weeks those who are suitable but have not established in labour spontaneously. If the labour is preterm (< 34 weeks), many clinicians would also consider delivery by caesarean section.

Labour

An epidural may be very useful in assisting the delivery of a second twin. The first stage is managed as for singleton pregnancies, with both twins monitored by CTG. An experienced team should be present for delivery and a Syntocinon infusion should be ready in case uterine activity falls away after delivery of the first twin.

After delivery of the first twin it is often helpful to have someone 'stabilize' the second twin by abdominal palpation while a vaginal examination is performed to assess the station of the presenting part. If a second bag of membranes is present, it should not be broken until the presenting part has descended into the pelvis. If twin II lies transversely after the delivery of twin I, external cephalic or breech version is appropriate. If still transverse (particularly likely if the back is towards the fundus), the choice is between breech extraction (gentle continuous traction on one or both feet through intact membranes) or caesarean section. There is an increased incidence of postpartum haemorrhage.

Triplets and higher multiples

Most clinicians would deliver those with triplets or higher-order gestations by caesarean section because of problems with malpresentation and difficulties with intrapartum fetal monitoring.

Multiple pregnancy

- It is essential to establish chorionicity early to help advise about prenatal diagnosis and stratify subsequent care.
- Monochorionic pregnancies have the additional risks of feto-fetal transfusion sequence, loss of co-twin problems, and twin reversed arterial perfusion sequence.

Breech presentation

Breech presentations account for 2–3% of all labours. The incidence falls with gestational age, being 20% at 28 weeks, 16% at 32 weeks, falling to 3–4% at term as most breeches will turn spontaneously. Therefore there is only a problem if premature labour ensues or the presentation persists. Up to 30% are undiagnosed by clinical examination. Breeches may be frank, complete or footling (Fig. 1).

Causes

Excluding prematurity, in which the incidence is increased, there are several possible reasons why breech presentations persist to term:

- extended legs preventing spontaneous version, by 'splinting' the body
- uterine anomalies
- something preventing engagement, placenta praevia, fibroid, head of twin
- fetal anomalies, especially hydrocephalus and anencephaly.

In the majority of cases no cause is found.

Antenatal management

External cephalic version (ECV)

Spontaneous version becomes increasingly unlikely with advancing gestational age. ECV is usually attempted at around 36–37 weeks with the intention of ensuring that the baby

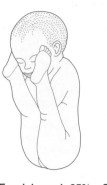

Frank breech 65%
Both legs extended

Complete breech 10%
Both legs flexed at knee and hip

Footling breech 25%
One foot up, one foot down
(more common in multiparae due to lax abdominal muscles)

Fig. 1 **Types of breech presentation.**

is cephalic before labour begins. The procedure results in a lower incidence of caesarean section. The success rate is quoted to be 46–65% (UK and US studies), although it has been reported to be as high as 80% in Africa.

Cases must be carefully selected (Fig. 2). A number of factors have been found to increase the likelihood of success, including multiparity, adequate liquor volume and the station of the breech above the pelvic brim. Although intended for the management of the uncomplicated

term breech, ECV has also been carried out after previous caesarean section and during early labour. Various interventions have been tried to further improve the success rate, e.g. vibroacoustic stimulation, amnioinfusion and epidural analgesia, but these are still under evaluation.

After the procedure mothers are reviewed weekly to check that the cephalic presentation persists. Some would advocate a second attempt at ECV if the presentation reverts to breech.

Elkin's manoeuvre

Some National Childbirth Trust (NCT) members may advocate attempting to influence the fetal presentation by natural means. The woman is instructed to adopt the knee–chest position for 15 minutes every 2 hours during the day for 5 days. Studies have failed to show significant benefits with this approach.

The persistent breech

If ECV is unsuccessful or not suitable, a decision has to be made on the mode of delivery – either by elective caesarean section or vaginal delivery.

The data for term breeches is irrefutable following the Canadian international multicentre randomized control trial, which showed perinatal morbidity three times higher in the group delivered vaginally compared to those delivered by elective caesarean section.

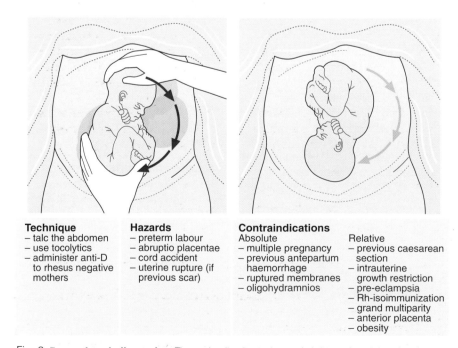

Technique	Hazards	Contraindications	
– talc the abdomen	– preterm labour	**Absolute**	**Relative**
– use tocolytics	– abruptio placentae	– multiple pregnancy	– previous caesarean
– administer anti-D to rhesus negative mothers	– cord accident	– previous antepartum haemorrhage	section
	– uterine rupture (if previous scar)	– ruptured membranes	– intrauterine growth restriction
		– oligohydramnios	– pre-eclampsia
			– Rh-isoimmunization
			– grand multiparity
			– anterior placenta
			– obesity

Fig. 2 **External cephalic version.** The mother lies flat and a tocolytic is used to ensure that the uterus is relaxed. The obstetrician disengages the breech with one hand and encourages the baby's head forward towards the pelvis with the other.

Therefore, each case must be judged carefully by an experienced obstetrician before a decision is made to allow a vaginal breech delivery. Abdominal palpation may reveal a baby that is obviously so large that elective caesarean section is required. An ultrasound is performed at 37 weeks to estimate the fetal birthweight (EBW) and more importantly the biparietal diameter (BPD) (Fig. 3). The scan will also indicate the degree of extension or flexion of the head and legs. The baby may have adopted a complete or footling presentation.

Vaginal delivery is safest in the case of a frank breech as there is an increased risk of cord prolapse with an ill-fitting presenting part. An attempt must also be made to assess the size of the pelvis. Clinically, this can be done by a gentle vaginal examination to estimate:

- the width of the subpubic angle
- the gap between the ischial spines
- the sacral curve.

An erect lateral pelvimetry X-ray may be helpful or magnetic resonance

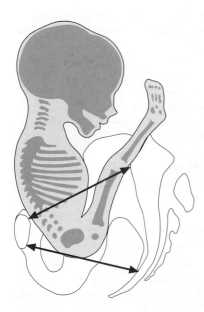

Fig. 3 **Assessment of mode of breech delivery.** In this case the biparietal diameter is close to size of outlet.

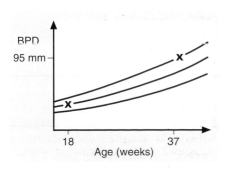

Table 1 **Indications for caesarean section for term breech even if vaginal delivery requested**
Elective caesareans
Pelvic
■ small pelvis, flat sacrum, bony abnormalities, e.g. rickets
Fetal
■ estimated birthweight 3.5 kg or over
■ Large biparietal diameter, e.g. hydrocephalus
■ Hyperextension of fetal head
Pre-existing obstetric problems
■ pre-eclampsia
■ bad obstetric history
■ placental insufficiency
Pre-existing maternal problems
■ history of infertility
■ older primigravida
■ diabetes
Emergency caesareans
Failure to progress in first stage
Failure of descent of breech in second stage

imaging (MRI) pelvimetry can be performed. It is essential to see the films as well as the measurements (ideally inlet: 13.5 × 11.5 cm, outlet 12.5 × 10.5 cm). A well-curved sacrum provides a large pelvic cavity; a flat sacrum limits the space available to the aftercoming head and may cause problems during a vaginal delivery, even if the inlet and outlet are adequate.

If obstetric or medical problems co-exist, operative delivery is necessary (Table 1).

Management of labour

Preterm labour

Prospective data are still unavailable. The poor outcome for very low birthweight infants is mainly related to prematurity and not the mode of delivery. Some labours advance too rapidly to allow delivery by caesarean section. The baby may fare better if it is delivered within its intact membranes, a caul delivery. The main concern with vaginal delivery of very small preterm infants is that the trunk and limbs will slip through an only

partially dilated cervix and that the cervix may clamp down on the fetal head. Immediate intravenous administration of tocolytics may be helpful. In extreme cases the cervix can be incised or the baby pushed upwards from below and delivered by caesarean section.

Labour of the term breech

The management of a breech labour is the same as for a cephalic presentation. The rate of cervical dilatation and descent of the presenting part are plotted on a partogram (see p. 50). Continuous fetal monitoring is usual. An epidural may be desirable as it prevents the mother pushing involuntarily before full cervical dilatation (a more common problem with breech than vertex presentations) and provides pain relief during the assisted delivery.

Augmentation with Syntocinon should be used with caution. The breech should descend easily into the pelvis. Fetal distress may intervene despite good progress in labour and should be dealt with in the same way as a vertex presentation.

Even at full dilatation the breech may not descend. The baby should be born by the mother's own efforts with a little assistance from the obstetrician at key points, an *assisted breech delivery*. The overriding priority is control of the aftercoming head. There is no time for moulding, and if the head is allowed to descend rapidly great pressure differences occur that may cause tentorial tears and intracerebral bleeds. Occasional difficulty is encountered with extended arms but there are special manoeuvres available to overcome this. There is no merit in strong traction to bring down an undescended breech, a breech extraction, because perinatal outcome is poor.

Most mothers will opt for external cephalic version. If this fails, most request caesarean delivery.

Breech presentation

- Most breeches spontaneously turn to the cephalic presentation by 36 weeks.
- Prematurity is associated with an increased incidence of breech presentation.
- ECV increases the chances of vaginal delivery.
- Careful selection must be made to decide which term breeches should be considered for an attempt at vaginal delivery.
- Selection involves assessment of the biparietal diameter and estimated birthweight of the fetus together with the size of the pelvis.
- Caesarean section may be best for some preterm babies.
- The most important aspect of an assisted vaginal breech delivery is careful delivery of the aftercoming head.

Venous thromboembolic disease

Obstetrics

Antenatal

In pregnancy the clotting system is altered towards clot formation. There are increased levels of fibrinogen, which lead to increased risk of clot formation. This is in part offset by an increase in fibrinolysis. Mechanical obstruction from the uterus leads to reduced venous return from the lower limbs and therefore venous stasis.

Venous thromboembolic disease is very rare in Africa and the Far East but is the commonest direct cause of maternal mortality in the UK. The reason for such wide racial difference remains unclear. The incidence of pulmonary thromboembolism (PTE) is between 0.3 and 1.2% of all UK pregnancies with just over 40% occurring antenatally, often in the first trimester. Over 80% of deep vein thromboses (DVTs) in pregnancy are left sided, probably because the left common iliac vein is more compressed by the uterus where it is crossed by the right common iliac artery. More than 70% are ileofemoral.

Risk factors include

- obesity
- age > 35
- high parity
- previous thromboembolism
- immobility
- pre-eclampsia
- varicose veins
- congenital or acquired thrombophilia
- intercurrent infection
- caesarean section (particularly emergency caesarean section).

DVT may be asymptomatic or, in addition to the traditional symptoms and signs, it may present with lower abdominal pain. It is essential to make a definitive diagnosis if possible, not just for management of the current pregnancy but because there are major implications for subsequent pregnancies as well. Duplex Doppler ultrasound is particularly useful for identifying femoral vein thromboses, although iliac veins are less easily seen (Fig. 1). It is safe and should be the first-line investigation. Venography is better, but has the disadvantage of radiation exposure and should be carried out if Doppler gives equivocal

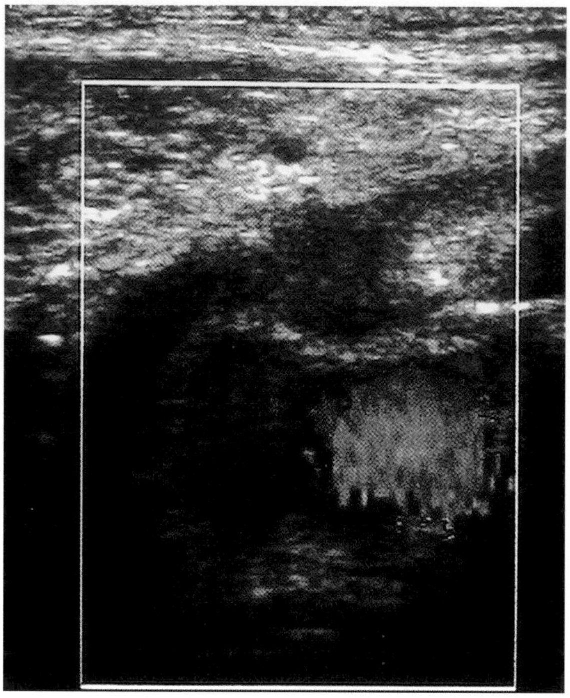

Fig. 1 **Normal Doppler flow in the femoral artery (red, right) with no flow through the occluded femoral vein (black, left).**

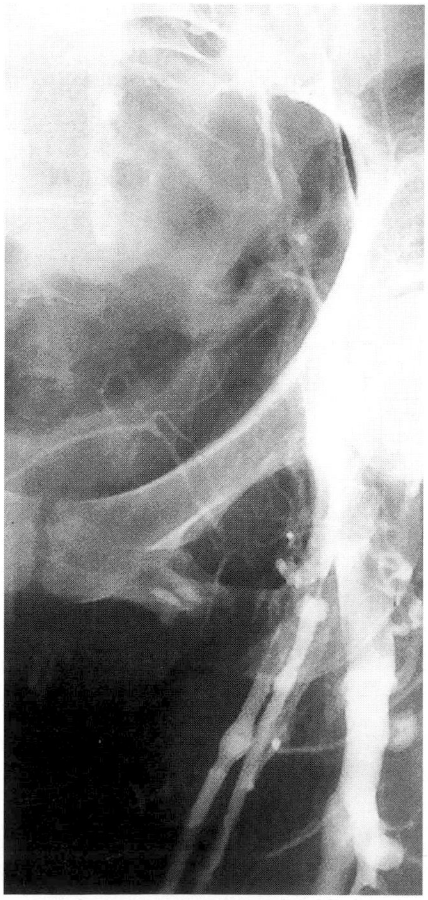

Fig. 2 **Thrombus occluding the left common iliac vein, with patent left femoral vein.**

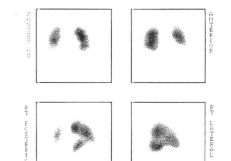

Fig. 3 **Positive Q scan – note the lack of perfusion in the right lower lobe.** The ventilation scan was normal.

Table 1   **Potential thrombophilias**
■ Activated protein C resistance (if present, test for the factor V Leiden mutation)
■ Antithrombin III
■ Protein C deficiency
■ Protein S deficiency
■ Lupus anticoagulant and antiphospholipid antibodies
■ Prothrombin gene variant
■ Hyperhomocystinaemia

results or is not available (Fig. 2). It is also essential to fully investigate a suspected pulmonary embolism, and pregnancy is not a contraindication to a ventilation–perfusion (VQ) scan – any risks are far outweighed by the benefits of accurate diagnosis (Fig. 3). A normal scan virtually excludes the diagnosis of pulmonary embolism.

Management of DVT or pulmonary embolism in pregnancy is with therapeutic subcutaneous heparin. Postnatally the patient may choose to continue with subcutaneous heparin or start warfarin, continuing anticoagulation for 6–12 weeks as decided by timing of onset and clinical severity. Once anticoagulants are stopped, the patient should be screened for thrombophilia.

Management of those with a previous thromboembolic history carries more uncertainties. Women who have had a single episode of DVT/PTE should be screened for thrombophilia (Table 1). If the screen is negative, and the event occurred outside pregnancy and was not severe, thromboprophylaxis may not be required. If positive, or there are other risk factors, antenatal and postnatal prophylaxis can be considered. Heparin treatment may induce thrombocytopenia and may also rarely lead to osteoporotic fractures.

Postnatal risk assessment

The risks of thromboembolism should be assessed in all patients who have undergone caesarean section (see Table 2). It is also essential to consider prophylaxis in those who have had vaginal deliveries, whether instrumental or not, who may be considered to be at increased risk.

Gynaecology

Venous thromboembolic disease accounts for around 20% of perioperative hysterectomy deaths. As prophylaxis is effective in reducing thromboembolism, all gynaecological patients should be assessed for risk factors and prophylaxis prescribed accordingly (Table 3). The incidence is higher in those with malignancy (35%), lower for 'routine' abdominal hysterectomy (12%) and lowest for vaginal hysterectomy.

As some prophylactic methods may be associated with side effects (e.g. wound haematomas and hypersensitivity reactions with heparin), the methods chosen must be based on some form of risk vs benefit assessment. The benefits to the patient of heparin in moderate/high-risk groups are felt to outweigh the approximately 2/100 risk of wound haematoma, which may be minimized by avoiding injection close to the wound. Graduated compression stockings would be an alternative, although compliance with stockings may be reduced in those who find them uncomfortable. In addition, they have not been shown to reduce the risk of fatal pulmonary thromboembolism. Dextran carries a significant risk of anaphylaxis.

Any benefits to stopping the combined oral contraceptive (COC) 4–6 weeks prior to surgery must be weighed against the risk of unwanted pregnancy. In the absence of other risk factors there is insufficient evidence to support a policy of routine COC discontinuation. It may be advisable to stop hormone replacement therapy (HRT) before major surgery.

Table 2 **Risk factors following caesarean section**

Low risk — early mobilization and hydration

Elective caesarean section — uncomplicated pregnancy and no other risk factors

Moderate risk — heparin (e.g. heparin 5000 U b.i.d. or enoxaparin 20 mg/day) and TED stockings

Age > 35 years
Obesity (> 80 kg)
Para 4 or more
Gross varicose veins
Current infection
Pre-eclampsia
Immobility prior to surgery (> 4 days)
Major current illness, e.g. heart or lung disease; cancer; inflammatory bowel disease; nephrotic syndrome
Emergency caesarean section in labour

High risk — heparin (e.g. heparin 5000 U t.i.d. or enoxaparin 40 mg/day) and TED stockings

A patient with three or more moderate risk factors from above
Extended major pelvic or abdominal surgery, e.g. caesarean hysterectomy
Patients with a personal or family history of deep vein thrombosis; pulmonary embolism or thrombophilia; paralysis of lower limbs
Patients with antiphospholipid antibody (cardiolipin antibody or lupus anticoagulant)

Table 3 **Risk factors for venous thromboembolic disease in gynaecology**

Group	Risk factors	Deep vein thrombosis (DVT)	Proximal vein thrombosis	Fatal pulmonary embolism (PE)	Suggestion for prophylaxis
Low risk	Minor surgery (< 30 minutes); no risk factors other than age Major surgery (< 30 minutes); age < 40; no other risk factors (as below)	< 10%	< 1%	0.01%	Early mobilization ± TED stockings
Moderate risk	Minor surgery (< 30 minutes) with personal or family history of DVT, PE or thrombophilia Major gynaecological surgery (> 30 minutes) Age > 40 years, obesity (> 80 kg), gross varicose veins, current infection Immobility prior to surgery (> 4 days) Major medical illness: heart or lung disease, cancer, inflammatory bowel disease	10–40%	1–10%	0.1–1%	Early mobilization + TED stockings + low-dose heparin
High risk	Three or more of above risk factors Major pelvic or abdominal surgery for cancer Major surgery in patients with previous DVT, PE, thrombophilia, or lower limb paralysis (e.g. hemiplegic stroke, paraplegia)	40–80%	10–30%	1–10%	Early mobilization + TED stockings + high-dose heparin

---

Venous thromboembolic disease

- Although pregnancy-related venous thromboembolic disease is very rare in Africa and the Far East, it is the commonest direct cause of maternal mortality in many western countries.
- Any symptoms should be investigated fully, even if this requires X-rays or isotope scanning.
- Prophylaxis is important in both obstetrics and gynaecological practice.

Psychosocial problems in antenatal care

Clinicians should be careful, when focusing on medical disorders of pregnancy, to be sensitive to psychosocial and cultural issues that may impact on care.

Teenage pregnancy

The UK has the worst record for teenage pregnancies in Europe. Over 90 000 teenagers become pregnant each year, including 8000 who are less than 16 years old. Teenage mothers are less likely to finish their education or find a good job and more likely to end up as single parents. The children run a greater risk of poor health and have a higher chance of becoming teenage mothers in their turn (Table 1). Certain risk factors have now been identified (Table 2). The risk for teenage motherhood is 10 times higher in social class V than in social class I. The risk is 3 times higher for a girl in local-authority housing than owner-occupied housing. There is a strong link between teenage pregnancy and not being occupied either in education, training or work between 16 and 17 years of age. High truancy rates and social exclusion at school are also factors.

Antenatal care

Teenage mothers achieve less good antenatal health care. There are a number of reasons for this:

- The majority of teenage pregnancies are unplanned, so preparations, e.g. prophylactic folic acid, are less likely.

Table 2 **Risk factors for teenage pregnancies**
■ Poverty
■ Children currently, or previously, in care are at higher risk
■ Children of teenage mothers
■ Low educational achievement
■ Low expectations
■ Previous sexual abuse
■ Mental health problems
■ Crime

Many young people share several of these risk factors and therefore have a very high chance of becoming a teenage parent (from UK Parliamentary Report on Teenage Pregnancy, June 1999).

- Teenagers present much later for booking and may miss accurate dating scanning and advice on health precautions.
- Nearly two-thirds of under 20-year-olds smoke before pregnancy and almost half during pregnancy.
- Pregnancy under the age of 16 can be complicated by poor fetal growth, independent of social circumstances including smoking and poor nutrition (teenage mothers are 25% more likely than average to have a baby weighing less than 2500 g).
- For many, formal planned antenatal care is very difficult as they face family conflict, relationship stress or breakdown, and moving home.

There is an increased incidence of anaemia, urinary tract infection and hypertension. Postnatal depression is three times as common and teenage mothers are half as likely as older mothers to breast feed.

Smoking

Numerous studies have shown that smoking reduces the birthweight by 13 g per cigarette smoked daily. Educational campaigns have succeeded in encouraging some women to stop smoking when they conceive but few interventions have been successful in women still smoking at booking. Some studies have shown that smokers reduced or stopped smoking when they were told that it caused a fetal tachycardia or if the effects of smoking were explained.

Alcohol

Fetal alcohol syndrome

Alcohol is a fetal teratogen. Chronic, heavy ingestion is associated with the fetal alcohol syndrome (FAS). Diagnosis requires signs in the following categories:

- central nervous system involvement including neurological abnormalities, developmental delay, intellectual impairment, head circumference below the third centile and brain malformation
- characteristic facial deformity, including short palpebral fissures, elongated mid-face and flattened maxilla.

Although the facial dysmorphic features may regress with age, the mental impairment does not.

Alcohol affects all fetal systems and FAS will occur in approximately one-third of children born to women who drink the equivalent of 18 units of alcohol per day. Other factors dictating susceptibility to alcohol include genetic factors, social deprivation, nutritional differences and the possibility of associated tobacco and drug abuse.

Social alcohol consumption

There is growing evidence that even as little as two units of alcohol a day has a small negative effect on intrauterine fetal growth, reducing the birthweight by 60–70 g. Impairment of neural development, however, seems to occur only at higher levels of consumption.

Alternative methods for screening for heavy alcohol consumption during pregnancy have been devised as the routine tests (serial mean corpuscular volume and gamma glutamyl transferase) are less reliable in

Table 1 **Teenage pregnancies**	
■ Teenage birth rates:	
The Netherlands	3.5 per 1000 girls 15–19 years
France	7 per 1000 girls 15–19 years
Germany	10 per 1000 girls 15–19 years
UK	20 per 1000 girls 15–19 years
US	55 per 1000 girls 15–19 years
■ Just under 30% of teenagers are sexually active by age 16	
■ 50% of these do not use contraception the first time	
■ Teenagers who do not use contraception have a 90% chance of conception within 1 year	
■ In one single act of unprotected intercourse with an infected partner there is:	
– 1% chance of acquiring HIV	
– 30% risk of genital herpes	
– 50% chance of gonorrhoea	
■ Of those who do get pregnant:	
– 50% under 16 opt for abortion	
– 30% of 17–18-year-olds opt for abortion, i.e. 15 000 abortions per year in under 18-year-olds	
■ 90% of teenage mothers have their babies outside marriage	
■ The mortality for babies born to teenage mothers is 6% higher than for babies of older mothers:	
– increased low birthweights	
– increased childhood accidents (especially poisoning or burns)	
– increased hospital admissions (mainly accidents or gastroenteritis)	

From UK Parliamentary Report on Teenage Pregnancy, June 1999 by the Social Exclusion Unit.

pregnancy. A full dietary and substance-abuse history should be taken. A more searching questionnaire for alcohol is the TACE questionnaire. A total score of two points or more is considered positive and correctly identifies approximately 70% of heavy drinkers.

Nutritional problems are common. Trace element deficiencies (e.g. zinc and copper) and vitamin deficiency states (folate, thiamine and pyridoxine) may exist.

Alcohol passes freely to the milk. Regular heavy drinking by the mother may impede psychomotor development of the breast-fed infant, although mental development is probably unaffected. Heavy binging may lead to neonatal sedation.

Specific counselling, referral for specialist treatment and a telephone contact number provide support.

Domestic violence

Most acts of domestic violence are directed by men against women, and are unrelated to social class. An estimated 835 000 incidents were reported in 1997. One woman in nine is subjected to severe beatings by her partner each year.

Violence against a partner is often linked to wider family problems. In three out of five cases where children suffered abuse, their mother was abused. Midwifery staff and health care workers should be vigilant for any signs of domestic violence. Self-help groups and one-parent hostel facilities may need to be considered.

Psychological issues

Depression and psychosis

Patients who have been previously treated with antidepressants or antipsychotics will need to be reassessed in the antenatal period. The social, economic and domestic factors that may have contributed to any depression will need to be reassessed and social service support provided early if deemed necessary.

It is preferable to try to withdraw any medication if possible, but if the mental condition is brittle, the dose should be reduced to the lowest possible to maintain stability, or a milder alternative substituted. It is better to use behavioural and psychotherapeutic treatments during pregnancy if possible.

Racial aspects

Every woman must be treated with respect and her religious and cultural views acknowledged wherever possible.

Female genital mutilation

Female genital mutilation (FGM) affects more than 80 000 women and children worldwide. The type of mutilation performed varies from Sunna (excision of the clitoral prepuce) to excision of the clitoris, labia minora and majora (in the most severe form) (Fig. 1). The age at which FGM is performed varies from birth to immediately prior to marriage, but most commonly is between 6 and 7

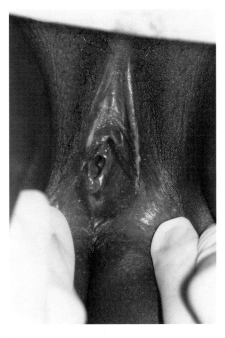

Fig. 1   **Female circumcision.**

years. Anaesthetic is rarely given and asepsis is limited. The raw edges of the labia are sutured together with catgut or more commonly thorns. The girl's legs are bound together and a small aperture is left to allow drainage of urine and menstrual fluids.

The practice is widespread in a band from the Horn of Africa through Central Africa to parts of Nigeria, and involves 90% of female children in Somalia and Ethopia. Immediate complications include severe haemorrhage and infection and there is a significant mortality. Long-term problems include recurrent urinary tract infections, dysmenorrhoea, non-consummation and lack of sexual enjoyment. Circumcision increases the marriage prospects within that society. Failure to undergo circumcision may lead to social rejection.

Women who have been victims of FGM and book for antenatal care should, if possible, be treated in a specific African Well Woman Clinic with access to a translator and psychologist if required. They should be encouraged to have the circumcision reversed in the second trimester under spinal anaesthetic between 20–28 weeks. This allows adequate examination vaginally to assess progress in labour. If a patient declines, reversal should be performed in the first stage of labour, to allow catheterization, examination and continuous fetal monitoring where required.

It is illegal under the terms of the 1985 Prohibition of Circumcision Act to resuture these women after delivery.

Psychosocial problems in antenatal care

- The USA has the highest teenage pregnancy rate.
- The UK has the worst record of teenage pregnancies in Europe.
- There is increased morbidity and mortality in babies born to teenage mothers.
- Smoking is implicated in low birthweight babies.
- Chronic heavy alcohol ingestion is associated with the fetal alcohol syndrome (FAS).
- Domestic violence continues to be the most common violent crime against women in England and Wales.
- Although victims of female genital mutilation should be advised to undergo de-infibulation between 20–28 weeks or certainly in the first stage of labour, this will depend on consent and consideration of cultural issues.

Mechanisms of normal labour

Labour is the process whereby regular uterine activity causes progressive cervical dilatation and usually results in delivery of the fetus. It is divided into three stages, each with defined normal progression which aids identification of problems.

Prior to the onset of labour it is usual for cervical effacement to occur. The cervix becomes shorter, softer and moves from its position in the posterior vaginal fornix towards the anterior vaginal fornix. If full cervical effacement has not been achieved before the onset of regular uterine activity there may be a prolonged latent phase when uterine activity (± pain) completes the process of cervical effacement but the patient is not in labour. Labour is diagnosed once the cervix starts dilating, so the diagnosis of the time of onset of labour has to be made retrospectively.

Spontaneous rupture of the membranes (SRM) may occur prior to the onset of labour but is more usual during the first stage. If labour has not begun after SRM, it is common practice to induce within the first 48 hours providing gestation is >37 weeks (see p. 19). Membrane rupture may be preceded by loss of the cervical mucous plug (show) which is often blood stained.

Mechanism of labour

The most common presenting part is the fetal head – 95%. The vertex is the area bounded by the parietal eminences, the anterior and posterior fontanelles. With the vertex presenting, the smallest presenting diameter occurs – suboccipito-bregmatic (Fig. 1). Any deflexion will result in larger diameters – the occipito-frontal and,

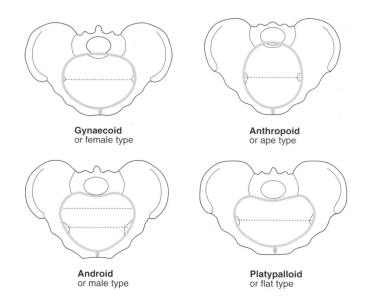

Gynaecoid
or female type

Anthropoid
or ape type

Android
or male type

Platypalloid
or flat type

Fig. 2 **The four pelvic types.**

with further deflexion, a brow. These presentations decrease the likelihood of a normal delivery.

The head has to pass through the bony pelvis and thus the shape of the maternal pelvis is important (Fig. 2). The commonest pelvic type is the gynaecoid pelvis, found in about 50% of women. It has parallel sides which allow passage of the fetal head. The anthropoid pelvis (25%) similarly does not cause problems by shape, whereas the android (male type) pelvis (20%) with its converging pelvic side walls gives increasing problems as the head descends. The fourth pelvic type, flat (5%), presents problems at the inlet but widens with further descent.

Initiation of labour

Possible mechanisms include a change in the progesterone : oestrogen ratio,

releasing uterine activity from progesterone inhibition, local release of prostaglandins stimulated by oxytocin or tissue trauma.

Stages of labour

First stage

Stage one is from the onset of labour until full cervical dilatation – usually 1 cm/hour in primigravidae and 1–2 cm/hour in parous women. Uterine activity during labour shows fundal dominance with spread of a wave of uterine contraction down towards the cervix (Fig. 3). As uterine muscle displays the property of retraction (shortening) the uterus is thus pulled towards the fundus dilating the cervix and encouraging descent of the fetus down the birth canal. Monitoring of labour progress is

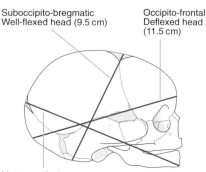

Suboccipito-bregmatic
Well-flexed head (9.5 cm)

Occipito-frontal
Deflexed head
(11.5 cm)

Mento-vertical
Brow presentation (14 cm)

Fig. 1 **The fetal skull.**

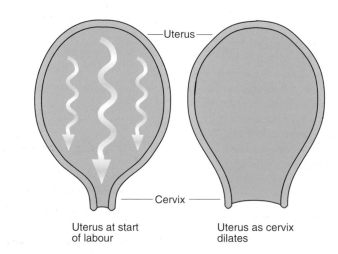

Uterus

Cervix

Uterus at start
of labour

Uterus as cervix
dilates

Fig. 3 **Contractions start from the fundus.**

Occurrence	Position of head
Engagement of head	OT
Descent to pelvic floor where guttering encourages rotation of head 90°	OA /OP
Further descent of head and occiput under symphysis	OA (or OP)
Head extends and face passes over perineum	
Restitution – head realigns with shoulders	OT

The anterior shoulder is then delivered under the symphysis with downward traction then an upward sweep to deliver the posterior shoulder carefully over the perineum. Finally, the infant is delivered onto the mother's abdomen.

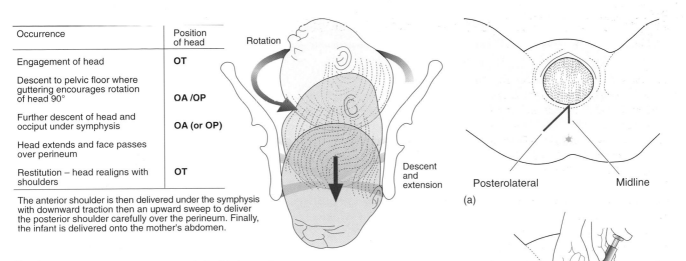

Fig. 4   **Movement of the fetus through the birth canal.**

facilitated by use of the partogram (see p. 51).

Second stage

Stage two is from full cervical dilatation until delivery of the infant – usually 1 hour or less in parous patients but may be 1–3 hours in primiparae. The second stage may be either passively managed, where the mother pushes when she feels the need, or with active encouragement to push with each contraction. There is no evidence that passive management is of benefit.

Third stage

Stage three is from delivery of the infant to delivery of the placenta – usually 15 minutes or less. Figure 4 shows the stages in the movement of the fetus through the birth canal.

The episiotomy

The need for an episiotomy is determined by signs of tearing or excessive blanching of the perineum. Infiltration with lidocaine (lignocaine) is performed prior to cutting the episiotomy, which is most commonly right posterolateral The cut is made at the start of the contraction during which it is considered the head will deliver. The episiotomy avoids uncontrolled tearing in a downward direction which might involve the rectal mucosa and rectal sphincters to the detriment of the mother's future bowel control (Fig. 5). A midline episiotomy does not offer sphincter protection.

Third stage

Signs of placental separation

These comprise:

■ lengthening of the umbilical cord

■ a gush of blood vaginally
■ firming of the fundus.

Once signs of separation have occurred the placenta may be delivered by controlled cord traction where the left hand is placed suprapubically holding the uterine fundus in the abdomen. The right hand is placed on the cord and gentle downward traction in the direction of the birth canal ensures delivery of the placenta. The mother may prefer to make expulsive efforts herself to deliver the placenta.

Active management of the third stage of labour is by prophylactically administering Syntometrine intramuscularly to the mother with the delivery of the anterior shoulder. This encourages contraction and retraction of the uterus with separation of the placenta and minimizes the blood loss during this stage. The practice of 'fundus fiddling' – trying to rub up a contraction of the uterus by massaging the uterine fundus – may encourage incomplete separation of the placenta with attendant haemorrhage.

If there are no signs of placental separation an infusion of Syntocinon may be set up or the baby put to the breast to encourage uterine contraction by release of oxytocin. Alternatively, gentle downward traction on the cord

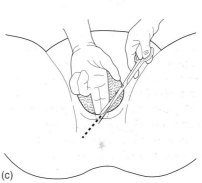

Fig. 5   **Performing an episiotomy.**
(a) Episiotomy incisions. **(b)** Local anaesthetic is infiltrated before the incision is made. **(c)** Midline episiotomy does not protect the sphincter.

while protecting the fundus may allow delivery of the placenta. However, it may also result in avulsion of the cord and the need for a manual removal of the placenta (see p. 60). Requests for a 'natural' third stage (no medication) are associated with a greater blood loss and are thus inappropriate in anaemic patients.

Mechanisms of normal labour

■ There are three stages of labour.

■ The shape of the maternal pelvis will affect the progress of labour.

■ The second stage of labour may be managed passively, but active encouragement to push is more usual.

■ Episiotomy is used only if needed.

Induction of labour and prolonged pregnancy

Induction of labour is indicated when the risks of continuing the pregnancy are felt to be greater than that of the induction itself. The induction is usually carried out in the interest of fetal well-being, occasionally for that of the mother, and only rarely for 'social' reasons. Labour should not be induced unless there are good medical reasons to do so. The decision is often difficult, particularly at preterm gestations, and many factors, including neonatal facilities, need to be considered.

Fetal indications

These include:

- Intrauterine growth restriction (IUGR) with risk of fetal compromise (based on estimated growth, biophysical assessment – including cardiotocograph (CTG) and Doppler studies). There may be associated pre-eclampsia. While it may, for example, be appropriate to induce for mild pre-eclampsia at term, the pre-eclampsia would need to be severe in a markedly preterm infant.
- Certain diabetic pregnancies.
- Worsening fetal abnormalities (very rare), e.g. cardiac lesions, hydrops or twin–twin transfusion syndrome.
- Deteriorating haemolytic disease of the newborn.

Maternal indications

- Pre-eclampsia. This is a condition in which both maternal and fetal interests are relevant.
- Deteriorating medical conditions (cardiac or renal disease, severe systemic lupus erythematosus).
- In rare situations in which treatment is required for malignancy.

Induction

The main risks of inappropriate induction are uterine hyperstimulation, increased obstetric intervention, and failed induction. The gestation should be checked, presentation confirmed and contraindications excluded (e.g. placenta praevia). Caution is required with previous caesarean section and uterine surgery (risk of uterine rupture), and grand multiparity or previous precipitate labour (risk of hyperstimulation).

The cervix should be assessed using the modified Bishop's scoring system (Table 1 and Fig. 1).

Prostaglandins

Intravaginal PGE₂ gel has fewer side effects than oral preparations and also has a lower failure rate than using the intracervical route (Fig. 2). The gel is inserted into the posterior fornix. If there is no uterine activity, the cervix is reassessed in 6 hours. If the Bishop's score is < 7, further gel is given and the cervix reassessed again 6 hours later. Further doses may then be given

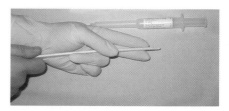

Fig. 2 **Prostaglandin gel is used to ripen the cervix.** Amniotomy may be performed when the cervix is favourable.

or the patient may be left for 12–18 hours (e.g. overnight). If at any stage the Bishop's score is > 6, artificial rupture of the membranes (ARM) may be performed, reassessment made in a further 2 hours and Syntocinon started if still no change. Gel should not be given if there is regular uterine activity.

Sustained-release preparations are also available in the form of a polymer-based vaginal insert, with retrieval thread, containing PGE₂. It is placed in the posterior fornix for 12 hours, after which it is removed. This technique has the advantage that the pessary can be removed if hyperstimulation develops, and trials indicate that it is probably safe. It has not been shown to be superior to gel.

Artificial rupture of the membranes (ARM)

ARM (amniotomy) is used to induce labour in those with a sufficiently favourable cervix and is also used for augmentation. Further, it allows assessment of the colour of the liquor (see Meconium, p. 51). Its routine use in early labour is surrounded by a degree of controversy, as it can be argued that there is less cushioning of the fetal head and therefore a greater incidence of fetal heart rate decelerations. Early ARM and Syntocinon probably do not confer benefit over conservative management in nulliparous women with mild delays in early spontaneous labour.

The fetal head should be well applied to the cervix to minimize the risk of cord prolapse. With asepsis, the tips of the index and middle fingers of one hand should be placed through the cervix onto the membranes (Figs 2 and 3). The amni-hook should be allowed to slide down the groove between these fingers (hook pointing towards the fingers) until the cervix is reached. The point is then turned upwards to break the membrane sac.

Table 1 **Bishop's scoring system for cervical assessment**			
Score	**0**	**1**	**2**
Cervical dilatation (cm)	< 1	1–2	3–4
Length of cervix (cm)	> 2	1–2	< 1
Station of presenting part in relation to the ischial spines (cm)	–3	–2	–1
Consistency	Firm	Medium	Soft
Position	Posterior	Central	Anterior

- If the score is < 7, the cervix should be 'ripened' with prostaglandins (gel or pessary).
- If > 6, consider either prostaglandins or ARM ± Syntocinon (there may be greater patient satisfaction with the former, but the latter may allow more control).

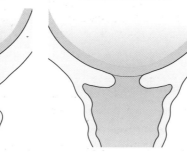

Unfavourable cervix — An unfavourable cervix is long, closed, firm and uneffaced

Favourable cervix — A favourable cervix is soft, effaced and admits a finger

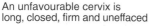

Fig. 1 **Unfavourable (low Bishop's score) and favourable (higher Bishop's score) cervix.**

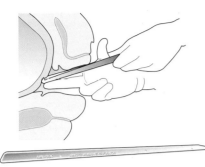

Fig. 3 **Artificial rupture of the membranes.**

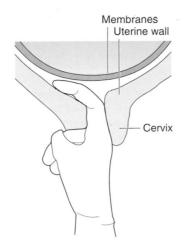

Fig. 4 **Sweeping the membranes.**

Liquor is usually seen, but may be absent in oligohydramnios or with a well-engaged head. Cord prolapse should be excluded before removing the fingers. The fetal heart should be rechecked. Absent liquor following ARM should be treated as meconium staining until proven otherwise.

Syntocinon

This may be used for induction following ARM with a favourable cervix, or for augmentation of a slow, non-obstructed labour. It should only be started if the membranes have been ruptured, and continuous CTG monitoring is mandatory. The dose should be titrated against the contractions, aiming for not more than 6–7 every 15 minutes with a reduced dose in highly parous women (> 5 labours).

For induction, the use of Syntocinon immediately following ARM reduces the time to delivery, the rates of postpartum haemorrhage (PPH) and the need for operative delivery. As labour will begin within 24 hours in 88%, however, it is unclear whether these advantages outweigh the maternal inconvenience of an intravenous infusion, restricted mobility and continuous fetal monitoring. An individual approach is advised.

Prolonged pregnancy (> 42 weeks)

This occurs in 10% of pregnancies and is associated with an increased perinatal mortality (perinatal mortality is 5 : 1000 between 37–42 weeks and 9.7 : 1000 after 42 weeks) owing to intrauterine death (IUD), intrapartum hypoxia and meconium aspiration syndrome. Dating the pregnancy by ultrasound before 18 weeks is more reliable than last menstrual period (LMP) in reducing the incidence of prolonged pregnancy.

Sweeping the membranes. If this is done once after 40 weeks it doubles the incidence of spontaneous labour over controls, especially in those with a low Bishop's score. The risk of infection is considered to be minimal but the procedure is uncomfortable (Fig. 4).

Routine induction of labour. Induction after 41 weeks reduces the incidence of fetal distress and meconium staining over those managed conservatively with monitoring. There is also a reduction in the caesarean section rate and no increase in the incidence of uterine hypertonus. It has been estimated, however, that 500 inductions may be required to prevent one perinatal death. Dissatisfaction with labour is strongly associated with

operative delivery, and does not seem to be associated with induction of labour.

Monitoring of postdates pregnancy. Monitoring with ultrasound and CTG confers no demonstrable benefit but is frequently performed.

Other methods of induction

Antiprogesterones

Mifepristone, a progesterone antagonist, has been studied in early pregnancy and has been shown to increase uterine activity and lead to cervical softening. Research into its use as an induction agent later in pregnancy has shown promising results, but it is not yet in clinical use.

Extra-amniotic saline

This involves passing a Foley catheter through the cervix and infusing normal saline into the extra-amniotic space. The infusion volume should be limited to 1500 ml. Success at cervical ripening has been shown to be similar to PGE2 but the process carries a small risk of introducing infection. It is a much cheaper technique than using PGE2 and this, together with the fact that PGE2 needs to be refrigerated, may make it a more suitable method for less affluent countries. It has not yet been compared in studies to misoprostol, a much cheaper prostaglandin preparation than PGE2.

Failed induction

Despite the above techniques, induction of labour is sometimes unsuccessful. The plan then depends on the reason for the induction. If it was for some significant fetal or maternal indication, there is probably little choice but to consider caesarean section. If, on the other hand, the induction was for some epidemiological reason then it may be reasonable to consider a more conservative approach. This would depend on an informed discussion with the patient and her partner.

Induction of labour and prolonged pregnancy

- Induction should only be carried out for medical reasons as it carries risks, particularly of hyperstimulation.
- Prostaglandins are useful to 'ripen' the cervix.
- Routine induction of labour after 41 weeks reduces the incidence of fetal distress, caesarean sections and meconium staining over those managed conservatively with monitoring.

Intrapartum fetal monitoring

Cardiotocography

Continuous electronic fetal heart rate monitoring – cardiotocography (CTG) – provides more information than intermittent auscultation with a fetal stethoscope. Abnormalities of fetal heart rate are used as a screening test for fetal acidosis and therefore poorer fetal outcome. There is no evidence that continuous monitoring reduces the risk of low Apgar scores or the rates of admission to special care nurseries.

Neonatal encephalopathy has been labelled hypoxic–ischaemic and thought to be due to fetal asphyxia during labour but evidence for this is surprisingly thin. A growing number of other significant non-asphyxial risk factors are being recognized. The abnormality to be detected is poorly defined and the screening test poorly assessed.

Interpretation of the CTG is a skill acquired over many years of practice but differing interpretations may be made by the same clinician on different dates or by different clinicians viewing the trace together. There are some basic rules to guide the uninitiated.

It is most important to interpret the CTG as part of the whole process of labour. For example, if there is meconium-stained liquor with an abnormality on the CTG this will be more likely to be significant than the same CTG abnormality with clear liquor draining. The stage the labour has reached will also influence decisions, with the same tracing needing different actions if the cervical dilatation has reached 3 cm or 10 cm. Initial assessment should follow a pattern designed to ensure that nothing is missed.

Baseline heart rate

Normally accepted limits are a rate between 110 and 160 bpm (beats per minute). A baseline rate above 160 bpm may be associated with a maternal tachycardia or pyrexia but other abnormalities of the tracing or progress of labour should be sought. Fetal blood sampling may be appropriate to determine whether there is fetal acidosis. Baseline rates below 110 bpm may suggest fetal distress.

Baseline variability

This is dependent on the fetus having an intact neurological system and a normal cardiac conducting system. Normal variability is more than five beats and gives the tracing a jagged appearance. Fewer than five beats' variation makes the tracing appear flat – almost a straight line. This can happen after opioid analgesia with acidosis or may be noted during phases of fetal sleep, which last for 20–40 minutes only.

Accelerations

An increase of more than 15 bpm for more than 15 seconds in response to fetal movement or a maternal contraction is termed an acceleration (Fig. 1). This shows development of good autonomic nervous system control and is indicative of a fetus that is not distressed. Absence of accelerations may be a sign of fetal distress and might warrant further investigation in the antenatal situation. During labour absence of accelerations as a sole sign would require continuation of the monitoring and observation for other indicators of problems such as loss of variability, presence of meconium-stained liquor, or development of decelerations.

Decelerations

A decrease in the fetal heart rate of more than 15 bpm below the baseline is a deceleration. They are divided into three categories – early, late and variable.

Early – these occur in time with the maternal contraction and are thought to be due to the fetal head being compressed, which stimulates the vagus and thus slows the fetal heart rate.

Late – these occur with their nadir beyond the peak of the maternal contraction and tend to be slow to recover to the baseline. They are suggestive of acidosis and if persistent warrant further assessment (e.g. fetal blood sampling) or delivery (Fig. 2).

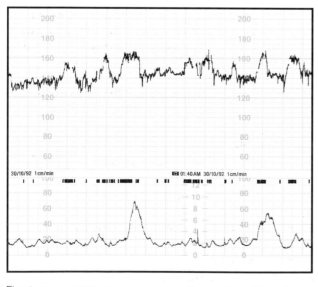

Fig. 1 **Normal CTG showing accelerations and good baseline variability.**

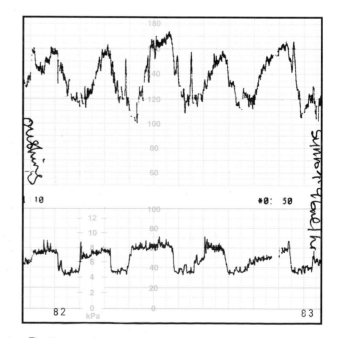

Fig. 2 **CTG showing late decelerations.**

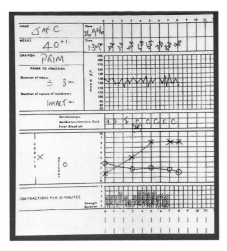

Fig. 3 **Partogram.**

Variable – these have a variable pattern and may be found in any relation to maternal contractions. They tend to conform to an M-shaped wave with an initial acceleration followed by a deceleration, then rebound acceleration. These occur with compression of the cord, the deceleration being found as the arteries are compressed. Changing the maternal position may see a resolution.

The partogram

Plotting the progress of labour on this chart (Fig. 3) allows, at a glance, an assessment as to whether labour is proceeding at an appropriate pace. Other recorded parameters enable the full picture to be clearly visualized. The progress of labour is determined by the rate of cervical dilatation and the corresponding descent of the head (or presenting part).

Latent phase

The latent phase is of variable length. In induced labour it can be shortened with use of prostaglandin gel to ripen the cervix.

Active phase

The active phase is when the minimum rate of cervical dilatation in a primigravid patient reaches 1 cm per hour. Multigravid patients are usually much quicker so a problem should be sought if the slope of this part of the partogram is less steep than illustrated.

Descent of the presenting part

When a primigravid patient enters labour the head is usually engaged but in highly parous patients engagement may not occur until the second stage of labour. There should be no head palpable abdominally before an assisted delivery is attempted.

Other parameters

Other parameters which should be recorded during labour are given in Table 1.

Liquor amnii

This fluid that surrounds the fetus is normally clear. Green or yellow discolouration suggests that the fetus has passed meconium (faecal material) which is a response to vagal stimulation and may be a sign of post dates or fetal distress. In a breech presentation the passage of the abdomen through the birth canal may cause passage of meconium which thus has less sinister significance.

Contractions

Assessment of the timing of contractions can be made from the CTG; however, this gives no information about their strength. An experienced midwife or intrauterine pressure monitoring will inform about the strength of contractions. The optimum is to aim for coordinated contractions lasting 1 minute with a frequency of 3 to 4 in 10 minutes. In the second stage of labour contractions lasting 1 minute with 1 minute space between are most likely to result in reasonable progress.

Fetal blood sampling (FBS)

In the presence of a non-reassuring CTG, a blood sample is taken from the presenting part – usually possible for an experienced operator by 3 cm dilatation. Analysis gives the fetal pH and the base excess (Table 2).

The base excess gives additional help by suggesting how much further buffering is available if the fetus continues to produce lactic acid (anaerobic metabolism). When the base excess is negative there is no further buffering for the lactic acid and the pH might be expected to fall rapidly so an earlier repeat FBS may be appropriate.

Indications for fetal blood sampling include:

Table 1	**Parameters recorded during labour**	
	Parameter	**Frequency**
Maternal	Pulse	15 mins
	Temperature	60 mins
	Contractions	Number per 10 mins
	Cervical dilatation	2–4 hours
	Urinary output	At least 4-hourly
	i.v. fluids	
	Drugs administered including Syntocinon	
Fetal	Heart rate	15 mins
	Liquor colour	15 mins
	Descent of presenting part	2–4 hours

Table 2	**Analysis of fetal blood pH**
pH value	**Action**
> 7.25	Observe CTG and if abnormality persists repeat sample in 1 hour
7.20–7.25	If delivery imminent, episiotomy or assisted delivery – if CTG changes persist repeat sample in 30 mins and act according to the value and clinical situation
< 7.20	Expedite delivery

- persistent late decelerations on CTG
- persistent loss of baseline variability
- persistent fetal tachycardia with no maternal tachycardia
- marked fetal bradycardia
- complicated CTG patterns (combining abnormalities)
- sinusoidal (saw tooth) pattern
- any CTG abnormality accompanied by meconium-stained liquor.

If fetal distress is suspected then:

- Stop Syntocinon infusion – this may decrease the frequency of the contractions and allow a greater time for the fetus to obtain oxygenated blood from the placental bed.
- Turn the mother onto her left side – which should relieve any aortocaval compression, again allowing the fetus to obtain oxygenated blood.
- Seek the cause for the problem and correct it or determine the optimum timing for delivery of the fetus.

Intrapartum fetal monitoring

- Labour can be very stressful for the fetus with interruption of the blood supply during maternal contractions.
- Continuous intrapartum electronic monitoring is only necessary for the high-risk fetus.
- If abnormalities of the fetal heart rate are noted during auscultation or the liquor becomes meconium-stained then this low-risk labour becomes high risk and warrants continuous electronic fetal monitoring.
- Labour management requires use of the partogram.
- Interpretation of cardiotocography is a skill that requires practice.
- Fetal blood sampling gives additional information to the cardiotocography about fetal well-being.
- pH correlates poorly with Apgar scores.

Abnormal labour

Abnormal labour

Although normal labour can be defined as that ending in a healthy mother and baby, it is more traditionally defined as beginning between 37 and 42 weeks, progressing at an acceptable rate and resulting in the spontaneous vaginal delivery (SVD) of a live non-distressed neonate in the occipitoanterior position. Deviation from this latter definition may therefore occur if progress is too fast (precipitate labour), or too slow (often in association with malposition or malpresentation).

Precipitate labour

This occurs especially with induction of labour, augmentation and grand multiparity. The risk is that excessively frequent or prolonged contractions reduce the blood supply to the baby and may lead to hypoxia and consequent damage. Such hypoxia may occur over a short period of time to an otherwise healthy fetus, so that the prognosis is usually good.

If prolonged contractions occur, Syntocinon should be stopped, and the fetal condition assessed with the cardiotocograph (CTG). If there is evidence of 'distress' a vaginal examination (VE) should be performed and consideration given to delivery. If not fully dilated, caesarean section should be considered. The uterine hypertonus may respond to a bolus of i.v. ritodrine or subcutaneous terbutaline.

Slow labour

There may be an initial and sometimes prolonged (hours/days) latent phase before true labour begins, but an acceptable rate of dilatation after 3 cm is 1 cm per hour in a primigravida and 1–2 cm an hour in a multigravida. Slow labour may be due to inadequate uterine activity or to cephalopelvic disproportion, i.e. too small a pelvis, or too big a presenting part. A partogram is very useful to assess progress (Fig. 1).

Inadequate uterine activity

In clinical practice, the strength of contractions is difficult to measure, and the diagnosis is usually made by excluding obstruction of whatever cause. Obstruction is suggested by malposition, caput (oedematous swelling on the fetal head) and moulding (1+ if the sutures of the fetal skull are aligned, 2+ if overlapping and 3+ if irreducible). If there is felt to be inadequate uterine activity, consideration may be given to augmentation with Syntocinon, but caution is required in parous women, particularly those with a previous caesarean section scar, owing to the risk of uterine or scar rupture.

Cephalopelvic disproportion (CPD)

The pelvis may be too small. This may occur following trauma to the pelvis, but is usually idiopathic. Worldwide, rickets and osteomalacia are the commoner causes (Fig. 2). The role of computed tomography or radiographic pelvimetry to measure the size of the outlet is probably very limited.

The presenting part may be too big. The baby's head may be large, particularly in association with macrosomia (e.g. diabetes). Only rarely is there hydrocephalus. More commonly, there may be relative disproportion, i.e. the head is extended or rotated in some unfavourable way (malposition), presenting a larger diameter to the pelvis than is ideal.

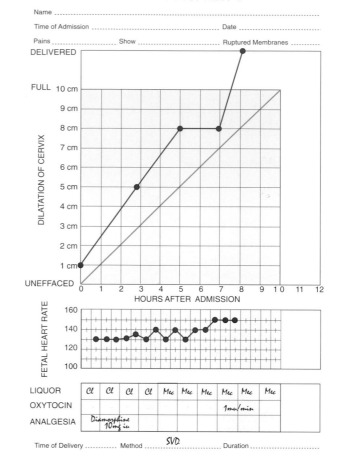

Fig. 1 **Partogram.** Progress was arrested at 8 cm and the baby was in right occipitoposterior position (i.e. relative cephalopelvic disproportion). As the patient was a primigravida and the CTG was reassuring, Syntocinon was commenced, the head rotated and there was an SVD.

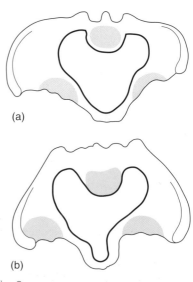

Fig. 2 **Pelvis in (a) rickets and (b) osteomalacia.** Pressure deforms the softened bones.

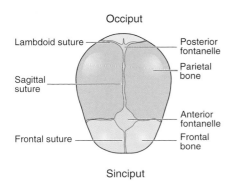

Occiput

Lambdoid suture — Posterior fontanelle

Sagittal suture — Parietal bone

Frontal suture — Anterior fontanelle

Frontal bone

Sinciput

Fig. 3 **Diagram of the fetal scalp sutures.**

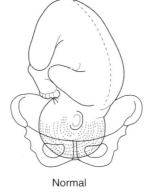

Normal   Malposition (OP)

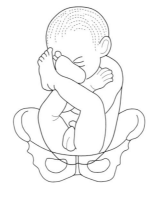

Malpresentation (Breech)   Malpresentation (Shoulder)

Fig. 4 **Malpresentation and malposition.**

Malpresentations and malpositions

(see also Breech, p. 40)
It is possible to establish the position of the fetal head at VE by palpation of the scalp sutures (Fig. 3).

Occipitoposterior (Fig. 4). Although the head usually rotates to occipitoanterior (OA) in normal labour, some arrest in the transverse position and a small proportion (≈ 10%) rotate to occipitoposterior (OP). There are usually longer first and second stages of labour with an increased chance of requiring a caesarean section, rotational forceps or ventouse delivery. If still OP and undelivered despite second stage pushing, a low/mid-cavity OP delivery, manual rotation, rotational ventouse, or Kielland's rotational forceps delivery will be required.

Face presentation (Fig. 5). Caution is required to avoid confusion with a breech presentation. Most face presentations engage in the transverse position and 90% rotate to mento-anterior so that the head is born with flexion. If mento-posterior, a caesarean section will be required unless very preterm or there has been an intrauterine death, as the extending head presents an increasingly wide diameter to the pelvis and worsening relative CPD.

Brow presentation (Fig. 6). The supraorbital ridges and the bridge of the nose are palpable. The head may flex to become a vertex presentation or extend to face presentation in early labour. If the brow presentation persists or there is no cervical dilatation, a caesarean section will be required.

Transverse/oblique lie. This usually occurs in multiparous women and is associated with multiple pregnancy, preterm labour and polyhydramnios. It may also occur with an abnormal uterus or placenta praevia. Vaginal

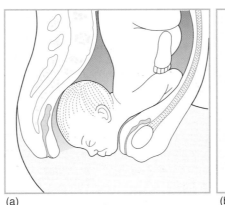 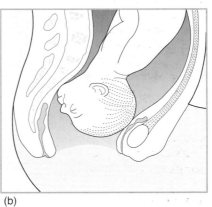

(a)   (b)

Fig. 5 **Face presentation. (a)** Mento-anterior – delivery possible. **(b)** Mento-posterior – delivery impossible.

delivery is not possible and there is a risk of cord prolapse. Pre-labour external cephalic version with or without induction or elective caesarean section is needed. Transverse lie (± arm presentation) following spontaneous rupture of the membranes is an indication for urgent caesarean section, which may require a vertical uterine incision to enable delivery of the fetus.

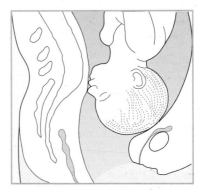

Fig. 6 **Brow presentation.**

Abnormal labour

- Slow labour may be due to poor uterine activity or fetal obstruction.
- Obstruction may be due to true cephalopelvic disproportion (i.e. the baby is too big or the pelvis too small). It may also be due to relative cephalopelvic disproportion (i.e. with malposition or malpresentation).

Operative delivery

Forceps and ventouse can be used to deliver a baby in the second stage of labour. Caesarean section can be used in both the first and second stages. Operative delivery may be indicated:

1. in the presence of fetal distress or
2. for 'delay' or failed progress despite good contractions and maternal effort.

Forceps delivery

There are three main types of forceps (Fig. 1):

- Low-cavity outlet forceps (e.g. Wrigley's), which are short and light.
- Mid-cavity forceps (e.g. Haig Ferguson, Neville Barnes, Simpson's) for when the sagittal

Table 1 Criteria for instrumental vaginal delivery

- The cervix fully dilated with the membranes ruptured
- The head at spines or below with no head palpable abdominally
- The position of the head known
- The bladder empty
- Analgesia satisfactory (perineal infiltration and pudendal blocks usually suffice for mid-cavity and ventouse deliveries but spinal or epidural analgesia is required for Kielland's)

suture is in the anteroposterior plane (usually occipitoanterior).
- Kielland's forceps for rotational delivery (the reduced pelvic curve allows rotation about the axis of the handle).

The most common indications for use of forceps are presumed fetal distress or second stage delay. The criteria listed in Table 1 should all be met before forceps delivery is attempted.

The most difficult part is often identifying the fetal position accurately. If there is a suspicion from palpation of the sutures that the baby is occipitotransverse, it is often helpful to try to feel for an ear anteriorly under the symphysis pubis (this is painful).

Low or mid-cavity non-rotational forceps (Fig. 2)

The mother should be placed in the lithotomy position with her bottom just over the edge of the bed (the bottom half of the bed needs to lift away). Using an aseptic technique, the perineum is cleaned and draped, the bladder emptied and the vaginal examination findings rechecked. A pudendal block and perineal infiltration is inserted if required, and the forceps assembled discreetly in front of the perineum before application, care being taken to ensure that the pelvic curve will be sitting over the malar aspect of the baby's head, convex towards the baby's face. The handle that lies in the left hand is inserted to the mother's left side by placing the right hand into the vagina to prevent injury and slipping the blade between the hand and baby's head between contractions (Fig. 2a,b,c). Opposite hands are used for the right blade and the blades are locked into position by lowering the handles and allowing articulation to occur gently (Fig. 2d).

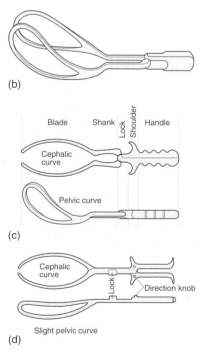

(a)

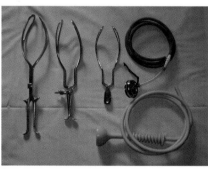

(b)

(c)

Blade Shank Lock Shoulder Handle

Cephalic curve

Pelvic curve

(c)

Cephalic curve

Lock

Direction knob

Slight pelvic curve

(d)

Fig. 1 **Types of forceps and ventouse cups.**
(a) Forceps: from left to right, Kielland's, mid-cavity, Wrigley's. Ventouse cups: metal (above), Silastic (below). **(b)** Wrigley's forceps. **(c)** Simpson's mid-cavity obstetric forceps. **(d)** Kielland's forceps.

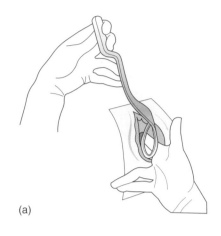

(a)

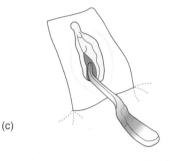

(c)

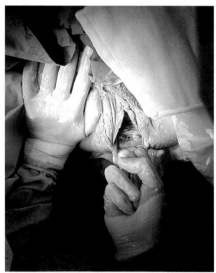

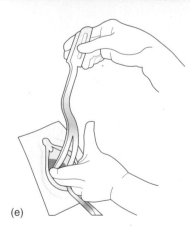

(e)

Fig. 2 **Mid-cavity forceps delivery** (see text).

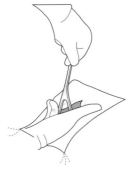

(b)

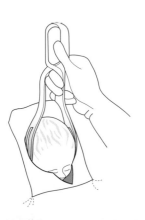

(d)

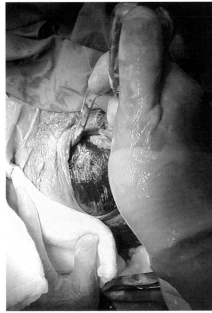

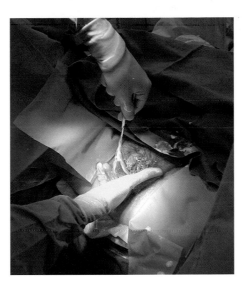

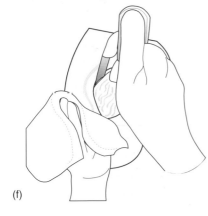

(f)

Traction is applied by pulling initially downwards at an angle of ≈ 60° (maternal pelvis to obstetrician's pelvis if sitting), with the direction of traction becoming horizontal and then upwards as the baby's head advances over the perineum (Fig. 2e,f). It is usual to perform an episiotomy as the vulva stretches, but occasionally this may not be necessary with a low-cavity lift-out in a parous woman. The forceps are removed after delivery of the baby's head, and the remainder of the baby is delivered as normal.

Rotational forceps (Fig. 3)

These lack the pelvic curve of non-rotational forceps and can be applied directly to the baby's head if it is occipitoposterior to allow rotation to occipitoanterior before traction. If the baby's head is occipitotransverse, the blades may be applied directly, or the anterior blade applied posteriorly, before being 'wandered' past the baby's face to the anterior position (Fig. 3a–d). After gentle rotation to occipitoanterior, delivery is as for the mid-cavity forceps. Rotational forceps require considerable skill, and may be associated with greater maternal injury than rotational ventouse. They should only be used by experienced obstetricians.

Manual rotation can be a useful alternative for correcting malposition as it may be possible to rotate the fetal head to occipitoanterior using digital pressure on the sutures (usually the lambdoid sutures). Some operators prefer to rotate during a contraction to minimize the risk of pushing the head up out of the pelvis.

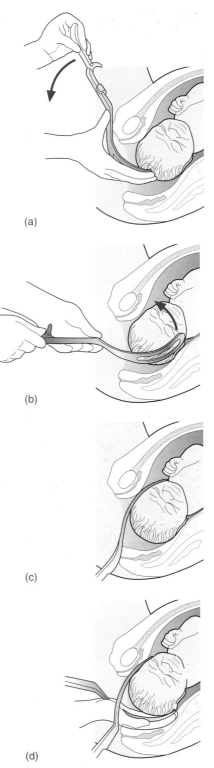

(a)

(b)

(c)

(d)

Fig. 3 **Rotational forceps. (a)** The forceps blade is inserted posteriorly. **(b)** It is then 'wandered' anteriorly over the baby's face. **(c)** It sits unsupported in this position. **(d)** The other blade is applied directly and locked to the anterior blade. The head can then be rotated to occipitoanterior before delivery by direct traction.

Ventouse (Figs 4,5,6)

Ventouse may be associated with less maternal trauma than are forceps. The same criteria for use apply to ventouse delivery as to forceps. The use of a soft Silastic cup rather than a metal vacuum extractor cup is associated with more failures but with fewer neonatal scalp injuries. Silastic cups are therefore often used for occipitoanterior deliveries and a metal occipitoposterior cup for transverse and posterior malpositions.

The cup is ideally placed in the midline overlying, or just anterior to, the posterior fontanelle (Fig. 5). Suction is applied, care being taken to ensure that the vaginal skin is not included under the cup. Traction is also applied downwards as for forceps, but delivery is much more likely to be successful if traction is timed with contractions and maternal effort. The risk of significant fetal injury is increased with use of metal cups (rather than Silastic), and duration of application.

Whether to use ventouse or forceps remains an area for debate, but depends to a significant degree on operator experience and familiarity. The use of ventouse compared to forceps is associated with an increased risk of failure, less regional/general anaesthesia, less maternal perineal or vaginal trauma, more cephalhaematomata, more retinal haemorrhages, and more low Apgar scores at 5 minutes. No differences between ventouse and forceps were found in the one study that followed up mothers and children for 5 years.

The vacuum extractor is contraindicated with a face presentation. Although it has been suggested that it should not be used at gestations of less than 36 weeks because of the risk of cephalhaematoma and intracranial haemorrhage, a case control study suggests that this restriction may be unnecessary. There is minimal risk of fetal haemorrhage if the extractor is applied following fetal blood sampling or application of a spiral scalp electrode. No bleeding was reported in two randomized trials comparing forceps and ventouse.

Forceps delivery before full dilatation of the cervix is contraindicated and ventouse before full dilatation should only be considered in special circumstances and with a very experienced operator.

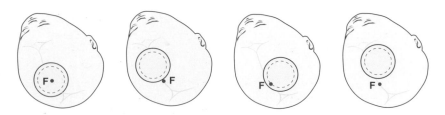

Fig. 4 **Ventouse – the 'flexing median' is the correct position for cup application.** The three other abnormal positions are much less likely to lead to a successful vaginal delivery and are more associated with fetal trauma.

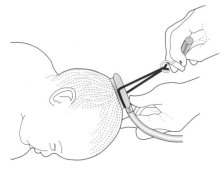

Fig. 5 **Ventouse – method of traction.** Note the finger–thumb position.

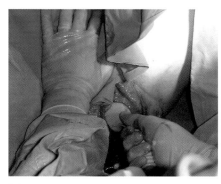

(a)

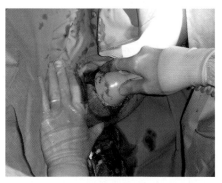

(b)

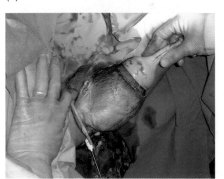

(c)

Fig. 6 **Ventouse delivery.**

Caesarean section (Fig. 7)

Caesarean section may be:

1. Pre-labour (i.e. 'elective') for many reasons, e.g. placenta praevia, severe intrauterine growth restriction (IUGR), severe pre-eclampsia, transverse lie or breech presentation unsuitable for vaginal delivery.
2. In labour (i.e. 'emergency'), usually for the reasons listed under 'Forceps delivery' if not fully dilated or suitable for vaginal delivery.

Maternal mortality is higher for emergency section than for elective section. Overall, there is also significant morbidity from thromboembolic disease, haemorrhage and infection. Lower uterine segment caesarean section is by far the most commonly used and has a lower rate of subsequent uterine rupture, together with better healing and fewer postoperative complications. A classical caesarean section (vertical uterine incision) will provide better access for a transverse lie following ruptured membranes, or with very vascular anterior placenta praevias, very preterm fetuses (particularly after spontaneous rupture of the membranes), or large lower segment fibroids. The chance of scar rupture in subsequent pregnancies following a vertical uterine incision is, however, much greater.

Preparation includes intravenous access, group and save, sodium citrate ± ranitidine (to reduce the incidence of Mendelson's syndrome), appropriate thromboprophylaxis and antibiotic prophylaxis, anaesthesia (spinal, epidural or general), and catheterization. The table should be tilted 15° to the left side (reduces aortocaval compression), and a lower abdominal transverse incision made, cutting through the fat and the rectus sheath to open the peritoneum. The bladder is freed and pushed down, and a transverse lower segment incision made (Fig. 7a–c).

The baby's head is encouraged through the incision with firm fundal pressure from the assistant (Wrigley's forceps are occasionally required). If the baby is a breech presentation, traction is applied to the pelvis by placing a finger behind each flexed hip (Fig. 7d) and, if transverse, a leg identified to deliver (i.e. internal podalic version). After delivery, Syntocinon is given i.v. stat. and the placenta delivered after uterine contraction. Haemostasis is obtained with straight artery forceps, a check made to ensure that the uterus is empty and that there are no ovarian cysts, and the incision closed with two layers of dissolving suture to the uterus (Fig. 7e,f), one layer to the sheath and one layer to the skin.

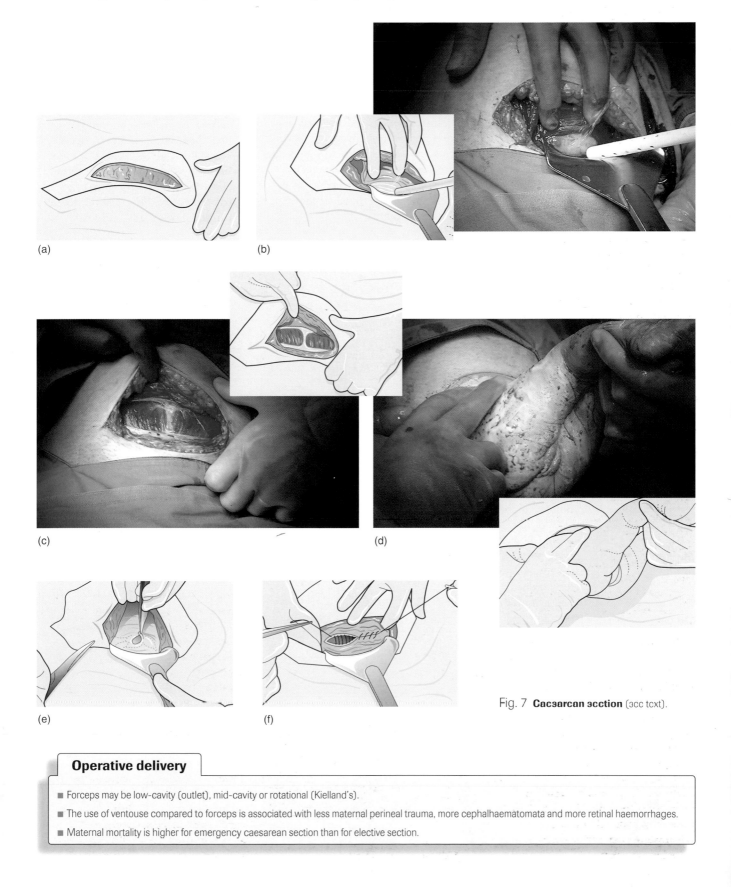

(a)

(b)

(c)

(d)

(e)

(f)

Fig. 7 **Caesarean section** (see text).

Operative delivery

- Forceps may be low-cavity (outlet), mid-cavity or rotational (Kielland's).
- The use of ventouse compared to forceps is associated with less maternal perineal trauma, more cephalhaematomata and more retinal haemorrhages.
- Maternal mortality is higher for emergency caesarean section than for elective section.

The perineum

Perineal tears

Perineal trauma affects women's physical, psychological and social well-being in both the immediate and long-term postnatal periods. It can also disrupt breast feeding, family life and sexual relations. In the UK, approximately a third of women will continue to have pain and discomfort for 10–12 days postpartum and 10% of women will continue to have long-term pain (3–18 months following delivery). Faecal incontinence and urinary incontinence can occur postpartum (see below).

It was previously felt that the use of episiotomy reduced the incidence of anal sphincter tears. There is, however, little good evidence to suggest that this is the case, and there is certainly no evidence to support routine episiotomy in all deliveries to prevent third- or fourth-degree tears. Midline episiotomy in particular offers little protection and right posterolateral episiotomy is preferred (see p. 47).

The rate of episiotomy has wide geographic variations from 8% in the Netherlands, 20% in England and Wales, 50% in the USA to 99% in some Eastern European countries. It is also high in many developing countries. It is therefore difficult to define what a 'good' episiotomy rate should be. Restricting the use of episiotomy to specific fetal and maternal indications leads to lower rates of posterior perineal trauma and healing complications. A tear may be less painful than an episiotomy and may also heal better.

There is controversy about whether the baby's head should be 'controlled' during delivery (i.e. a hand used to slow the head as it delivers). A controlled head is likely to tear the perineum less, but may increase the blood flow and distract the mother in her pushing.

Spontaneous tears are defined as:

- first degree involving skin only
- second degree involving perineal muscles
- third degree involving partial or complete disruption of the anal sphincter
- fourth degree involving complete disruption of the external and internal anal sphincters and anal mucosa.

Although there is some dispute as to the most useful classification for perineal tears this system allows a differentiation to be made between injuries to the anal sphincter and those involving the anal mucosa. Anterior perineal trauma is defined as any injury to the labia, anterior vagina, urethra or clitoris and is associated with less morbidity.

Repair of perineal tears should be with an absorbable synthetic material (Dexon or Vicryl), using a continuous subcuticular (possibly non-locking) technique to minimize short- and long-term problems. Good perineal toilet post-delivery is likely to aid healing, and the use of ice packs and analgesia may be useful to control symptoms.

There is some evidence to support the use of perineal massage in women completing their first pregnancy as a preventive measure to reduce the incidence of trauma.

Repair of episiotomy or first- or second-degree tear (Fig. 1)

1. Infiltrate with 1% lidocaine (lignocaine) (unless an epidural is in situ or the perineum has been infiltrated prior to delivery) (Fig. 1a).
2. Find the apex of the vaginal incision or tear and place the first suture above this level (but note that the rectum is just posterior to the vaginal wall) (Fig. 1b).
3. Use a continuous locking suture to appose the vaginal wall, continuing until the hymenal edges are apposed. The suture can then be tied, or more simply locked, and the needle threaded between the apposed vaginal edges a few centimetres back ready to close the perineal body.

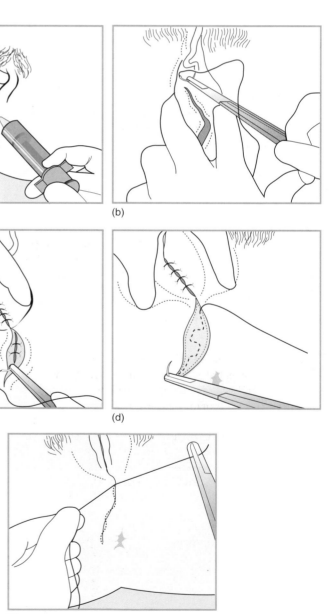

(a)

(b)

(c)

(d)

(e)

Fig. 1 **Repairing an episiotomy** (see text).

4. The perineal body sutures should be interrupted, and then a continuous finer suture used for the skin (Fig. 1c–e). It is possible that not closing the skin (i.e. leaving the skin edges approximately 5 mm apart) reduces postnatal pain. Check instruments and swabs (a retained swab is a common cause of litigation in obstetrics).

Repair of third- or fourth-degree tears

This should ideally be by an experienced clinician in a theatre with good analgesia and light. The edges of the sphincter should be approximated or overlapped, with the knots tied in the lumen of the bowel rather than buried in the perineal tissues. Antibiotics, laxatives and fibre are important to allow healing. If secondary breakdown occurs, it may be necessary to perform a defunctioning colostomy before re-repairing.

Postnatal urinary tract problems

In the first year after delivery, 3–5% of women experience urinary tract infection and about 5% report urinary frequency for the first time after delivery. The possibility of low-grade urinary tract infection should be kept in mind, especially after catheterization.

At least 20% of women suffer from stress incontinence for up to 3 months after delivery, mostly from neuropraxia, although this commonly resolves spontaneously. Some will still be incontinent a year later without treatment. Postnatal exercises may be of help. It is possible that targeting women who are still incontinent at 3 months may help, but this needs further research.

Bowel problems

Up to 20% of women report constipation after delivery, which may in part be due to narcotic analgesia in labour. Haemorrhoids affect around 20% of women, and these frequently last long term. They are more common in primiparous women and after instrumental delivery.

Anal incontinence

Inability to control flatus or faeces occurs in around 4% of women after delivery. Because of its embarrassing nature, women often fail to report it. New evidence has demonstrated that 35% of primiparae have demonstrable damage to the anal sphincter, although many of the women with damage do not have symptoms (Fig. 2). Both direct trauma and nerve damage following spontaneous vaginal or instrumental delivery contribute to this problem. Proper investigation and treatment are essential.

Elective caesarean section on request

In view of the potential risks of vaginal delivery to the perineum as outlined above, together with the potential for fetal injury, a small proportion of women may request an elective caesarean section despite a normal antenatal course.

Performing such a caesarean section when it is not clinically indicated has traditionally been considered inappropriate, but views may be changing. Elective caesareans under regional blockade with antibiotic cover and appropriate thromboprophylaxis are relatively safe, and short-term

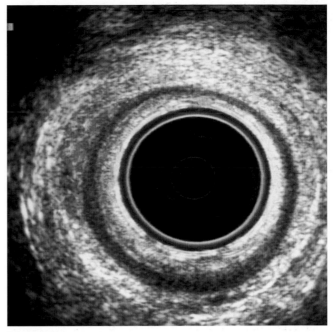
(a)

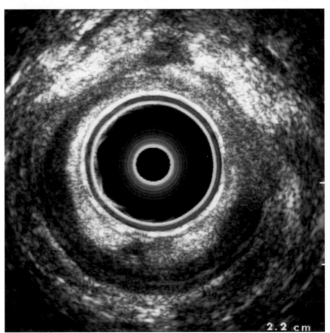
(b)

Fig. 2 **Anal sphincter damage on endoanal ultrasound. (a)** Normal anal sphincter scan. **(b)** Anterior anal sphincter defect exceeding one quadrant.

neonatal complications from transient tachypnoea and respiratory distress syndrome are reduced by delaying the operation until 39 weeks of pregnancy. Nonetheless, all surgery carries risks and the longer-term possibilities of adhesions, scar rupture, visceral damage and the potential for more difficult future gynaecological surgery need to be considered.

The perineum

- There is no evidence to support routine episiotomy – a tear may be less painful than an episiotomy and may also heal better.
- Right (or left) posterolateral episiotomy is preferable to a midline episiotomy.
- Perineal damage may affect bladder, bowel and sexual function.
- Third- and fourth-degree tears need to be repaired by experienced clinicians.

Postpartum haemorrhage and abnormalities of the third stage of labour

Postpartum haemorrhage (PPH) can be sudden, dramatic and life threatening and is one of the obstetric emergencies. *Primary* PPH is the loss of more than 500 ml of blood from the genital tract in the first 24 hours after the delivery. *Secondary* PPH is excessive blood loss from the genital tract between 24 hours and 6 weeks postpartum (see p. 66).

The usual mechanism for control of uterine blood loss following delivery of the placenta is for contraction with retraction of the uterine muscle. This means shortening of the fibre length and the muscle fibres maintaining this shortened length. Due to the interlacing nature of the muscle fibres this retraction will stem the bleeding that has been supplying the placenta (Fig. 1).

Causes of postpartum haemorrhage

The main causes of PPH are given in Table 1.

Primary postpartum haemorrhage

Uterine atony is the commonest cause (~ 90%) of primary PPH and may be due to many differing factors (Fig. 2).

Trauma is the second most common cause of primary PPH (~ 7%), with coagulation disorders making up the remainder. Caesarean section may be associated with blood loss greater than 500 ml and therefore constitutes a PPH. Additional bleeding will occur if the uterine incision extends laterally to the uterine artery or down towards the cervix.

Caesarean section for an anterior placenta praevia is highly likely to be

Table 1 Causes of primary and secondary postpartum haemorrhage	
Primary	**Secondary**
Uterine atony – common	Retained products of conception
Cervical lacerations – rare	Infection
Vaginal lacerations – rare	
Uterine tear/rupture – very rare	
Coagulation disorders	

associated with excessive blood loss, particularly in the presence of a previous caesarean section scar as placenta accreta or percreta may have occurred. Placenta accreta is abnormal adherence of all or part of the placenta to the uterine wall – termed placenta increta where there is placental infiltration of the myometrium or placenta percreta if penetration reaches the serosa.

Tears of the cervix or vagina may result in considerable blood loss and need suturing. A spiral vaginal tear is classically described associated with a rotational forceps delivery (see p. 55).

Management of primary postpartum haemorrhage

Active management

With the adage that prevention is better than cure, active management of the

third stage of labour reduces blood loss by 50% – although it leads to a slightly increased risk of retained placenta (see below). In some high-risk conditions an intravenous infusion of oxytocin is used in addition to the bolus dose. High-risk conditions would include prolonged labour, known placenta praevia, polyhydramnios, twin pregnancy, high parity, uterine fibroids, abruptio placentae or previous PPH.

Retained placenta

The placenta is usually separated from the uterus during the process of uterine retraction and maternal effort or controlled cord traction used to expel the placenta and membranes from the uterus.

If the placenta does not separate or only partially separates and there is bleeding, removal needs to be facilitated. Controlled cord traction may encourage delivery of the placenta. If this measure fails, manual removal of the placenta will be required. During this procedure prevention of infection is important, thus obstetric antiseptic cream is used, the hand and arm being covered. The gloved hand is placed into the uterus and the placenta and membranes removed. The hand is allowed to be placed back into the uterus on one

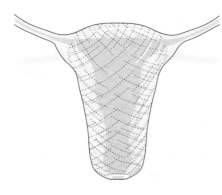

Fig. 1 **The usual mechanism for control of uterine blood loss following delivery.** The mesh-like network of smooth muscle fibres, on contraction and retraction, controls bleeding.

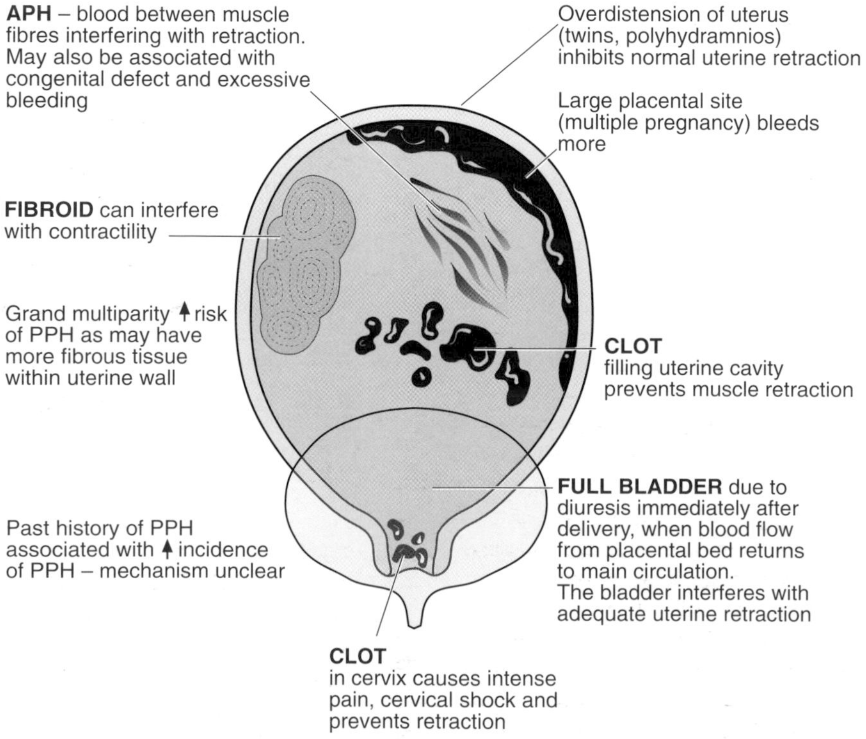

APH – blood between muscle fibres interfering with retraction. May also be associated with congenital defect and excessive bleeding

FIBROID can interfere with contractility

Grand multiparity ↑ risk of PPH as may have more fibrous tissue within uterine wall

Past history of PPH associated with ↑ incidence of PPH – mechanism unclear

Overdistension of uterus (twins, polyhydramnios) inhibits normal uterine retraction

Large placental site (multiple pregnancy) bleeds more

CLOT filling uterine cavity prevents muscle retraction

FULL BLADDER due to diuresis immediately after delivery, when blood flow from placental bed returns to main circulation. The bladder interferes with adequate uterine retraction

CLOT in cervix causes intense pain, cervical shock and prevents retraction

Fig. 2 **The main causes of uterine anatomy.**

further occasion to check that all products have been removed. This procedure is usually done under regional blockade and only rarely under general anaesthesia, unless in the presence of a PPH.

For practical management of primary PPH:

- summon senior help
- summon an anaesthetist
- keep ahead of the blood loss
- rub up a contraction and catheterize to ensure bladder empty and allow monitoring of urinary output
- gain intravenous access with two large venflons; run in crystalloid or colloid and cross-match 6 units of blood
- give Syntocinon intravenously
- remove placenta if possible; ensure no blood clot distending the cervix
- if apparent uterine atony, further intravenous Syntocinon and carboprost intramuscularly or intramyometrially
- if bleeding possibly due to trauma, general anaesthetic (not regional block) is required before repairing lacerations
- in the face of persistent bleeding consider internal iliac artery ligation, hysterectomy or radiological embolization
- intensive therapy unit support and central monitoring; correct coagulopathy as disseminated intravascular coagulopathy (DIC) is likely – fresh frozen plasma and uncross-matched or group-specific blood may be transfused; monitor for development of acute renal failure and adult respiratory distress syndrome.

Secondary postpartum haemorrhage

Distinguishing between retained products of conception and infection allows effective management of secondary PPH. Pyrexia, raised WBC, offensive lochial discharge and a closed cervical os are found with endometritis which will require antibiotics particularly covering anaerobic organisms. Intravenous therapy for 24 hours and bed rest will usually see a rapid improvement.

Bleeding, maybe with passage of tissue, an open cervical os and failure of uterine involution leaving the uterus larger than usual for the number of postpartum days are all features of secondary PPH due to retained products of conception. The patient will be taken to theatre for evacuation of the uterus under anaesthesia. Antibiotic cover may

prevent the development of endometritis. Syntocinon or ergometrine are used to control blood loss. It is usually unnecessary to request uterine ultrasound to make the diagnosis.

Third stage problems

These may include:

- failure of placental separation
- incomplete placental separation
- postpartum haemorrhage – due to retained portion of placenta
- uterine atony – leading to excessive blood loss
- tear of genital tract
- collapse (may be due to excessive blood loss, eclamptic fit, amniotic fluid embolus, cardiac failure, pulmonary embolus, cerebral haemorrhage, diabetic coma)
- uterine inversion (p. 63).

Collapse in the third stage needs prompt action to ensure maternal well-being. Epilepsy and diabetes would be known about from the history and there may be a relevant cardiac history. Blood loss would be obvious. Amniotic fluid embolus, cerebral haemorrhage and pulmonary embolus would all be associated with sudden collapse of the mother needing resuscitation and investigation to distinguish between the pathologies.

Sheehan's syndrome

This is an especial problem in obstetrics if there is profound hypotension that remains uncorrected. During pregnancy the pituitary gland increases in size predisposing it to circulatory problems if there is blood loss. It has end arterial blood supply which means no collateral supply, and hypotension may result in an avascular pituitary gland. If this is not corrected quickly enough the pituitary gland will undergo avascular necrosis (Sheehan's syndrome) (Fig. 3).

The consequences of this depend on which area of the pituitary gland is inactivated. If the anterior lobe is lost then no follicle-stimulating hormone (FSH), luteinizing hormone (LH), thyroid-stimulating hormone (TSH), growth hormone (GH), prolactin or adrenocorticotropic hormone (ACTH) will be produced resulting in secondary amenorrhoea, atrophy of breasts and genital organs, osteoporosis, hypothyroidism and Addisonian symptoms.

The importance of adequate and urgent blood and fluid replacement in postpartum haemorrhage is thus obvious.

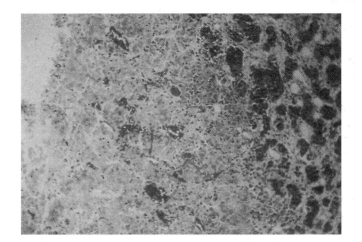

Fig. 3 **Histology of pituitary gland in Sheehan's syndrome.**

Postpartum haemorrhage

- Postpartum haemorrhage can be life threatening.
- Uterine atony is the commonest cause of primary postpartum haemorrhage.
- Emergency management includes ensuring contraction of the uterus and adequate fluid replacement.
- If the uterus is well contracted check for trauma to the genital tract and that blood is clotting.
- Active management of the third stage of labour reduces the incidence of primary postpartum haemorrhage.
- Retained products of conception are prevented by a thorough check of the completeness of the placenta and membranes at delivery.

Obstetric emergencies

Amniotic fluid embolism

This rare complication occurs when amniotic fluid suddenly enters the maternal circulation during labour or delivery. It carries a high maternal mortality (up to 80%) and is associated with multiparity, precipitate labour, uterine stimulation and caesarean section. Clinically there is sudden dyspnoea, fetal distress and hypotension, followed within minutes by cardiorespiratory arrest with or without seizures. It is often followed by haemorrhage from disseminated intravascular coagulation (DIC) and uterine atony, and may lead to acute renal failure (ARF) and adult respiratory distress syndrome (ARDS; Fig. 1). It is often diagnosed by exclusion (Table 1), but is ideally identified by the presence of fetal squamous cells on a blood film from a central line.

Management includes cardiopulmonary resuscitation (CPR) with high-flow O_2, with or without ventilation if required, and consideration given to urgent delivery. Two large-bore i.v. lines are inserted and the patient is rapidly infused with a combination of crystalloid and colloid until the blood pressure approaches normal. This is then stopped to minimize the risk of ARDS. As uterine atony is common, oxytocics are given postnatally. Bloods are sent for clotting, screen and cross-match to anticipate DIC. Cardiogenic shock, ARDS and ARF are managed as appropriate.

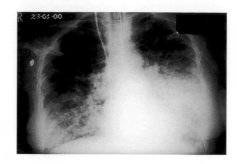

Fig. 1 **ARDS.** There is bilateral alveolar consolidation.

Fig. 2 **Cord prolapse.**

Cord prolapse

This may occur especially when membranes rupture (or are ruptured) with a high or poorly fitting presenting part (Fig. 2). The risk is of cord occlusion with pressure from the presenting part, or of vessel spasm and constriction following exposure to the lower temperature of the air, leading to hypoxia and possibly death. It is also more likely to occur with twins, polyhydramnios, breech or transverse lie.

- If the cord is palpated before artificial rupture of the membranes ('cord presentation') then caesarean section is required.
- If cord prolapse occurs, the presenting part should be displaced upward with a hand and the hand kept there until delivery. If the cervix is fully dilated and easy delivery is anticipated, then an immediate forceps or ventouse delivery should be carried out. If not, then the patient should be instructed to adopt the knee–chest position (kneeling with head down) and transferred to theatre for an immediate caesarean section under general anaesthesia or rapid spinal anaesthesia.

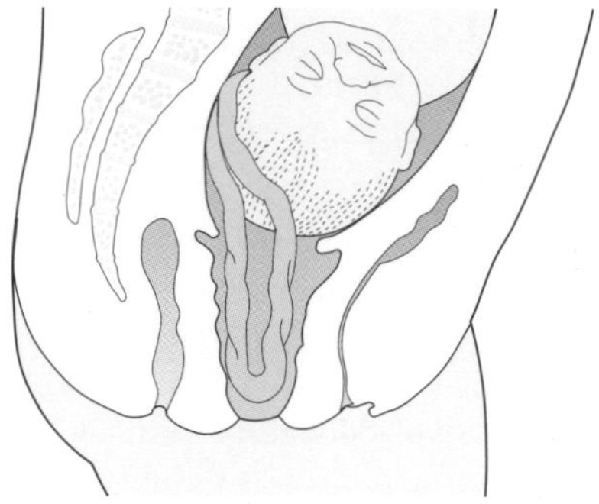

Mendelson's syndrome

This is due to pulmonary injury following inhalation of acid gastric contents, and is more likely during obstetric anaesthesia than routine anaesthesia because of pressure from the gravid uterus and reduced competence of the gastro-oesophageal sphincter. There is rapid onset of cyanosis, bronchospasm, tachycardia and pulmonary oedema. Cricoid pressure should be used with induction of general anaesthesia to minimize the risk.

If inhalation occurs, the patient should be given 100% O_2, tilted head down and turned onto her left side. The pharynx should be aspirated. Antibiotics may prevent secondary infection. Further management is with ventilation if required, physiotherapy and rarely bronchoscopic aspiration of mucous plugs.

Shoulder dystocia

The shoulders are stuck in the anteroposterior (AP) plane with the anterior shoulder behind the symphysis pubis (Fig. 3). Prompt, calm action is vital, as the baby will become rapidly asphyxiated and will die without appropriate action. The diagnosis is made after failure to deliver shoulders with the *first* downward pull of the head.

Management

The acronym 'PALE SISTER' summarizes the management of shoulder dystocia.

Table 1 **Causes of sudden collapse**	
Problem	**Discussion**
Amniotic fluid embolism	Is associated with multiparity, precipitate labour, uterine stimulation and caesarean section. There is **sudden dyspnoea**, **fetal distress** and **hypotension**, followed within minutes by cardiorespiratory arrest ± seizures
Anaphylaxis	There may be **cyanosis**, **hypotension**, **wheezing**, **pallor**, prostration and tachycardia ± urticaria
Cerebrovascular accident	May be history of severe pregnancy-induced hypertension or past history of intracranial problems (e.g. previous subarachnoid haemorrhage). **Nausea and vomiting with headache**
Eclampsia	There is a **tonic–clonic seizure** (differentiate from epilepsy and amniotic fluid embolism on the basis of the history)
Myocardial infarct	May be past history of heart disease. **Chest pain**, **sweating**, **pallor**
Tension pneumothorax	There is sudden onset of **pleuritic chest pain** (differentiate from pulmonary embolus) and diminished breath sounds
Pulmonary embolism	There may be apprehension, **pleuritic chest pain**, **sudden dyspnoea**, cough, haemoptysis and collapse (differentiate from pneumothorax) ± antecedent risk factors
Uterine inversion	Occurs in the third stage only. It may lead to **profound hypotension** (there may be only a partial inversion and therefore the diagnosis may not be obvious)

The most important symptoms and signs are in bold type.

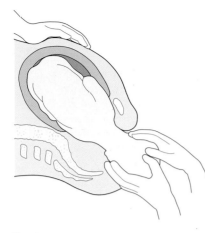

Fig. 3 **Shoulder dystocia.** The anterior shoulder is behind the symphysis pubis.

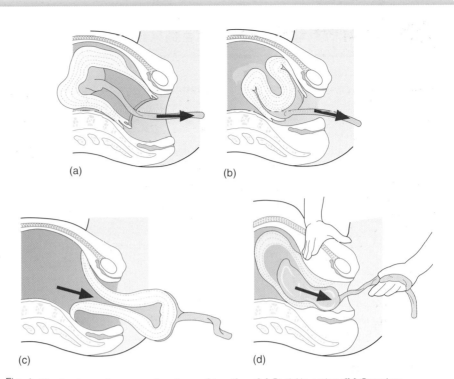

Fig. 4 **Uterine inversion secondary to cord traction. (a)** Partial inversion. **(b)** Complete inversion. **(c)** Complete inversion with prolapse. **(d)** Position of the hands to avoid uterine inversion in the third stage.

P **Prepare**. There should be a plan, and the team should know the plan.

A **Assistance**. Experienced help should be sent for, and management started immediately.

L **Legs into McRobert's position** (femora abducted, rotated outwards and flexed such that the thighs touch the abdomen). This straightens the sacrum relative to the lumbar spine, rotating the symphysis anteriorly, and allows the anterior shoulder to enter the pelvis.

E **Episiotomy** (make it large).

S **Suprapubic pressure**. An assistant should apply suprapubic pressure with 'CPR' hand posture over the anterior shoulder both laterally (towards the direction the baby is facing) and posteriorly (to rotate it under the symphysis), while gentle traction is applied from below. It should be abandoned after 30–60 seconds.

I **Internal rotation**. Traction should be continued and a hand inserted to push the anterior shoulder forwards with counterpressure on the posterior clavicle to rotate the trunk to oblique. It should be abandoned after 30–60 seconds.

S **Screw manoeuvre**. Pressure is applied to the posterior aspect of the posterior shoulder, attempting to place the shoulder into oblique. This may disimpact the anterior shoulder. It should be abandoned after 30–60 seconds.

T **Try recovering posterior arm**. An attempt should be made to deliver the posterior shoulder by pulling the posterior arm down, flexing it across the chest. It should be abandoned after 30–60 seconds.

E **Extreme measures**. The choice is to either:

- try the above again
- fracture the clavicle (it may already be fractured after the above manoeuvres)
- push the baby's head back up and perform a caesarean section (Zavanelli manoeuvre) or perform a symphysiotomy, using a scalpel to divide the symphysis pubis to increase the size of the pelvic outlet.

R **Repair, record details, relax**. Make comprehensive notes.

Uterine inversion

This is usually an iatrogenic problem caused by pulling on the cord before separation and should be suspected if there is profound shock without obvious explanation (Fig. 4). It may be partial or total.

The placenta should not be detached until the uterus is replaced and contracted. If the prolapse is easily reducible, it should be reduced. If the reduction is unsuccessful, hydrostatic reduction (O'Sullivan's) is used. The inverted uterus is held within the vagina by the operator and the introitus sealed with the two hands of an assistant. Two litres of warm saline are infused rapidly (through a wide-bore tube). If all this fails, a laparotomy may be necessary.

Uterine rupture

This may occur if there has been a previous caesarean section (risk with lower segment incision < 1%, classical or De Lee 5–10%). It may also occur with obstructed labour in multiparous patients and with use of prostaglandins or Syntocinon. It is virtually unheard of in primigravidae.

Classically there is maternal tachycardia, shock, cessation of contractions, disappearance of the presenting part from the pelvis and fetal distress. Pain may be minimal or may be severe and there is variable bleeding per vaginum (bleeding is intraperitoneal if there is a complete rupture). It may present postpartum with a continued trickle or bleeding in the absence of another cause.

An immediate laparotomy under general or rapid spinal anaesthesia is required for delivery.

Obstetric emergencies

- It is important to practise emergencies in advance: who will be called to do what, how will they do it, what will they do, what will they do next and what if that still does not work.
- Amniotic fluid embolism may lead to ARDS, DIC or acute renal failure and carries a high maternal mortality rate.
- Cord prolapse may occur with artificial membrane rupture with a high head.
- Shoulder dystocia requires a calm approach and working through a practised protocol.

The normal puerperium

It is important to understand the normal process of the puerperium in order to be able to recognize complications when they occur, with the increasing trend towards early discharge from hospital, often before lactation is established.

Physiological changes

Physiological changes occur rapidly in the first week postpartum.

Structural

Immediately postdelivery the fundus of the uterus is just below the umbilicus. It should be impalpable abdominally by the end of the first week and almost normal size on bimanual assessment at 6 weeks. The lochia is the normal discharge from the genital tract in the puerperium. It is red for the first 3 days, then pink and becomes yellow/brown by the end of week one, diminishing in volume over 3–6 weeks.

Endocrine

Serum progesterone and oestradiol fall to non-pregnant levels by 72 hours. Human placental lactogen (HPL) levels fall rapidly in the first 48 hours but are still detectable at the end of the first week. Thyroxine and thyroid-binding globulin fall slowly to normal over 6 weeks. Fasting plasma, insulin and the insulin response curve are normal 2 days postpartum.

Body weight

On average a woman will lose 6 kg through labour and parturition (water loss and products of conception). Body weight stabilizes by 10 weeks postdelivery. A diuresis commences within the first 3 to 4 days postnatally. The haemoglobin level is lowest on day 4 to 5 postdelivery and then rises slowly until 8 weeks postpartum. Changes in platelet levels and other coagulation factors produce a relative hypercoagulability, persisting for approximately 8 weeks. During the first 4 weeks postnatally, there is a 50-fold increase compared to the non-pregnant state.

Milk

The suckling stimulus releases prolactin and oxytocin – the former stimulates lactogenesis, the latter controls milk ejection. Initially, milk rich in colostrum is released. Milk production commences by day 3.

Routine care

Routine observations carried out postpartum include pulse rate, blood pressure and temperature. If these are normal, daily recordings of the pulse rate and temperature will suffice. If the blood pressure has previously been elevated, 4-hourly readings are continued until it settles. The fundal height is checked daily to ensure that involution is occurring normally. The lochia is inspected and the volume, colour and odour noted. Very offensive lochia will require further investigation.

It is important to check the urine output, as retention can occur postnatally secondary to a painful perineum, after an epidural, or following surgery. A full bladder will increase the apparent fundal height and may retard uterine contraction. Perineal toilet after each bowel action should prevent infection of the episiotomy and subsequent breakdown. The perineum is often swollen and painful and many women develop haemorrhoids secondary to the expulsive efforts of labour. Adequate analgesia, laxatives and rectal suppositories may be required.

There must be adequate time for supervision and support of the mother following delivery. She must become familiar with nursing and bathing her infant with confidence, and the method of feeding to be adopted. Supervision of these processes may begin in hospital or be initiated in the community.

Breast feeding

Most women have made the decision to breast feed prior to delivery. Many units have a breast-feeding counsellor to offer guidance. There are some obvious advantages to breast feeding (Table 1). Consistent advice should be given by health care professionals to avoid confusion and demotivation.

The correct positioning of the baby on the breast is vital to prevent chewing of the nipples, causing sore or cracked nipples which can predispose to infection and discomfort (Fig. 1). Milk production requires a good fluid intake. Many mothers feed their babies 'on demand', others introduce a 3- to 4-hourly feeding regime. Supplementary and complementary feeds have not been shown in any randomized controlled trials to be of benefit to healthy term breast-fed infants. Extra fluids are no longer recommended for jaundiced babies. The best management is demand feeding. All babies will initially lose weight until lactation is fully established.

Human milk delivered at a rate of 750–800 ml a day (in a healthy, well-nourished mother) contains calcium at

Table 1 **Advantages of and contraindications for breast feeding**	
Advantages	**Contraindications**
■ Balanced nutritionally	■ Breast implant (breast augmentation)
■ Passive immunity	■ Previous surgery for breast abscess (relative contraindication)
■ Enhanced bonding	
■ Reduced infections of	■ Maternal phenylketonuria
– middle ear	■ Drugs taken by mother
– respiratory system	– lithium
– urinary tract	– cytotoxic drugs
– gastrointestinal tract	– immunosuppressants
■ Reduced incidence of cot death	■ Very poor maternal health
■ Reduced atopy, e.g. eczema	■ Puerperal psychosis – in some cases
■ Reduction in childhood insulin-dependent diabetes mellitus (by 50%)	■ HIV positive status
■ Reduced problems of prematurity	
– necrotizing enterocolitis	
– suboptimal neurological development	
■ Cheap and readily available	
■ Easy to deliver (no sterilization of equipment involved)	
■ Reduced incidence in the mother of premenopausal breast cancer	
■ Mother more likely to lose weight naturally	
■ Babies with cleft palate can be fed with special appliances.	

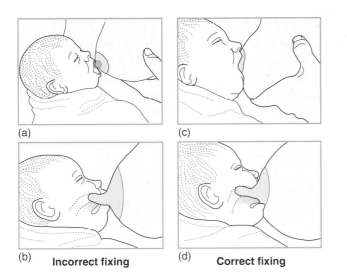

(a)

(c)

(b) **Incorrect fixing**

(d) **Correct fixing**

Fig. 1 **Positioning of the baby on the breast.**

Table 2 Situations requiring lactation suppression

- Bereavement (if the mother wishes)
  - mid-trimester miscarriage
  - stillbirth
  - neonatal death
- The mother is adamant she wishes to bottle feed but has a history of mastitis or breast abscess
- Breast feeding is contraindicated for whatever reason
- The child is to be given up for adoption
- The mother is HIV-positive

Bromocriptine is used, initially 2.5 mg daily increasing to 5 mg a day once it is seen to be tolerated or cabergoline 1 mg a day stat. It must be initiated soon after delivery to be effective as milk production commences on day 3. Bromocriptine is contraindicated in hypertensive women and those with coronary artery disease. The blood pressure should be monitored during treatment.

Table 3 Contraceptive needs and breast-feeding status

- Amenorrhoeic women who are fully breast feeding have a 98% protection for 6 months
- 2% of mothers who do not breast feed will ovulate before 28 days
- 33% of mothers who do not breast feed will ovulate before their first period
- Ovulation does not occur provided full lactation is maintained, i.e. reduced intervals between feeds, preferably 2-hourly feeds, and 2- to 4-hourly feeds by night – and complete amenorrhoea
- Once supplementary feeds are introduced 50% of women will ovulate within 3 months, even if lactation is maintained
- All progestogen-based contraception can be used by breast-feeding mothers, e.g. progestogen-only pill, depot injections, Implanon, Mirena
- The optimum time to start the contraceptive pill in non-breast-feeding mothers is 3 weeks postpartum; prior to this there is a significant risk of thromboembolism

---

a concentration of around 34 mg/dl. The loss of calcium from the mother is substantially more during lactation than during pregnancy. Bone density studies indicate a loss of bone mineral density over 6 months, but this is recovered after feeding ceases.

Bottle feeding

The mother should be taught how to sterilize the bottle correctly, either by boiling or immersing in a dilute solution of hypochlorite (Milton) or using a steam sterilizer. Bottle-feeds mimic breast milk as closely as possible. Cow's milk is used in artificial feeds and contains more protein (casein) and less sugar (lactose) than is found in human milk. The fat content is similar. The higher levels of casein make cow's milk less digestible. Milk feeds are fortified with additional iron and vitamins.

The volume of milk given commences at 20 ml/kg per day and builds up to 150 ml/kg per day by the seventh day. If babies exhibit an allergy to cow's milk, soya milk can be substituted. It may sometimes be necessary to suppress milk lactation (Table 2).

Postpartum contraception

The spacing of pregnancies is essential for the health of the mother and child. Severe anaemia may result if pregnancies follow each other too closely.

For breast feeding alone to be effective contraception, lactation must be complete (Table 3). Progestogen-based contraception does not suppress lactation and may be used by breast-feeding women. For the bottle-feeding mother, the combined oral contraceptive pill is the most effective method of contraception. Hypertension in pregnancy is not a contraindication to the combined oral contraceptive pill as long as the blood pressure has returned to normal. Women who intended to breast feed but stopped will need to be reminded to revise their contraception.

The coil is traditionally fitted at the 6-week postnatal visit. Risk of uterine perforation is slightly higher during lactation and following caesarean section. Laparoscopic clip sterilization carries a higher risk of failure in the immediate postpartum period than when it is performed as an interval procedure. If the previously used contraception was the diaphragm, it will need to be re-fitted 6 weeks postpartum.

The postnatal visit

Following uncomplicated normal vaginal deliveries, the postnatal visit is traditionally performed at 6 weeks at the general practitioner's surgery. Following difficult forceps deliveries and caesarean sections the visit may be performed at the hospital. Certainly, if there were complications at the time of delivery it is important that the parents have a chance to discuss the issues with the consultant.

Clinicians should be alert to the possibility of postnatal depression.

It is now thought unnecessary to perform a routine vaginal examination, which is reserved for symptomatic women, or in cases where a smear is due or a coil is to be inserted. Most women will already have resumed coitus without difficulty.

The normal puerperium

- A hypercoagulable state exists until approx. 8 weeks postpartum, increasing the risk of venous thromboembolism.
- Breast feeding supplies passive immunity to the infant and reduces the risk of atopy and cot death.
- Breast milk has a high carbohydrate, but low iron content – it is rich in calcium.
- Bottle milk has a higher protein content, but has less sugar – it is fortified with iron.
- Contraception is an important issue to allow spacing of pregnancies.

The abnormal puerperium

Problems occurring in the puerperium can be immediate, intermediate or late. The most serious complications are haemorrhage, infection and thromboembolism.

Haemorrhage

The incidence of postpartum haemorrhage is approximately 7%. Haemorrhage may be primary or secondary (Table 1). Most severe haemorrhages occur within the first few hours of delivery. The initial management of primary haemorrhage is discussed on page 60.

The most likely cause of secondary haemorrhage is retained products of conception. Clinically the uterus feels large, soft and tender and the cervical os is open. An ultrasound scan may be useful to confirm the presence of retained products if the clinical presentation is less obvious. The patient will need to return to theatre for evacuation of the uterus under antibiotic cover. Suction curettage is the safest approach. Until full culture and sensitivity results are available broad-spectrum antibiotics should be used that cover both aerobic and anaerobic organisms.

Infection

A puerperal pyrexia is defined as any febrile illness where the temperature is 38°C or higher during the first 14 days postpartum. This is no longer a notifiable illness but still needs to be taken seriously. Examination should include chest, breasts, abdomen, perineum and legs. Cervical swab, blood cultures and sputum may all need to be sent for culture and a mid-stream urine sample sent for microscopy and culture (Table 2).

Breast engorgement occurs in the first 2–3 days and can be associated with a mild pyrexia. This should improve spontaneously within 24–48 hours, particularly if breast feeding is encouraged. Mastitis is clinically obvious and prompt treatment should avoid abscess formation. If an abscess occurs the treatment of choice is drainage. Lactation need not be suppressed. The patient should continue to breast feed on the unaffected side expressing from the infected breast initially.

Thromboembolism can present with pyrexia (see below).

Urinary tract infections are the commonest cause of puerperal pyrexia. It is always important to repeat the urine sample at the end of the course of antibiotics to ensure that the infection has been eradicated.

Endometritis is more frequent following caesarean section than after vaginal delivery. Many centres now advocate the use of prophylactic antibiotics to cover a surgical delivery, especially in cases of prolonged labour or prolonged rupture of membranes. Cefuroxime or Augmentin are usual. Endometritis can be delayed and occur secondary to retained products of conception.

Venous thromboembolism

This is still one of the leading causes of maternal mortality. Clinical diagnosis of venous thromboembolism (VTE) can be difficult. Clinical signs are not always clear and initial investigations can be normal. Venography or duplex Doppler blood flow assessment of the femoral veins may be necessary. A ventilation–perfusion scan is required if pulmonary embolism is suspected.

The most frequent incorrect diagnosis is one of chest infection. Treatment is mainly with subcutaneous, high-dose, twice-daily heparin to achieve anticoagulation

Table 1 **Postpartum haemorrhage**

Type	Timescale	Presentation	Predisposing factors
Primary haemorrhage	In the first 24 hours	Fresh bleeding, often severely heavy. Uterus may be soft and poorly contracted with the fundus still above the umbilicus	Uterine atony (90%) Trauma, vaginal or cervical lacerations, labial tears (Fig. 1) Coagulation disorders
Secondary haemorrhage	After 24 hours and up to 6 weeks	May be fresh loss or old, altered blood, often malodorous. The uterus may feel soft, poorly contracted and possibly tender, with the cervical os open	Retained products of conception Endometritis Dysfunctional bleeding

Postpartum haemorrhage is defined as a blood loss greater than 500 ml from the genital tract after delivery of the baby.

Table 2 **Causes of puerperal pyrexia**

Site	Timescale	Presentation	Predisposing factors
Breast			
Breast engorgement	2–3 days postnatal	Can cause a transient pyrexia	Physiological
Mastitis	2–3 weeks postnatal	Spreading erythema (cellulitis) over the breast, lymphangitis, nipple discharge, malaise, fatigue and swinging pyrexia	Milk stasis secondary to engorgement with bacteria entering the milk ducts via cracked nipples (usually *Staphylococcus aureus*)
Breast abscess	2–3 weeks postnatal	Brawny oedema of overlying skin with fluctuating swelling	Poorly treated mastitis
Genital tract			
Endometritis	Variable	Very unwell, high temperatures (approx. 38°C) tachycardia, bulky tender uterus ± purulent vaginal discharge	Repeated vaginal examinations in labour (> 4) after rupture of membranes Prolonged rupture of membranes Chorioamnionitis Caesarean section Episiotomies and tears Retained products of conception
Infected episiotomy/tear	3–4 days postnatal	Very tender stitch line, often breaking down with oedema, haematoma and discharge	Poor surgical technique Poor perineal hygiene
Wound infection (post LSCS)	4–7 days postnatal	Tense, tender, erythematous stitch line, occasional abscess formation	Rectus sheath haematoma Poor surgical technique Staphylococcal carrier

Respiratory and urinary tract infections and thromboembolism may all produce pyrexias and would represent differential diagnoses (see p. 42).

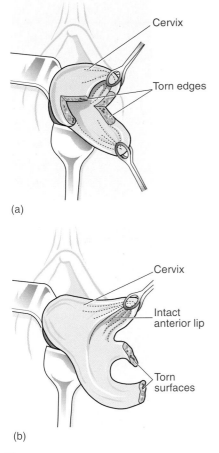

(a)

(b)

Fig. 1 Cervical tears. (a) Lateral.
(b) 'Bucket handle'.

(intravenous heparinization is rarely used) until symptoms are resolved. Initial treatment is followed by carefully monitored warfarin treatment for 3–4 months.

Musculoskeletal problems
Divarication of the recti can occur antenatally due to the enlarging uterus and effects of raised progesterone levels. It is painless but unsightly. Treatment is based on improving the tone of the abdominal muscles by exercise.

Pregnant pelvic arthropathy (see p. 77) may persist postnatally. Treatment involves bed rest, non-steroidal anti-inflammatory analgesia and a support girdle. A zimmer frame may be necessary. The condition is self-limiting and should improve within the first week postnatally. Severe cases may continue for several months.

Bladder and bowel problems
Urinary retention or voiding difficulties may occur postnatally secondary to painful episiotomies or use of epidurals in labour. Decompression by an indwelling catheter for 24–48 hours and careful observation of bladder function once the catheter has been removed is usually all that is required.

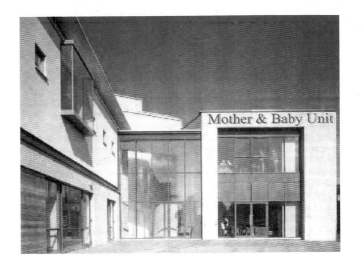

Fig. 2 Mother and baby unit.

Incontinence can also occur in the immediate postnatal period but usually improves after a course of pelvic floor exercises. Pudendal nerve latency conduction studies have shown delayed conduction up to 6 weeks postnatally but most have returned to normal when the test is repeated at 6 months and 1 year. In a small proportion of women, permanent pelvic floor weakness may occur which deteriorates over subsequent pregnancies.

Haemorrhoids are a common problem after childbirth, exacerbated by bearing down during the second stage of labour. Local application of lidocaine (lignocaine) gel or anusol cream may help, together with bulking agents to soften the motions. Occasionally, thrombosed piles will occur but these usually regress after 5–6 days.

Puerperal affective disorders
There are a range of presentations from transient tearfulness to the frankly psychotic. Puerperal depression and psychosis are often not detected as early as they should be.

The 'blues' classically present on the fourth or fifth day after delivery and may be preceded by 24 hours of euphoria and elation. Support from health care professionals and family should be adequate and it will resolve spontaneously.

Postpartum depression usually presents within the first 2 weeks, often with low mood, inappropriately poor sleep, lack of pleasure in motherhood, undue anxiety about the baby and feelings of unworthiness with restlessness and agitation. It is often associated with a prior history of depression or with traumatic delivery, e.g. caesarean section.

Antidepressants, either tricyclic or serotonin re-uptake inhibitors, are commonly used. Progesterone has been suggested but without good evidence. Oestrogen has been shown to be effective therapy, as it is in premenstrual and perimenopausal affective disorders. Specialist psychiatric help should be obtained early if necessary. Management is preferred in a dedicated mother and baby unit (Fig. 2). Compulsory admission to hospital under sections of the Mental Health Act is rarely required.

Puerperal psychosis is rare (1 in 800 deliveries) and resembles manic depressive psychosis. It first presents at 3–7 days and the peak incidence is at 2 weeks. Auditory and visual hallucinations are common features and a prior history is not uncommon. Lithium prophylaxis in subsequent pregnancies may be effective. Urgent specialist psychiatric involvement is necessary as there is a real risk of suicide and infanticide. Psychotherapy, neuroleptics and electroconvulsive therapy may be indicated.

The abnormal puerperium

- Secondary haemorrhage presents after the first 24 hours postpartum; the most common cause is retained products of conception.
- Venous thromboembolism is still a leading cause of death, and diagnosis can be difficult.
- Breast engorgement can cause a transient pyrexia in the first 2–3 days postpartum.
- Breast feeding may continue on the contralateral side if a breast abscess develops.
- Puerperal depression presents within the first 2 weeks; it may be severe and is frequently unrecognized and hence neglected.

Alternative approaches to delivery

Looking at the history of childbirth through time the commonest position adopted is the upright or ambulant position. This prompted work in the 1980s to study the effect of change in posture on uterine activity, blood loss during labour and pregnancy outcomes. There was much popular pressure for a change in the routine practice found in hospitals in the western world of pregnant patients lying in bed during labour and delivery.

Figures 1–4 show a variety of birthing positions that may be adopted. There is little good evidence that posture during labour or delivery has a major effect on the outcome for mother or baby.

Water birth

There have been many trends in delivery type. The Leboyer delivery in a darkened room is supposed to allow a more calm experience for the mother and to be less traumatic for the baby at delivery. The French obstetrician Michel Odent advocated delivery upright and had many supporters. He was the first person to present data on delivery into water (Fig. 5).

The perceived advantages and disadvantages (Table 1) to mother and neonate have not been subjected to rigorous study but are presumed from physiological principles.

Birthing cushion (Fig. 6), chair and stool

All these have been used in an attempt to achieve a more upright position for the mother. Work assessing blood loss shows a rather higher loss at delivery in mothers who use the birthing chair, with a higher incidence of low haemoglobin and an increased need for blood transfusion. This is likely to be due to perineal trauma exacerbated by obstructed venous return.

The fetus benefits from a maternal upright position with less abnormal fetal heart rate patterns seen and a higher arterial pH noted in studies comparing upright versus recumbent posture for the second stage of labour. The lateral position seems to have similar benefits for the fetus. Mothers may also prefer to adopt an upright position for the second stage of labour and sometimes report less pain.

In situations when fetal monitoring would be considered necessary, this can be more difficult unless telemetry

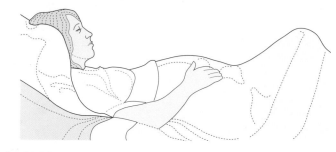

Fig. 1 **Supine birthing position.** Overall reduction in uterine activity, supine hypotension and resultant fetal hypoxia.

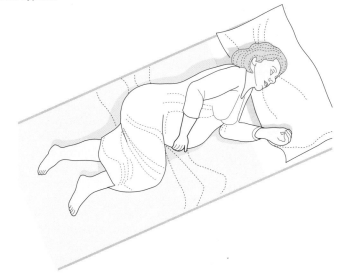

Fig. 2 **Side birthing position.** Contractions of less frequency but greater intensity.

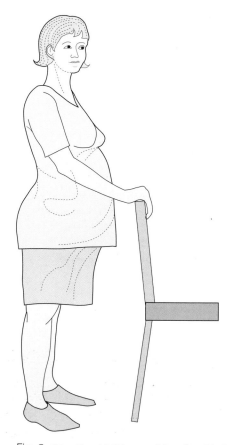

Fig. 3 **Standing birthing position.** Possible increased pressure on the cervix, increasing the dilating effect.

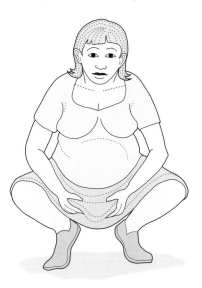

Fig. 4 **Squatting birthing position.** The 28% increase in pelvic outlet may have benefits for second stage but greater blood loss is noted if delivery is from an upright position.

is available. Continuous electronic fetal monitoring allows limited maternal mobility but the mother may not find this acceptable. Intermittent auscultation allows sampling of the fetal heart rate for only 7% of the time, although it should be remembered

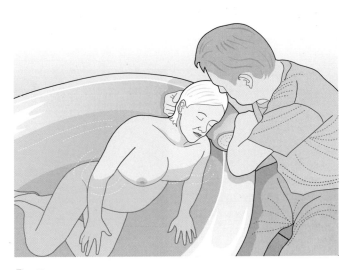

Fig. 5 **Water bath.**

Table 1 **Advantages and disadvantages of water birth**	
Advantages	**Disadvantages**
To the mother	**To the mother**
Pain relief from the warm water	Vasodilatation with circulatory redistribution, especially to the skin
Relaxation with the water buoyancy	Fatigue due to decreased muscle tone
	Fluid loss due to perspiration in the warm water
	Increased hydrostatic pressure against which to deliver
	Possible increase in blood loss due to hyperaemia with warmth
	Difficult, physically, to get out if emergency arises (and disappointment)
To the neonate	**To the neonate**
Gentle exit from the uterus	Respiratory depression due to warmth and immersion in water – the exposure to a cold stimulus before cessation of oxygen from the placenta is negated
	Infection hazard – maternal organisms in the water from vagina and bowel may be aspirated
	'Wet lungs' if the neonate aspirates and difficulty initiating breathing
	Adequate fetal monitoring is difficult

Maternal choice

Patients wish to be involved in decisions regarding their treatment. This extends to pregnancy when some women wish to choose an elective caesarean section as their mode of delivery. The mode of delivery may be determined by medical events either which necessitate caesarean section on a mechanical basis or where a better fetal outcome is associated with delivery by caesarean section. If there is no medical indication for caesarean section then the risks of vaginal delivery and caesarean section for both the mother and fetus need to be assessed.

The risk of vaginal delivery for the fetus is unpredictable but in those with growth restriction the risk is likely to be less with caesarean section. However, the fetus benefits from vaginal delivery by a lower incidence of respiratory distress syndrome compared to infants of the same gestation delivered by caesarean section.

From the maternal side, elective caesarean section increases the mortality risk for the mother by 50% compared with a vaginal delivery in a healthy woman but numerically this is still a very small risk. There is an increased need for blood transfusion after caesarean section and increased infection risk, though this has been reduced with the use of prophylactic antibiotics. If we could predict the women most likely to have a long and difficult labour, elective caesarean section would probably be safer and more acceptable for them than the trial of labour.

Some women may prefer an elective caesarean section with a small risk of mortality and serious morbidity as a way of avoiding the disabling complication of incontinence and the discomfort of labour. Many see the element of predictability and control of an elective procedure as important advantages with about 50% saying they would request another caesarean section in a future pregnancy. Looking at what is an ideal caesarean section rate perhaps the correct answer is the rate which gives maximum maternal satisfaction for the least risk.

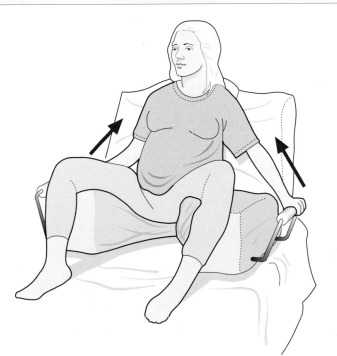

Fig. 6 **Birthing cushion.**

that fetal heart rate monitoring in low-risk women has not been proven to improve neonatal outcomes, but increases the chance of operative delivery.

Alternative approaches to delivery

■ Safe delivery of the mother and her baby are most important and how this is achieved may be varied to obtain maximum maternal satisfaction.

■ The upright posture for delivery may be more efficient at dilating the cervix.

■ Use of birthing chairs or cushions may be associated with greater perineal damage.

■ Maternal choice regarding mode of delivery should be carefully discussed and all risks and benefits considered.

Analgesia in labour

The level of pain experienced by women in labour varies considerably and is influenced by previous experience, antenatal preparation, length of labour and strength of contractions. The value of antenatal preparation is largely unproven, but as the experience of pain is related to the mental state of the patient a lot of time is invested in antenatal classes to ensure adequate knowledge of the process of labour, thereby decreasing the stress of the unknown. The various methods of analgesia are shown in Table 1.

Non-pharmacological approaches

There are many accepted non-pharmacological methods of relieving labour pain, some deriving from long usage and others from more recent understanding of pain and its perception.

Massage – including aromatherapy

Massage, especially to the lower back, may work by the same principle as TENS (transcutaneous electrical nerve stimulation – see below) with incoming nerve impulses modifying transmission along pain fibres. Massage may also relieve 'stress'. The 'stress' hormones (adrenaline (epinephrine) and noradrenaline (norepinephrine)) are thought to interfere with the coordination of uterine contractions and so relaxation techniques may enhance the progress of labour. Aromatherapy may work in a similar way and the use of lavender oil has found favour with some mothers.

Acupuncture and acupressure

Acupuncture may also have a role, with use of specific points to provide pain relief and possible additional electrical current to augment these analgesic effects. Acupressure, where the fingers are used to press over the

acupuncture point, may be easier to apply in labour and does not restrict mobility.

Mobilization

Labouring women, if left unrestricted, adopt a wide variety of positions. Sitting, standing and walking may all be used during labour. Patients with low back pain often adopt a forward-leaning position that may relieve pressure on the sacroiliac joint. Control of breathing patterns is widely taught in antenatal classes – this may work by diverting the mind away from the pain but is also a technique used to relieve stress.

Hydrotherapy

Many women already know the soothing effect of warm water on the uterine cramping pain experienced during menstruation. In the past, obstetric care tended to confine labouring women to bed but with greater freedom many select a warm bath or shower during the first stage of labour. The mode of action of any analgesic effect is unclear but over the centuries hydrotherapy has been used for many painful conditions so the expectation of a soothing effect may be its main method of action. In the mid-1950s abdominal decompression found a role in labouring women and immersion in water may be found to act similarly by relieving external pressures on the uterus and allowing it to assume a more rounded position.

Transcutaneous electrical nerve stimulation

TENS uses the gate theory of pain control and, by application of an electrical current to the nerves carrying the painful stimuli, transmission of pain is partially blocked. Skin surface electrodes (Fig. 1) are used to apply a low voltage electrical current, which is modified by the patient. These are usually applied across the lower back covering the T10–L1 nerve roots (the

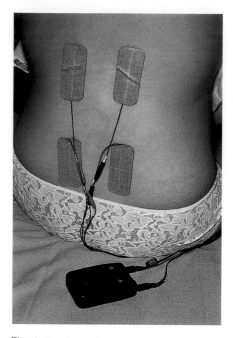

Fig. 1 **Uterine pain can be relieved by the application of TENS to the lower back.**

innervation of the uterus) early in the first stage for optimum effect. Although concern has been expressed about the use of TENS applied over the lower abdomen as the electrical activity may theoretically have an effect on the fetal heart, no adverse effect has been documented.

'Audioanalgesia'

Music can reduce stress and enhance other pain-relieving measures. White sound has been used during contractions and may block external stimuli. Studies of the use of so-called 'audioanalgesia' have suggested a trend towards decreased use of analgesic medication.

Pharmacological approaches

Inhalational analgesia

This has the benefits of long usage and thus familiarity whilst also being controlled by the patient in both timing and dose. Entonox is most commonly used and contains a 50 : 50 mix of oxygen and nitrous oxide. This would be expected to have a powerful analgesic effect as a 20% mixture is equipotent to 15 mg subcutaneous morphine, but in reality it is a poor analgesic. Despite its widespread use – it is the most widely used agent in labouring mothers in the UK – no major side effects have been noted. An excess may theoretically lead to

Table 1 **Methods of analgesia in labour**	
Non-pharmacological	**Pharmacological**
Massage – including aromatherapy	Inhalational analgesia
Acupuncture and acupressure	Opioid analgesia
Mobilization	Regional analgesia, including epidural and spinal
'Audioanalgesia'	Pudendal nerve block
Hydrotherapy	
TENS	

demyelination and megaloblastic anaemia but these effects have not been observed. Many women experience light-headedness and nausea, and hyperventilation may lead to hypocapnia and eventually tetany.

Narcotic analgesia

Pethidine was introduced in 1939 by the Germans who found it to be useful in treatment of war wounds. By 1950 it was generally accepted and in use by midwives for pain relief in labour. Unfortunately it is a rather poor analgesic, being associated with a 20% reduction in pain score, but it has powerful sedative effects on the mother at the expense of nausea and vomiting. In as many as half of all mothers there is no analgesic effect and, as it acts to delay gastric emptying, it should probably be used in labour in conjunction with ranitidine.

All opiates have a depressant effect on the neonate. This has led to attempts to develop other opioid analgesics with better pain-relieving properties and less respiratory depression in the neonate. Though neonatal respiratory depression is noted it need not limit the use of pethidine, as naloxone will rapidly reverse the respiratory effects, after delivery.

Diamorphine is used for its enhanced pain-relieving effect though some mothers experience considerable nausea and vomiting with it.

Epidural analgesia

This developed from the need for analgesia without neonatal respiratory depression and acts by affecting the spinal opioid receptors directly. Epidural analgesia has indications besides simple pain relief during labour:

- pregnancy-induced hypertension – to control hypertension which may worsen during labour (exclude coagulopathy)
- trial of scar – the epidural has not been found to mask the pain of a scar dehiscence but will give adequate analgesia
- preterm labour – there may be positive advantages in these cases as epidural analgesia has been shown to be associated with a reduced neonatal mortality rate among low birthweight babies
- breech presentation – to ensure a controlled delivery, by preventing the urge to push prior to full cervical dilatation – a problem in the preterm breech
- multiple pregnancy – delivery may be complicated and the presence of an epidural allows intervention as necessary
- incoordinate uterine activity – pain relief in this situation is associated with improved uterine action.

Correct placement of the catheter in the epidural space is confirmed by loss of resistance as the catheter finds the space and the absence of cerebrospinal fluid running from the catheter end (Fig. 2). Confirmation of correct placement is vital before giving the full dose of local anaesthetic down the catheter or a 'total spinal' (i.e. a high block) may result, with rapidly rising numbness and dyspnoea which may require ventilation until the effect wears off.

Alternatively, the catheter may be located intravascularly and during the test dose the patient will note light-headedness and tingling in the lips and fingers. If further anaesthetic is given, convulsions and cardiac dysrhythmias may ensue, necessitating resuscitation.

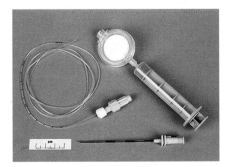

Fig. 2 **Equipment used for correct positioning of the epidural.**

Methods of administration

Intermittent doses. These are given as the mother requires, which may be at an approximate hourly rate. This may mean that pain relief is not complete and the midwife has to check with each dose whether the mother experiences any side effects. Patients are in bed and immobile.

Continuous infusion. This allows for more smooth pain relief and, if problems arise, a lower dose of the anaesthetic has been administered. Better analgesia, however, may be at the expense of an increased instrumental delivery rate or caesarean section and immobilization.

Spinal opioids. By acting on the spinal opioid receptors these enhance the analgesic effect of the epidural. They are short acting (2–4 hours) with a better analgesic effect in a more even distribution. They may be associated with pruritus.

Mobile epidural. These developed from the wish to overcome the immobility associated with standard epidural techniques. The pain-carrying nerve fibres are smaller than the motor nerve fibres and by giving appropriate anaesthetic mixes it may be possible to achieve blockage of only the smaller fibres.

Pudendal nerve block

This technique is used in the second stage of labour to obtain analgesia for an instrumental delivery. It blocks the pudendal nerve (S2,3,4) and is usually combined with perineal infiltration to allow episiotomy. The pudendal needle is guarded so that it can be advanced into the vagina in the region of the ischial spine. The needle is then advanced in turn and lidocaine (lignocaine) is introduced around the nerve. Once both sides are blocked the analgesia achieved should allow outlet forceps but would not give complete pain relief for a mid-cavity instrumental delivery.

Analgesia in labour

- Pain is an integral part of the process of labour.
- Adequate pain relief is associated with lower levels of maternal catecholamines ('stress' hormones which inhibit co-ordinated uterine activity).
- Non-pharmacological methods are widely used – both before the patient presents to hospital and in hospital.
- Entonox and opioids have a role but up to 30% may select an epidural.
- Excessive volumes of local anaesthetic can cause convulsions, hypertension and bradycardia.

The changing face of maternity care

In the last decade there has been a considerable change in attitude on how maternity care should be delivered. The driving force for change is specific to the individual countries' problems. In the UK it was felt that the current system was too rigid. Important conclusions were made:

- the policy of encouraging all women to give birth in hospitals cannot be justified on grounds of safety
- a more flexible system based on the community, not in the hospital, should be established
- midwives should have their own caseload
- the present imposition of a rigid pattern of frequent antenatal visits was not grounded on any good scientific basis.

Women should be placed at the centre of maternity services.

In less well-developed countries, the stimulus to change has been the high maternal morbidity and mortality. Almost 600 000 die each year from complications of pregnancy or delivery. In addition, approximately 40% of women suffer long-term complications.

Different approaches to care

United Kingdom

The old model of care in the UK sharply divided the community from the hospital midwife. Women were booked in hospital with a consultant as lead clinician and a routine number of antenatal visits. The general practitioner would see the woman at the surgery in between as part of shared antenatal care. In designated high-risk cases, hospital visits were more frequent.

The Cumberlege Report, 'Changing childbirth – how maternity services should be delivered', aims to provide a more flexible system of care in the UK (Table 1). Midwives are now rotated

Table 1 The Cumberlege Report: indicators of success
■ All women should be entitled to carry their own notes (Fig. 2)
■ Every woman should know one midwife who ensures continuity of her midwifery care – the named midwife
■ At least 30% of women should have the midwife as the lead professional
■ Every woman should know the lead professional who has a key role in the planning and provision of her care
■ At least 75% of women should know the person who cares for them during their delivery
■ Midwives should have direct access to some beds in all maternity units
■ At least 30% of women delivered in a maternity unit should be admitted under the management of the midwife
■ The total number of antenatal visits for women with uncomplicated pregnancies should be reviewed in the light of the available evidence and of Royal College of Obstetricians and Gynaecologists guidelines
■ All front-line ambulances should have a paramedic able to support the midwife who needs to transfer a woman to hospital in an emergency
■ All women should have access to information about the services available in their locality

Table 2 Different models of midwifery care
■ Caseload model
■ Midwifery teams
■ Midwife-only delivery units
■ Needs-based community services
■ Midwife-managed services in acute hospital trusts
■ Midwives based in primary care settings

through day and night shifts, through clinics into labour ward, and from labour ward into the community (Fig. 1). This ensures that all midwives are fairly exposed to high-pressure, high-risk areas of clinical practice. They are encouraged to keep up to date and have, through their professional development training, to be re-certified at regular intervals. They are encouraged to enhance their skills and take on new roles.

In some cases midwives employed in the community have become part of an integrated hospital/community team (Table 2). In other areas midwives have linked with general practitioners and have become the lead professional. Hospital-based midwifery staff may adopt their own caseload and follow women throughout the entire pregnancy, including postnatal visits in the community. Others may wish to develop their skills so that they form a core of labour ward midwives with specialist expertise providing intrapartum care for high-risk patients.

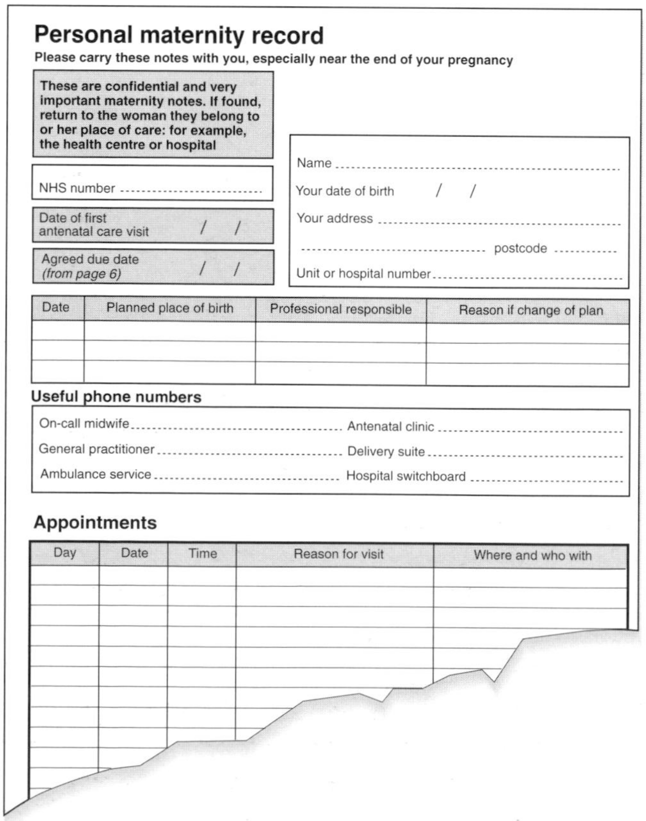

Personal maternity record

Please carry these notes with you, especially near the end of your pregnancy

These are confidential and very important maternity notes. If found, return to the woman they belong to or her place of care: for example, the health centre or hospital

NHS number ....

Date of first antenatal care visit   /   /

Agreed due date (from page 6)   /   /

Name ....
Your date of birth   /   /
Your address ....
.... postcode ....
Unit or hospital number...............................

Date	Planned place of birth	Professional responsible	Reason if change of plan

Useful phone numbers

On-call midwife............................... Antenatal clinic...............................
General practitioner .... Delivery suite...............................
Ambulance service .... Hospital switchboard...............................

Appointments

Day	Date	Time	Reason for visit	Where and who with

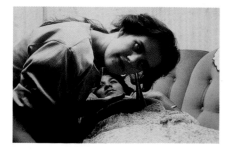

Fig. 1 **Antenatal home visit.**

Fig. 2 **Patient hand-held notes.**

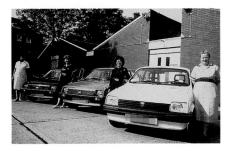

Fig. 3 **Community midwives.**

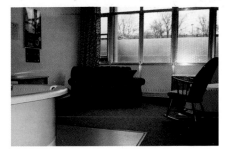

Fig. 4 **Low-risk midwife-run delivery unit.**

The rural setting

Maternity care must adapt to local circumstances. Where there are few hospital units, often many miles away, community midwives (Fig. 3) are highly experienced and will conduct a higher rate of home deliveries, having carefully screened out those pregnancies with potential problems.

General practitioner obstetricians still continue to offer intrapartum care in some cases, delivering their patient at home, in a low-risk community unit, or in the labour suite of the local hospital. Nevertheless, many general practitioners feel that they are involved in deliveries too infrequently to maintain their skills. This is particularly true of neonatal intubation, one area where midwives are expanding their skills and undergoing specific training.

Europe and the USA

The majority of the original work on independent midwifery practice was undertaken in the UK. Care models differ considerably between countries. Holland and especially New Zealand are excellent examples of the independent midwifery role. In the former there is a high rate of home confinements; in New Zealand the money truly follows the patient. The midwife is booked and can move freely from community to hospital sectors, allowing follow-through of care.

By contrast, the system in Spain is hierarchical. Only 50% of hospitals allow midwifery-led care, even in normal pregnancy and delivery. In the rest, care is doctor-led. There is a high epidural rate, women are delivered in theatre suites in the lithotomy position and all have episiotomies. Most women remain in hospital for 5 days after a normal delivery and there are very few community midwives. Postnatal care after discharge from hospital is provided by an obstetrician based at a community health clinic.

Midwives in the USA are still not allowed to practise in certain states. Where practice is permitted, they must be nurse-midwives and have a Master's degree. They are independent practitioners but frequently work within a group practice with obstetricians. Due to litigation, forceps deliveries are rarely practised and the elective caesarean section rate is high.

Developing countries

It was felt that improving the standard of women's education was as important as improving health services. The latter required improvement in community health services, better transportation for emergencies and improved referral centres. Women should not be left to give birth alone and birth attendants with training in at least basic hygiene should be present. This forms the basis of the WHO Safe Motherhood initiative.

Audit of progress has shown that the training of traditional birth attendants does not have an impact on maternal mortality unless it is combined with accessible units/hospitals where essential obstetric services are available. The attendants must learn to take an obstetric history to assess risk factors, to be alert to complications and to advise women to stay near basic obstetric centres.

Specific models of care

The Domino scheme

The same midwife who saw the patient in the community setting delivers the baby in the hospital maternity unit, and if all goes well mother and baby go home within 6 hours.

Midwifery-run delivery units

These units (Fig. 4) offer women a less technological, more relaxing environment located near the communities most likely to use them. The women must be assessed as being low risk. The unit must have a minimum of two midwives as core staff. No delivery should take place without two trained professionals being present.

Despite screening, statistics are fairly constant across a number of studies:

- 28–34% of women booked will develop antenatal complications, which will necessitate transfer to the local maternity unit
- 12–16% are transferred intrapartum, of whom approximately one-third will deliver by caesarean section
- 12% of breeches are not diagnosed until labour.

Consequently, the numbers of women delivering in these units are always less than the projected figures. Midwife-managed intrapartum care for low-risk women appears to result in more mobility and less intervention with no increase in neonatal morbidity.

Needs-based community services

Targeting women with needs means developing innovative ways of dealing with maternity care:

- extending services offered in local clinics, e.g. sickle cell support services
- ensuring that advocacy and language services are readily available
- providing culturally sensitive services
- allowing time for the complexity of the health needs
- ready access to housing and social benefit services.

Maternity care

- Severely high maternal mortality rates in underdeveloped countries have prompted the WHO Safe Motherhood initiative.
- The introduction of birth attendants trained in basic hygiene must be complemented by efficient access to obstetric units.
- In the UK the Cumberlege Report stressed the need for women-centred care.
- The woman should have a choice of carer and place of delivery and be offered continuity of care.
- The Domino scheme offers continuity of midwife and 6-hour discharge from hospital.
- The low-risk midwifery-run delivery unit offers an alternative venue for delivery.

Drug misuse and physical abuse

Drug misuse

The prevalence of drug misuse is on the increase, particularly in women of childbearing age. Serious problem misuse (especially i.v.) and poly-drug misuse are associated with socio-economic deprivation and an increase in obstetric complications including miscarriage, antepartum haemorrhage (APH), intrauterine growth restriction (IUGR), intrauterine death (IUD) and preterm labour. Care must usually be directed firmly towards social factors before any impact on obstetric problems can be achieved. Pregnancy may provide a window of opportunity to provide real help, often breaking a cycle of poor parenting leading in turn to further problems in the next generation.

The history should cover:

- type of drug(s) (see Table 2)
- street drugs, e.g. heroin, amfetamines
- pharmacological preparations (usually illicitly obtained), e.g. benzodiazepines, buprenorphine and analgesics, particularly DF118 and other codeine compounds
- prescribed preparations, usually methadone
- pattern of use, dose, route, frequency and method of financing supply
- available social support, the other children, partner, family, friends, social work involvement, clothing, food, shelter and transport
- impending legal problems
- risks of infection including HIV, hepatitis B/C counselling ± testing

- domestic violence – a common occurrence with all groups of pregnant women. All women should be asked about this (surprisingly, it is not any more common with socio-economic deprivation). Female drug misuse is often a consequence, rather than a cause, of violence.

There may be poor self-esteem following a lack of trusting relationships, loss of positive body image and concerns about their own abilities to be a parent.

Management

Social factors

Illegal drugs are expensive and addicts are often forced into theft (and therefore problems with the police and courts) or prostitution (with its risks of violence and sexually transmitted diseases including HIV). In addition, lifestyle may be erratic and pregnancy outcome is compounded by various additional nutritional and social factors. Attendance for antenatal care may often compete with more immediate problems (e.g. seeing the social worker, lawyer, or getting money/drugs, etc.) but if such care can be delivered locally with truly flexible access and be combined with confidentiality, non-judgmental consistency, access to social workers and legal aid, then fuller and more holistic care can be achieved.

Table 2 Drugs of misuse in pregnancy

Drug	Effect on fetus
Alcohol	There is no clear dose relationship. Fetal alcohol syndrome is rare (IUGR, microcephaly, craniofacial abnormalities and mental retardation). Consumption of even small amounts of alcohol has been associated with a reduction in birthweight and intellectual impairment
Amfetamines	No increased risk has been demonstrated
Benzodiazepines	'Floppy infant syndrome' may occur if high doses have been given within the 15 hours prior to delivery. Neonatal withdrawal occurs following prolonged use
Ecstasy	No increased risk has been demonstrated
Cannabis (hash, marihuana)	There have been no demonstrable teratogenic effects, but there is an association (?indirect) with IUGR
Opiates/opioids (e.g. heroin, methadone, DF118, buprenorphine)	There are associations with anovulation, IUGR, preterm labour, lower Apgar scores, and neonatal withdrawal difficulties
Cocaine and crack	Cocaine has been associated (rarely) with genitourinary, limb/body and brain abnormalities (probably because of vasoconstrictive vascular accidents)
Nicotine	There is an association with IUGR, preterm labour, perinatal death and delayed development. Tobacco use, if heavy, may lead to neonatal withdrawals
LSD	No increased risk has been demonstrated

Table 1 Therapeutic drugs in pregnancy

Class of Drug	Risk to fetus
General anaesthetics	Any risks are probably related to risks of hypoxia itself
Analgesics	Low-dose aspirin use OK, but analgesic doses may lead to impaired platelet function and an increased risk of haemorrhage. Indometacin causes impaired renal function. Paracetamol is thought to be safe
Antacids	Are thought to be safe. Cimetidine may have anti-androgenic effects
Antibiotics	Aminoglycosides carry a risk of fetal ototoxicity. Chloramphenicol is potentially harmful and the sulfa component of co-trimoxazole may displace bilirubin and cause kernicterus. Tetracyclines cause dental discolouration. Erythromycin, the penicillins, metronidazole and the cephalosporins are thought to be safe
Anticonvulsants	All carry risks of teratogenesis, though data are limited on the newer preparations (gabapentin, lamotrigine and vigabatrin)
Antidepressants	Lithium should be avoided if possible but, if used, monitor serum levels closely. The risks are probably low with SSRI and tricyclic antidepressants
Antihypertensives	Methyldopa and β-blockers probably safe. ACE inhibitors and diuretics should be avoided
Antihistamines	Chlorphenamine (chlorpheniramine) is thought to be safe in pregnancy. There is little experience with the newer preparations
Antimalarials	For prophylaxis, chloroquine is preferred. In treatment of malarial infection, benefits far outweigh the risks
Antipsychotic drugs	No consistent teratogenic effect has been demonstrated
Bronchodilators	All inhaled preparations, including inhaled steroids, are considered safe in pregnancy
Retinoids	High risk of fetal malformation sufficient to consider TOP
Steroids	No consistent teratogenic effects demonstrated in humans
Vaccines	There is a theoretical risk of teratogenic problems from vaccines but on principle, avoid

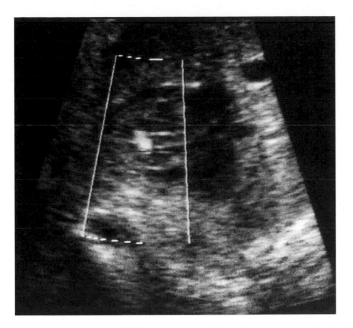

Fig. 1 **Ventricular septal defect (VSD) associated with anticonvulsants.** Note the Doppler flow across the interventricular septum.

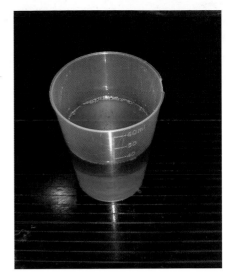

Fig. 2 **Those stabilized on methadone alone probably have a lower neonatal mortality than those still taking heroin.**

Transfer to methadone

Consideration should be given to transfer to methadone (slower metabolism therefore more stable levels and less prone to the risks of fetal distress and preterm labour associated with sudden withdrawals or fluctuations in serum opiate levels). Those stabilized on methadone alone probably have a lower neonatal mortality than those still taking heroin (Fig. 2). There may also be improved antenatal attendance.

Detoxification

There are theoretical fetal risks from very rapid detoxification but in practice the true fetal risks from even 'cold turkey' detoxification are relatively small. It has been suggested that the risks of detoxification (whether rapid or gradual) may be higher in the first and third trimesters, but practical experience does not bear this out. The goal should be to reduce drug use to a level compatible with stability (e.g. with methadone), not necessarily aiming for abstinence. It is more acceptable for the mother to top up with more of the same substance (e.g. smoking heroin) than adding additional preparations (especially if the addition is with benzodiazepines or codeine compounds). Patients should ideally be managed on an obstetric unit, or at least under the close supervision of an obstetrician.

Neonatal complications

There is an increased incidence of IUGR, meconium aspiration and sudden infant death syndrome (SIDS). Withdrawal is particularly associated with benzodiazepines, and is worse if they have been used in conjunction with other drugs. Severity is dose related and timing depends on the rate of drug metabolism, e.g. heroin and morphine are metabolized rapidly and signs develop within 1–2 days, whereas methadone is metabolized more slowly and signs occur between 5–7 days. Babies are classically hungry, but feed ineffectually. There is CNS hyperexcitability (increased reflexes and tremor), gastrointestinal dysfunction (finger sucking, regurgitation, diarrhoea) and respiratory distress. Treatment options include replacement (e.g. with methadone or oral morphine).

Physical Abuse

Violence against women can take the form of physical or sexual abuse. In some cultures, violence against women is accepted and societal norms blame the woman for the violence perpetrated against her. These attitudes may also occasionally be held by healthcare workers, sometimes resulting in an inadequate or inappropriate response to women who seek help. In most other cultures, where violence against women is not considered to be acceptable, there is still a surprisingly large problem.

Around 1 in 4 women worldwide will suffer from domestic violence at some stage in their lives and, in many countries, statistics suggest that more than 50% of women who are murdered are killed by their intimate partner. In other studies, more than 95% of women who are raped already know their assailant. In addition, violence against women can have both short- and long-term health consequences including sexually transmitted infections, and unwanted pregnancies which may in turn lead to unsafe abortions. Women living with partners may not feel able to make their own decisions about contraceptive issues, or even about staying or leaving the relationship, and the psychological implications are immense: victims of rape are 11 times more likely to experience clinical depression and are at greater risk of drug- and alcohol-related problems, and suicide.

It is important to bear in mind these issues when meeting patients. A history of such problems is unlikely to be volunteered spontaneously and considerable tact may be required to explore these areas.

Drug misuse and physical abuse

- All drugs are potential teratogens.
- Drug misuse is common.
- Serious problem misuse may be the end-point of multiple social factors which must be addressed.

Common problems in pregnancy

Most women feel well during pregnancy.

Minor ailments do occur (Table 1) and symptomatic relief is occasionally possible. Women should be encouraged to discuss these ailments with their health care professionals as apparently minor symptoms may be symptomatic of more serious conditions, e.g. pruritus of acute cholestasis of pregnancy, or leg oedema of venous thromboembolism.

Varicosities

Varicose veins may appear for the first time in pregnancy and if already present they are likely to deteriorate. Varicosities may appear in the legs, vulva, abdominal wall and also as haemorrhoids. They are probably due to impaired venous return secondary to back pressure from the expanding gravid uterus. Varicose leg veins can ache and itch intensely, especially by the end of the day. They are best helped by elastic support tights or stockings. These may be uncomfortable, particularly in high temperatures and the only alternative may be to sit down whenever possible with the legs elevated.

Anterior abdominal wall varicosities are unsightly but do not cause any real problem. They always disappear after delivery. Very rarely a patient may present with a large groin swelling in the third trimester which is a varicocele of the round ligament of the uterus. This may be misdiagnosed as an inguinal hernia.

Vulval varicosities can be very dramatic in their appearance and can cause considerable discomfort. There is unfortunately no useful intervention other than suggesting that the area is kept dry and well aerated to minimize itching. Controlled delivery minimizes bleeding. Vulval varicosities almost always disappear postnatally.

Haemorrhoids can be very troublesome and may cause considerable discomfort and even bleeding. Steps must be taken to avoid constipation. Local anaesthetic–steroid combination creams may be applied during the day and suppositories used for night-time relief. Application of ice packs may be helpful. A thrombosed pile may need incision and clot evacuation under local anaesthetic but a local anaesthesic gel may provide some relief.

Constipation

Constipation is common in pregnancy because of reduced bowel motility and increased colonic absorption of water. It can be helped by increasing dietary fibre and fluid intake. Regular exercise may also help. Bulking agents and a stool softener may be prescribed. Some iron preparations exacerbate constipation.

Dyspepsia

Dyspepsia ('heartburn') is due to a combination of reduced peristalsis and relaxation of the gastric smooth muscle sphincter predisposing to regurgitation of gastric content into the lower oesophagus. Women should be encouraged to eat regular small meals and may find relief from sleeping propped up at night rather than lying flat. Antacids may prove helpful.

Nausea and vomiting

Nausea and vomiting are very common in early pregnancy. The symptoms usually diminish by the 16th week but can occasionally continue throughout pregnancy. Vomiting is usually worse in the early morning but it can occur throughout the day. The majority of women respond to simple measures such as eating frequent, small, non-fatty, dry, high-calorie meals and avoiding spicy food.

Severe excessive vomiting in the first trimester is termed hyperemesis gravidarum. Hospital admission is necessary if there is dehydration, persistent ketosis, profound weight loss or impaired renal or liver function. Rehydration by intravenous infusion is the most effective therapy.

The majority of cases of hyperemesis are idiopathic but urinary tract infections, multiple and molar pregnancies should be excluded. If the symptoms do not settle with rehydration and dietary adjustment, medication should be considered (an antiemetic or phenothiazine preparation).

Recurrent or prolonged hyperemesis may indicate an underlying psychosocial problem (see p. 44). Unresolved hyperemesis may lead to Wernicke's encephalopathy, due to vitamin B1 deficiency, or pontine myelinosis, due to sodium depletion.

Urinary symptoms

Most women develop increased frequency of micturition in early pregnancy, related to vascular engorgement and the progestogenic effects on urinary tract smooth muscle. Frequency usually diminishes by the 12th week but recurs towards the end of pregnancy due to the pressure of the presenting part on the bladder.

Urinary tract infections are more common in pregnancy. Asymptomatic bacteriuria may be found in 10% of pregnant women and of these, 20–30% will develop ascending pyelonephritis if left untreated. Regular urine analysis is important throughout the antenatal period and asymptomatic bacteriuria should be treated with antibiotics.

Table 1	Common complaints in pregnancy
Complaint	**Cause and management**
Vomiting	Common in first trimester especially, but often persists through pregnancy
Constipation	Due to progesterone effect relaxing the gut – managed with mild laxatives and increased fluid intake
Heartburn	Also thought to be due to progesterone relaxation of the gut – managed with antacids
Backache	Due to the effect of relaxin on ligaments causing abnormal strain with lumbar lordosis – managed with physiotherapy
Abdominal pain	Often due to stretching of the round ligament – analgesia if severe
Fainting	Due to postural hypotension – advise standing up slowly and possibly the use of support stockings
Varicose veins Haemorrhoids	Due to pressure on the venous side by the gravid uterus – managed with support stockings for veins, anaesthetic steroid creams for haemorrhoids
Carpal tunnel syndrome	Due to oedema causing pressure on the median nerve as it passes under the flexor retinaculum – managed with splints and postural drainage of the hands, possibly surgery – usually postdelivery

Vaginal discharge

Normal physiological vaginal discharge increases during pregnancy. If the discharge is clear and non-offensive the woman can be reassured. Fungal infections (particularly candidiasis), *Trichomonas vaginalis* and bacterial vaginosis are more common in pregnancy. The treatment can be difficult as clinical response tends to be slower and recurrences are common. Topical antifungal treatment with imidazoles or nystatin can be given as either a vaginal pessary or a cream.

Bacterial vaginosis carries a five- to seven-fold increased risk for late miscarriage and preterm labour. Treatment is with metronidazole or, preferable in pregnancy, topical clindamycin.

Backache

The commonest cause of backpain is the increasing lumbar lordosis adopted to prevent toppling forward (Fig. 1). Pregnancy can exacerbate pre-existing back problems, particularly disc prolapse. A support corset may be helpful and flat shoes should be advised. It is advisable to keep the woman as mobile as possible in labour. Consideration should be given to route of delivery and types of analgesia.

Pregnant pelvic arthropathy

Normally the pubic symphysis and sacroiliac joints are fixed (Fig. 2). In pregnancy the ligaments become more lax and the symphysis pubis will separate to some extent. This is desirable as it allows the antero-posterior diameter available for the fetus to increase but in extreme situations the hemi-pelvices can be widely separated causing severe pain. Walking can be very difficult. Milder cases can be treated with analgesia and the use of a tight girdle or orthopaedic belt. In severe cases a zimmer frame and bed rest may be necessary. The condition is self-limiting and slowly improves after delivery.

Carpal tunnel syndrome

Pain may radiate up the forearm. The patient is often woken in the early hours of the morning with severe pain. Her fingers feel stiff and useless and she will often drop things.

Explanation and reassurance are usually all that are needed. In more severe cases the woman is advised to sleep with her hand slightly elevated and may be fitted with night splints to

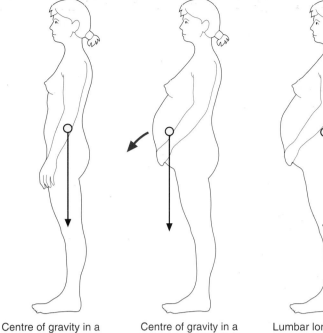

Centre of gravity in a non-pregnant woman goes through the knees

Centre of gravity in a pregnant woman is in front of the knees – uncorrected she will fall over

Lumbar lordosis corrects situation – centre of gravity now re-established

Fig. 1 **Lumbar lordosis in response to the body's change in centre of gravity.**

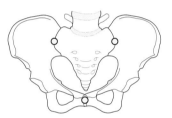

In the non-pregnant state the pubic symphysis and sacro-iliac joints are rigid and fixed

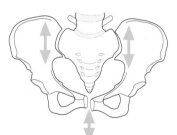

In the pregnant state ligaments are lax, sheering movements of one hemi-pelvis against the sacrum or the opposite half can occur

Fig. 2 **The pubic symphysis in pregnancy.**

dorsiflex the wrist and reduce the pressure on the median nerve.

Other aches and pains

Pain in one or both groins is common. Aetiology is unproven but has been attributed to stretching of the round ligaments of the uterus. Analgesia and reassurance are appropriate.

Tenderness over the intercostal muscles can occur in late pregnancy due to the enlarged uterus elevating the diaphragm and the subsequent alteration in the shape of the rib cage.

Abdominal pain

There are many causes of abdominal pain in pregnancy ranging from something as mild as viral gastroenteritis to acute fatty liver of pregnancy, a condition that is more severe.

Acute appendicitis is often higher and more lateral in pregnancy and localizing signs are reduced. Red degeneration of a fibroid can cause severe pain. Maximum tenderness is over the fibroid but, if right-sided, can be confused with appendicitis.

Common problems in pregnancy

- Most women feel well during pregnancy.
- A number of minor ailments do occur, for which symptomatic relief may be possible.
- Women should be encouraged to discuss minor symptoms with their health care professionals as they might indicate a more serious condition.

Vital statistics

Maternal mortality

Audit of clinical practice is important in the identification of areas for improvement. The maternal mortality report run in the UK is a good example of clinical audit. Data have been collected since 1952 and reports are produced every 3 years. The last four reports cover the UK as a whole. The maternal mortality rate has officially been approximately 10 per 100 000 maternities for the past decade but may have been ~ 12/100 000 due to missed cases. The major causes of death are thromboembolism, pregnancy-induced hypertension, amniotic fluid embolism, early pregnancy complications and sepsis. In the 1994–1996 report these accounted for 85% of direct maternal deaths (Fig. 1).

The problem globally is much bigger with the annual pregnancy-related death rate at 585 000. The estimated maternal mortality in each continent (Fig. 2) shows wide variation:

- Africa 640/100 000
- Asia 420/100 000
- Latin America 270/100 000
- all developed countries 30/100 000
- Northern and Middle Europe ~ 10/100 000.

Figure 3 shows the main causes of maternal mortality worldwide. An assessment of the causes of maternal mortality makes it clear what steps are needed to reduce the mortality:

- oxytocic drugs and blood transfusion
- antibiotics
- anticonvulsants
- partograms
- contraception.

Comparison of the causes of maternal death between the worldwide list and that in the the UK report reveals that haemorrhage and obstructed labour do not feature as major causes of death in the UK. Looking back to the figures from the 1950s (Fig. 4), it is obvious that deaths from haemorrhage have reduced considerably due to the use of oxytocic drugs and blood transfusion and an awareness of this as a major problem. Tackling the issues posed by maternal mortality globally will require health care provision and effort directed specifically at the areas of major concern. The loss of a mother in childbirth leaves the child orphaned and the other children of the family needing care. Money directed at the problem of maternal mortality would thus be well spent and might reduce money needed in other areas.

In 1987 the 'Safe Motherhood' initiative called for a halving of maternal deaths within a decade. Fifteen actions were suggested, mostly multifaceted approaches to problems identified as contributing to the high maternal mortality in developing countries. Ten years later the reduction had not been achieved, with obstetric disorders still a leading cause of death. The relationship between discrimination against women and maternal morbidity and mortality has been questioned, since countries that do discriminate do not have the highest mortality rates.

Promotion of family planning to reduce maternal mortality is questionable when most maternal deaths occur after wanted pregnancies. Antenatal care is also unlikely to offer a major reduction in deaths when most complications of childbirth arise in low-risk pregnancies. Training of traditional birth attendants has not shown any effect on the mortality rate. Further advances will necessitate the provision of accessible care for obstetric emergencies by trained staff with appropriate facilities – a costly necessity.

Perinatal mortality

This is another indicator of the level of health care provision and annual figures are available for many countries (Fig. 5). In the UK the perinatal mortality rate (PMR) is defined as the number of stillbirths plus the deaths in the first week of life per thousand births (live and still), but variations in other countries include stillbirths from 20 weeks and loss for

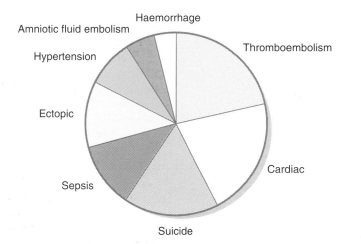

Fig. 1 **Causes of maternal deaths in the UK 1997–1999.**

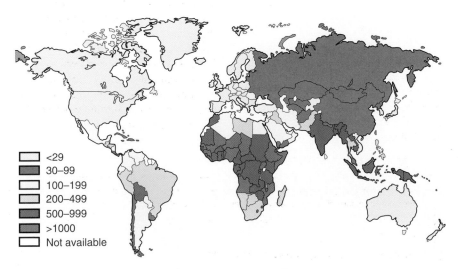

	<29
	30–99
	100–199
	200–499
	500–999
	>1000
	Not available

Fig. 2 **Worldwide maternal mortality rates in 1990.**

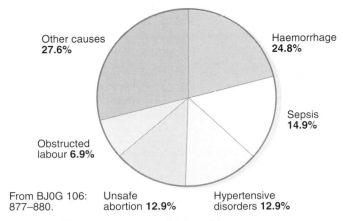

Fig. 3 **Main causes of maternal deaths worldwide 1990.**

From BJOG 106: 877–880.

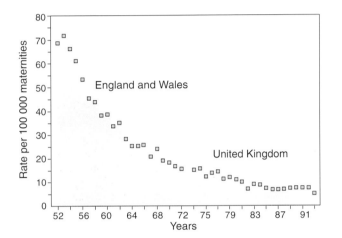

Fig. 4 **UK maternal mortality rates 1952–1993.**

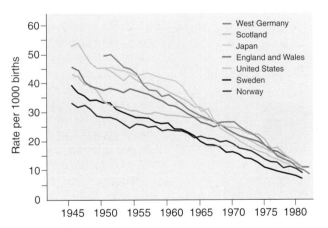

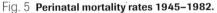

Fig. 5 **Perinatal mortality rates 1945–1982.**

be active in the neonatal period. Factors associated with a raised perinatal mortality rate are:

- preterm delivery – 5% of babies deliver preterm but this accounts for 70% of perinatal deaths
- congenital abnormality
- small for dates
- social class – IV and V rates are higher than I and II
- teenage and older (> 40) mothers
- multiple pregnancy.

Prevention of preterm delivery could dramatically affect the PMR but depends on a better understanding of the process of initiation of labour. Current methods of arresting labour are ineffective and the diagnosis of preterm labour is also difficult (see p. 18). Congenital abnormality can sometimes be detected antenatally with ultrasound but little can then be done if the condition is known to be lethal. Prevention of the small for dates infant is again dependent on a better understanding of what controls fetal growth.

The factors active in social class discrepancy are known but require great social change and are unlikely to undergo dramatic improvement without major funding. The incidence of multiple pregnancy is increased in association with assisted conception techniques. Management includes feto-reduction to try to improve the chances of the surviving infant(s) but this raises ethical questions.

The role of audit

The major 'vital statistics' are maternal and perinatal mortality but, in developed countries, every hospital audits their obstetric figures looking at the mode of delivery, complications including deaths, how analgesia is given, and many other factors. This allows changes to be made in the delivery of care to ensure best outcomes. In less-developed countries basic levels of health care need to be introduced but audit infrastructure must be added to ensure that the local community can continue to detect where to direct their efforts for maximum benefit.

up to the first month of life. Differing definitions hamper direct comparisons between countries. A dramatic reduction in the rates noted in the UK over the past five decades is seen with 62.5/1000 in 1930–1935 compared to 12–14/1000 during the 1990s.

Again, audit of the figures, by making an assessment of the factors leading to death in each case, can contribute to changes in clinical practice that may lower the PMR.

Numerous attempts have been made to classify the causes of perinatal death to improve preventive measures. The Wigglesworth classification centred on

division into the time when preventive action might be taken – congenital abnormality and antepartum stillbirths have factors present in the antenatal period, asphyxia occurs during labour and delivery, whilst immaturity must

Vital statistics

- Maternal mortality has reduced in developed countries due to use of blood transfusion, medication to control haemorrhage and antibiotics for sepsis.
- Worldwide reduction in maternal mortality requires adequate health care provision – a costly necessity.
- Perinatal mortality rate is not uniform in its definition.
- Prematurity accounts for 70% of perinatal mortality in western countries.

The newborn

Separation of the placenta means the infant must adapt to extrauterine life. The physiological changes are many and need to be immediate as the infant takes over oxygen exchange for itself. Acidosis in the baby and a fall in paO_2 will result in failure to breathe – if of short duration there is usually a rapid response to resuscitation; a slower response suggests anoxia of longer duration. The newborn has large glycogen stores in the brain, liver and heart which enable survival up to 20 minutes with no oxygen. Thus resuscitation is always worthwhile.

Adequate equipment (Fig. 1) in the delivery room to deal with infant resuscitation includes:

- radiant warmer
- resuscitation bags and masks
- endotracheal tubes
- laryngoscope
- stethoscope
- oxygen source and suction
- naloxone.

All high-risk deliveries should be attended by someone skilled in infant resuscitation but it is recognized that in approximately half of all cases

Table 1 **Assessing the Apgar score**			
	Score		
	0	**1**	**2**
Colour	Pale	Blue	Pink
Respiration	Nil	Gasps	Regular
Heart rate	Absent	< 100	> 100
Tone	Flaccid	Present	Good
Response to stimulation	Nil	Present	Brisk

requiring resuscitation the need for resuscitation is not recognized prior to delivery. It thus is necessary for those involved in delivery to be able to initiate and continue infant resuscitation.

Assessment of the infant immediately after delivery is usually by means of the Apgar score (Table 1).

Resuscitation

Most infants require only removal of mucus from the oropharynx, drying and handing to the mother or, preferably, delivery straight onto the mother's abdomen. The ambient temperature in a delivery room is high to ensure that there is minimal cooling of the infant. Neonates maintain their body temperature in a cool environment at the metabolic cost of increased energy expenditure. Ways to

Table 2 **Advantages and disadvantages of nasopharyngeal suction**	
Advantages	**Disadvantages**
Improved air exchange	Bradycardia
Decreased likelihood of aspiration of secretions	Laryngospasm and pulmonary artery vasospasm
Less acquisition of pathogens from amniotic fluid or birth canal	

reduce the postnatal fall in temperature include:

- skin-to-skin contact with the mother
- drying the neonate
- radiant heater
- covering the head ± body with insulated material.

The indications for resuscitation are:

- heart rate < 100 bpm after birth – needs oxygen administration
- generalized cyanosis – needs oxygen administration
- inadequate chest excursion and poor breath sounds – bag and mask
- poor response to bag and mask ventilation – needs endotracheal intubation.

Proper ventilation of the infant is the single most important aspect of neonatal resuscitation. Observation of the chest distending with squeezing the bag indicates a proper head position and a clear airway. A rise in the heart rate is an indicator of the success of the resuscitation. Enough pressure on the bag to produce chest excursion is needed as well as an adequate inspired oxygen concentration.

Nasopharyngeal suction has benefits and risks (Table 2) but in a delivery complicated by passage of meconium, nasopharyngeal suction before delivery of the chest may be useful. The use of routine intubation in these cases is accompanied by the risks of hypoxia, bradycardia and increase in intracranial pressure.

Medication

Routine administration of certain medications to the neonate is standard practice. Vitamin K is offered routinely for all newborns to prevent development of haemorrhagic disease of the newborn (HDN) which has an incidence of 0.25–0.5%. The vitamin K level in breast milk is considerably lower than in infant formula feeds and puts the infant at risk of serious

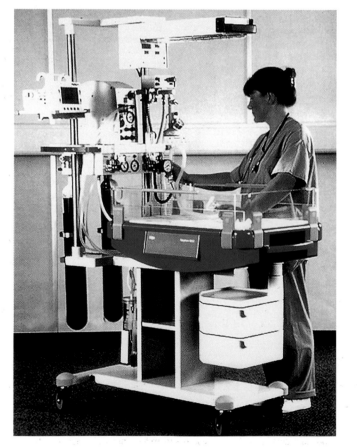

Fig. 1 **Resuscitation equipment.**

bleeding (e.g. intracranial haemorrhage). Thus a policy of giving routine vitamin K to all breast-fed babies seems reasonable. Recent work comparing vitamin K administered orally with that given intramuscularly (i.m.) suggested an increased rate of childhood cancers in the group who had had i.m. administration of the vitamin. This has subsequently been disproved but some parents may refuse i.m. vitamin K and thus oral doses should be administered.

Surfactant

The immediate postnatal administration of surfactant can reduce morbidity and mortality of infants born before pulmonary maturation has occurred. Administration decreases the likelihood of moderate or severe respiratory distress syndrome (RDS), pneumothorax and periventricular haemorrhage.

Naloxone

This narcotic antagonist may be given to a neonate who is slow to establish spontaneous respiration when this is thought to be due to narcotic analgesics given to the mother before delivery (see p. 71). As the role of endogenous opiates in the newborn is unclear, but thought to be important, it seems wise to restrict the use of naloxone to infants exposed in utero to narcotic analgesia who also require active resuscitation after delivery.

Examination

The examination of the newborn is important to establish normality and to allow the parents to discuss any worries they may have. In order to avoid missing anything it is important to have a clear plan which is followed during every examination (Table 3). The examination plan should be:

- colour
- tone
- head – fontanelles, eyes, ears, palate
- chest – heart, breasts
- abdomen – cord insertion, femoral pulses
- genitalia and anus
- hips
- feet
- neurological responses.

The skin colour will vary with the maturity of the infant, that of the premature baby being more red as the skin is more translucent. Peripheral cyanosis is common at delivery. Tone can readily be assessed by ventral

Examine	Signs to look for	Comment
Colour	Cyanosis, plethora	Examine in good light – cyanosis is easy to miss
Cranium	Large/small head circumference	Hydrocephalus/microcephaly
Face	Dysmorphism	Try to identify the specific abnormal features
Eyes	Red reflex	Use ophthalmoscope – red reflex is absent if cataract or retinal disease is present
Mouth	Cleft palate	Use little finger to feel the hard and soft palate
Neck	Sternomastoid 'tumour'	Head movement may be restricted
Pulses	Brachials and femorals	Absent femorals represent possibility of coarctation
Hands	Shape, creases, nails, accessory digits	
Chest	Shape, resp. rate, recession, auscultation	Heart murmurs
Abdomen	Palpable masses	Liver is always palpable and kidneys usually
Umbilicus	Discharge, flare around	Suspect cord sepsis
Genitalia	Boys: testes / Girls: labia and vaginal orifice	Cremasteric reflex may be very brisk
Anus	Check that it is present	Recto-vaginal fistula may allow the passage of meconium without an anus
Hips	Subluxation/dislocation	
Feet	Mobility	
Reflexes	Moro, grasp, sucking	
Tone	Posture during sleep / Posture on ventral suspension	

Table 3 **Checklist for neonatal examination**

After Field, D. et al. 1997. Paediatrics An Illustrated Colour Text, Churchill Livingstone, Edinburgh, p. 5.

suspension of the infant; normal tone is associated with arching of the back. This also allows examination of the spine. Normal head circumference in a term infant is 33–37 cm. The fontanelles should not be bulging or abnormally sunken. The eyes need to be opened to look for cataract and to elicit a red reflex. Examination of the ears and palate for normality and observation of the scalp for signs of trauma from a scalp electrode or ventouse delivery complete the examination of the head.

Listening to the heart sounds may elicit a heart murmur but this is common in the newborn so further assessment at a later stage is appropriate (Fig. 2). The breasts may appear engorged from the effect of stimulation due to the mother's hormone levels or vaginal discharge may be noted. Inspection of the cord insertion will exclude exomphalos. The femoral pulses are palpated to rule out coarctation of the aorta and the abdomen palpated for presence of masses. The genitalia should be inspected, looking especially for hypospadias or bifid scrotum which may call into doubt the allocated gender of the infant. Patency of the

anus should be confirmed, then the hips examined to exclude congenital dislocation (Fig. 3). The feet are inspected and their mobility assessed. Finally, neurological response may be checked by tapping the cot and a Moro reflex is usual – startle response.

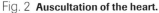
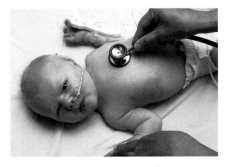

Fig. 2 **Auscultation of the heart.**

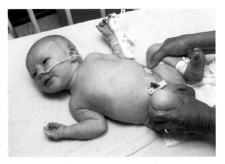

Fig. 3 **Examination of the hips of a newborn infant.**

The newborn

- The need for resuscitation of the neonate is not predictable in approximately half of all cases.
- Keeping the newborn warm after delivery improves survival, especially in the preterm infant.
- Adequate ventilation should move the infant's chest.
- The first routine examination of the newborn is to exclude identifiable abnormality.

Problems in the first week of life

A newborn baby must adjust very rapidly to extrauterine life. While cardiorespiratory changes are the most obvious, the thermoregulatory, gastrointestinal, and immune systems are also important.

Prematurity-related problems

Survival increases from approximately 5% at 23 weeks' gestation to 95% at 31 weeks. About 25% of these survivors have some disability – including cerebral palsy, short stature, respiratory difficulties, visual impairment and poor school performance. It is now well established that corticosteroids given to mothers who subsequently deliver preterm are effective in reducing the incidence of respiratory distress syndrome (RDS) by around 50% as well as the risk of periventricular haemorrhage. Whether or not to start resuscitation with an extremely premature (less than 24 weeks) infant can sometimes be a difficult question and, ideally, discussions with the prospective parents should have taken place beforehand in order to be able to gauge their wishes.

Heat loss

Preterm infants have a very high surface area to mass ratio and thin skin, and are extremely liable to hypothermia. This means that it is vitally important to deliver in a warm room with heated towels for drying and some method to keep the baby warm during resuscitation, e.g. an overhead heater. Survival is directly related to the temperature of the infant on admission to the neonatal intensive care unit.

Respiratory support

At 23–24 weeks the respiratory epithelial cells start to differentiate into type 1 (gas exchange) and type 2 (surfactant production) pneumocytes. Surfactant levels are very low but can be increased by antenatal glucocorticoids. Support at this gestation is often by mechanical ventilation, either conventional ventilation or with high-frequency oscillation. Exogenous surfactant can be administered via the endotracheal tube. A large proportion of extremely preterm infants develops chronic lung disease of prematurity (or bronchopulmonary dysplasia) with continuing requirements for respiratory support.

Central nervous system

The subependymal germinal matrix lies close to the ventricular space and contains the developing brain cells of the premature infant. Bleeding from this very vascular area may occur with preterm delivery, giving rise to periventricular haemorrhage, cortical damage and hydrocephalus. The extremely preterm infant is also prone to ischaemic brain injury from low arterial oxygen tension, hypotension, or reduced cerebral blood flow. Subsequent periventricular cysts (periventricular leukomalacia) may form and long-term neurological sequelae are common.

The gastrointestinal system

Structurally, the bowel is well developed by the end of the second trimester but there is functional immaturity. Motility and food absorption are both reduced and early enteral feeding may not be tolerated. Parenteral nutrition may be needed during the early days and weeks, but this may lead to numerous problems, from both the need to maintain adequate venous access and the tolerability of the amino acid and lipid solutions.

Sepsis

Sepsis is a major problem in the extremely preterm baby. Relative immunocompromise and frequent use of multiple, broad-spectrum antibiotics render the tiny baby prone to infection, particularly with sub-pathogenic bacteria, such as *Staphylococcus epidermidis*, and fungi, especially *Candida albicans*.

Retinopathy of prematurity

Early vasoconstrictive damage to the retina occurs as a result of high oxygen pressure and other factors. The incidence of this is reduced by using ventilation at lower pO_2 levels. Secondary proliferation of weaker, potentially haemorrhagic, vessels occurs. Regular ophthalmological review is vital as early laser or cryotherapy treatment of these new vessels can preserve vision.

Cerebral damage

Although commoner in premature infants, cerebral damage may be found in term infants and may lead to mental impairment and/or cerebral palsy (a non-progressive motor deficit). Probably less than 10% of cerebral palsy is related to intrapartum problems, the remainder being caused by some often unidentifiable antenatal event.

Apgar scores are a reflection of the level of resuscitation required but are a very poor predictor of long-term outcome. Neonatal encephalopathy grading is a better guide to long-term outlook:

- Grade 1: hyper-alert, reduced tone, jittery, dilated pupils: usually resolves in 24 hours
- Grade 2: lethargic, weak suck, fits: 15–27% chance of severe sequelae
- Grade 3: flaccid, no suck, no Moro reflex, prolonged fits: nearly 100% chance of severe sequelae.

The prognosis is generally good if the baby does not develop grade 3 encephalopathy, or if grade 2 encephalopathy lasts < 5 days. Further clinical evaluation may be available from electroencephalography (EEG; incidence of death or handicap low if normal or near normal), computed tomography (CT; good prognosis if normal or only patchy hypodensities) or ultrasound scan (USS; incidence of impairment correlates with intracerebral hypoechogenic areas of necrosis). Intracerebral haemorrhage is also an adverse sign (Fig. 1).

Congenital anomalies

The incidence of major anomalies in a low-risk unscreened population is

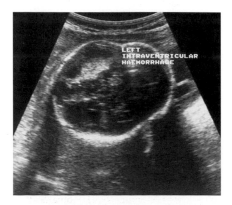

Fig. 1 **Spontaneous intracerebral bleed following preterm delivery, occluding the lateral ventricle on the right.**

around 2%. The incidence is higher in those exposed to potential teratogens (e.g. anticonvulsants) and with certain medical conditions (e.g. pre-existing diabetes). The incidence of live births with severe anomalies is lower in those countries which have some form of screening programme and which allow the option of pregnancy termination.

Trauma

Caput succedaneum (oedema caused by pressure over the presenting part) is common and resolves within a few days. Cephalhaematoma (a subperiosteal haematoma) is much rarer, but is significantly commoner following vacuum extraction compared to forceps delivery. Subgaleal (subaponeurotic) haemorrhage occurs when there is bleeding into the potential space beneath the aponeurosis of the scalp – this is a large space and can accommodate a large volume of blood. Although rare, it can be life-threatening (Fig. 2). Forceps are more likely to cause craniofacial injuries, including bruising, linear skull fractures and facial nerve palsies.

Fractured clavicle and brachial plexus injuries are more common following shoulder dystocia. Erb's palsy is a C5–6 lesion in which the arm is held loosely at the baby's side with internal rotation of the shoulder and extension of the elbow (waiter's tip). In Klumpke's palsy there is impairment of C8–T1. There is often very good, if not necessarily complete, recovery of palsies within the first few months, and physiotherapy may be offered to prevent contractures. A fractured clavicle will heal spontaneously. Other orthopaedic injuries, including spinal injury, are rare.

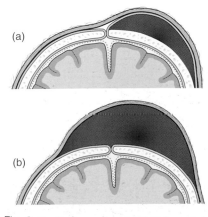

Fig. 2 **Cephalhaematoma (a) and subgaleal (subaponeurotic) haematoma (b)**. Note that the potential subgaleal space can hold a much greater volume of blood than the smaller potential space under the periosteum.

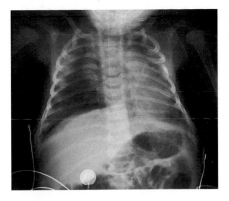

Fig. 3 **Respiratory distress syndrome following emergency caesarean section.** The mother had diabetes which predisposes to respiratory distress syndrome. Note the ground glass appearance of the lungs.

Scalp damage may occur from a scalp ECG clip. Rarely, this can be severe and associated with secondary infection and long-term scarring.

Respiratory distress syndrome (RDS)

This is caused by a deficiency of surfactant and is commoner in preterm infants (0.1% at term vs 30% at 28 weeks). Surfactant, a complex lipoprotein consisting largely of phosphatidyl choline, is synthesized by type II pneumocytes within the alveoli and is important in allowing the alveolus to expand. Hypoxia, acidosis and hypothermia reduce surfactant production; antenatal steroids increase production and thereby reduce the incidence of RDS. Clinically, there is tachypnoea, grunting and intercostal recession commencing within the first 4 hours of life, and the chest X-ray demonstrates a generalized reticulogranular appearance referred to as like 'ground glass' (Fig. 3). Treatment is with oxygen ± supportive ventilation and often includes giving artificial surfactant through an endotracheal tube.

Meconium aspiration syndrome

In utero, meconium is usually retained within the colon. Although it may be passed through the sphincter under physiological conditions, particularly

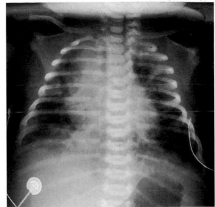

Fig. 4 **Meconium aspiration syndrome.** Note the widespread patchy shadowing in both lungs.

after 40 weeks, it also has an association with fetal hypoxic stress. Meconium is irritant to the neonatal lungs and may lead to a pneumonitis, the meconium aspiration syndrome (Fig. 4). Clinical features range from mild neonatal tachypnoea to severe respiratory compromise. Treatment is with oxygen, mechanical ventilation and, if very severe, extracorporeal membrane oxygenation.

Seizures

The immature central nervous system is particularly prone to seizure activity, which is the brain's common response to differing pathologies. They may be a feature of neonatal encephalopathy (see above) but can also occur with focal cerebral infarction, cerebral malformation, meningitis (e.g. with group B β-haemolytic streptococci), hypoglycaemia, hypocalcaemia, maternal drug misuse and inborn errors of metabolism.

The commonest timing of onset is between 12 and 48 hours. The resulting membrane damage of seizure activity releases excitotoxic substances such as glutamate, which can trigger further seizure activity, and investigation and treatment are therefore of great importance. In particular, prolonged fits can cause cerebral hypoxia and cerebral oedema.

Problems in the first week of life

- Prematurity is the commonest cause of fetal morbidity and mortality.
- Probably less than 10% of cerebral palsy is related to intrapartum problems.
- Neonatal encephalopathy is a better guide to long-term prognosis than Apgar scores.
- Respiratory distress syndrome responds well to surfactant administration.

Bereavement in obstetrics and gynaecology

There are few harder things to come to terms with than the loss of one's child at whatever gestation.

Obstetric bereavement shares many of the features of the mourning process common to other situations:

- accept the reality of the loss
- experience the pain of grief
- adjust to the environment
- reinvest in the future.

During the first two phases there are issues of blame, disbelief, acute sadness and an attempt to search for explanations. These negative emotions gradually disappear with time but levels of distress are higher in situations where there is a lack of opportunity to discuss the events surrounding the loss. Older women and particularly those who have had previous children are less likely to suffer depression.

It is a mistake to rush into another pregnancy to try to compensate for the loss of a previous child. The grieving process must be worked through in its entirety before the couple is emotionally and psychologically strong enough to undergo another pregnancy, and to be able to deliver the quality of bonding and parental care required by the new offspring.

Miscarriage

There is a risk that the miscarriage, or early pregnancy loss, is managed only medically with a failure to recognize that for the woman concerned, and her partner, the grief of a lost early pregnancy can be as real as the loss of a child at term.

The most appropriate care is in an early pregnancy assessment unit or gynaecological ward. The woman should be admitted and treated promptly, as long waits may enhance anxiety.

Parents should be given the opportunity to discuss the miscarriage with a counsellor and a suitable clinic appointment should be made. Information leaflets and contact numbers should be available. They may well wish to involve a religious adviser even at this early gestation. A Certificate of Non-Viability will need to be completed together with a Notification of Miscarriage Form in England. This is sent to the antenatal clinic to avoid the distress of an

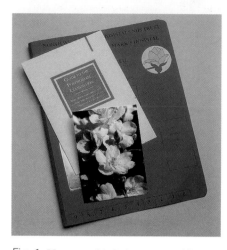

Fig. 1 **Memento birth document with name, photo, footprint, etc.**

inappropriate appointment being sent. Under 16 weeks the fetus will be sent to the histopathology laboratory. Anti-D should be prescribed, as appropriate, to the mother.

In the case of late second trimester miscarriages, i.e. those > 16 weeks' gestation but under 24 weeks' gestation, the mother might wish to see the baby or have a photograph (Fig. 1). This is not always the case and her wishes must be respected. It is also important to discover whether she would like a visit from the hospital chaplain or a blessing or naming ceremony for her baby. Gathering of mementoes, etc. may also be important.

When a histopathology examination is required in these later miscarriages a

consent form should be signed. If the family do not agree to a full autopsy, a limited autopsy may be performed. In order to help parents make a decision, the government leaflet entitled 'Guide to the Post Mortem Examination' is available in many different languages. A Certificate of Non-Viability and a clinical information form must be completed.

Intrauterine death (IUD) and stillbirth (SB)

When an IUD is diagnosed the parents should be offered a choice of admission for induction immediately or they may prefer to wait a day or two which will allow them the chance to mourn in private. It is important to keep the number of midwifery and medical staff to a minimum to provide continuity of care.

If the evidence suggests that the baby has been dead for longer than 4 weeks a clotting screen is performed, as disseminated intravascular coagulation can occasionally intervene. Induction of labour during the third trimester is usually undertaken with prostaglandin pessaries or gel similar to a normal induction (see p. 48). Cervagem or extra-amniotic prostaglandin infusions can be used for second trimester IUDs. Many units now use mifepristone.

Most hospitals will have an active policy for the management of

Table 1 Checklist for intrauterine deaths, stillbirths and neonatal deaths
■ Mother and partner informed of death
■ Parents offered a chance to see and hold their baby
■ Other relatives requesting to see and hold baby with parents' consent
■ Photograph of baby, two for parents if wanted, one for notes
■ Memento offered, cot card, name band, footprints, locks of hair
■ Religious leader notified if wished after discussion with parents
■ Father given the opportunity to stay in hospital overnight
■ Postmortem discussed and requested, consent obtained or refused
■ Clinical information and postmortem form completed
■ Certificate of Non-Viability (< 24 weeks) or stillbirth certificate completed
■ Consultant obstetrician informed
■ Consultant paediatrician informed, if neonatal death
■ General practitioner informed
■ Patients Officer informed regarding funeral/disposal arrangements and birth registration
■ Parents given appropriate booklets/access to videos
■ Any special clothing or items to be placed on baby
■ Discussion on suppression of lactation
■ Family planning advice offered
■ Community midwife informed
■ Health visitor informed
■ Medical social worker informed if necessary
■ Appointment made for appropriate consultant's clinic
■ Parent education classes cancelled
■ Antenatal appointments cancelled
■ Counselling offered

Table 2	**Investigations for late fetal loss (intrauterine deaths and stillbirths)**

Maternal
- TORCH screen (check if done antenatally)
- Kleihauer test
- Lupus anticoagulant test
- Anticardiolipin antibodies
- Syphilis serology screening (check if done antenatally)
- Random blood glucose
- Thyroid function tests
- Rhesus antibody titre (if mother is Rhesus negative)
- High vaginal swab and endocervical swab
- Parvovirus titre (if ultrasound evidence of hydrops)
- Genetic studies (if indicated)

Placental
- Histology
- Swab – or culture

Fetal
- Photograph ± X-ray
- Postmortem
- Chromosomal analysis

bereavement. A checklist (Table 1) is usually helpful for the midwifery and medical staff involved, who are often distressed themselves. Some mothers regard lactation as a tangible link with the child they have lost, others are horrified by the prospect and bromocriptine should be prescribed immediately to prevent lactation occurring. Advice regarding family planning should be offered as soon as is practicable.

Often no satisfactory cause is found but every attempt should be made to do so (Table 2) and consent to a postmortem may be useful. If this is refused, clinical photographs and X-rays of the baby can be substituted. Genetic counselling may be indicated when fetal malformation is detected. Chromosomal analysis on fetal material is required. Most areas run a regional congenital malformation register and a Notice of Malformation should be completed and sent appropriately. For gestations less than 24 weeks a stillbirth certificate will need to be completed.

Neonatal deaths

It is important to recognize the family as a unit and to involve the parents as much as possible in the care of the terminal baby. They should be encouraged to handle their child and to have photographs of the baby whilst alive. In the case of twins, photographs of the two babies together should be encouraged. Children need to grieve for their lost brother or sister and this process is facilitated if the sibling is actively involved from the beginning.

Parents must never be left to feel that they alone made the decision to withdraw intensive care support. Adequate provision of privacy for the parents to be with their child to allow them to say goodbye is very important.

Arrangements for cremation and burial

There is no legal requirement to bury or cremate a baby lost before 24 weeks' gestation, as it was non-viable, and no legal requirement for the parents to be involved. However, staff should be aware that parents could, if they so wish, take the body away for burial. Usually, they prefer the hospital to make appropriate arrangements. A book of remembrance is often kept in the hospital chapel and parents can enter their baby's name and an inscription of their choice regardless of the gestation. Often chapels will hold an annual service of remembrance for all bereaved parents.

In the case of stillbirths and neonatal deaths, there is a legal requirement for the baby to have a proper burial or cremation. Parents may make their own private arrangements or the hospital can arrange for a funeral. It is vitally important that carers are sensitive to the religious and cultural needs of the bereaved relatives. For members of the Jewish and Muslim faiths it is important that burial takes place, if possible, within 24 hours of the baby's death.

Continued support

Most units now have a special bereavement suite where the couple can stay overnight. Usually the mother is inclined to go home as quickly as possible after delivery. Counselling should be continued and often a counsellor will offer to call on the mother at home. She will not have worked through all the bereavement issues prior to leaving hospital. There are a number of useful support agencies (Table 3) and there are excellent information leaflets, books and videos available (Fig. 2).

Table 3	**Chromosome analysis**

Indications
- Malformed or dysmorphic baby
- Any baby significantly small for dates
- Significantly macerated stillbirths (although may be difficult to obtain karyotype)

Specimens required
- Blood sample by cardiac puncture (2–3 ml of blood in lithium heparin suitable from fresh stillbirth and early neonatal deaths)
- Skin biopsy (a full thickness 0.5 cm ellipse from the lateral border of the thigh if blood sample difficult)
- Placental tissue (sample of membranes and placental disc sent dry in a universal container if maceration is significant)

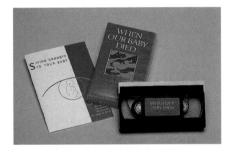

Fig. 2 **'When our Baby Died' video and 'Grieving after the Death of your Baby' accompanying booklet.**

Table 4	**Useful support agencies**

- The Miscarriage Association
- Stillbirth and Neonatal Death Society (SANDS) (Jewish Baby Bereavement Support affiliated to SANDS)
- ARC (Antenatal Results and Choices) (formerly Support Around Termination for Abnormality, SATFA)
- The Compassionate Friends
- The Asian Bereavement Counselling Service
- Bereaved Parents Mutual Support Group
- The Twins and Multiple Births Association (TAMBA)
- The Bereavement Clinic, The Lone Twin Network from the Multiple Birth Foundation
- Foundation for Study of Infant Deaths (FSID) (Cot Death Helpline 24-h service – run by FSID)
- Child Death Helpline (run by Great Ormond Street & Alderhey Children's Hospitals)
- The Child Bereavement Trust

Bereavement

- Couples often feel the loss of a miscarriage as greatly as the loss of a baby.
- A longstanding intrauterine death may result in clotting abnormalities and a clotting screen should be taken on admission.
- Even if a postmortem is refused, clinical photographs and X-rays of the baby can be useful to identify the cause of death.
- The parents should be encouraged to be involved in nursing a terminal baby.
- It is unwise to rush into another pregnancy to compensate for a lost child due to the greater risk of depression.

Gynaecological assessment of the patient

Basic facts about the patient are usually summarized in one sentence which is given at the start and at the end of the gynaecological history presentation, e.g. Mrs Jones is a 33-year-old with pelvic pain and deep dyspareunia. History starts with the patient's presenting complaint first, going thoroughly into such gynaecological details as may be relevant to this particular complaint. Whatever the complaint, it is usual to ascertain the length of the history, salient features such as the nature of pain, location and character of a mass, the timing of bleeding history, or length of infertility suffered. Thus many aspects of the gynaecological history may be covered under presenting complaint and further history discussed later.

Patient history

Menstrual history

Table 1 outlines the history to be elicited. The volume of blood lost during menstruation is usually gauged from the amount and type of sanitary protection, passage of clots and flooding bedding and outer clothes.

Vaginal discharge

Physiological discharge is usually off-white and varies in amount. This increases in mid-cycle when the nature also changes to that of a stringy mucous discharge at the time of ovulation. Questions concerning the volume of the discharge, the timing of it in relation to the menstrual cycle, the association with pruritus, and the odour of the discharge all need to be determined.

Non-physiological discharge may be associated with intense itching as caused by candidiasis, where the discharge would be thick and curdy. A frothy yellow/ green offensive discharge might be caused by *Trichomonas* (see also p. 104).

Pain

Dysmenorrhoea may be primary, noted at the onset of menses and relieved with the establishment of flow, or secondary, associated with other pelvic pathology (see p. 123). Dyspareunia is pain during sexual intercourse which may be experienced superficially (at the introitus – look for obvious cause) or be deep (within the pelvis – may be associated with endometriosis or pelvic infection). Pelvic pain may be colicky, due to uterine contractions, or more constant. Unilateral pain may suggest an adnexal problem but infection causes bilateral pain. Vulval pain is intense with an initial herpetic attack – look for blisters. Vulval itching in postmenopausal women is found with vulval dystrophies.

Sexual intercourse

A detailed history is appropriate in infertility patients (see p. 130).

Urinary symptoms

The five classic symptoms to enquire about are stress incontinence, urgency, urge incontinence, frequency, and nocturia. A detailed urinary history is appropriate if the presenting complaint is vaginal prolapse. Usually described as a lump in the vulval region, it may be associated with pain or difficulty in defecation. In some gynaecological complaints, subspecialty interest clinics have been developed where a specialised history is used – for example, infertility (see p. 130) and urogynaecology.

Table 1 **History taking**	
Term used	**Meaning**
Menarche	Age at first menstruation
Amenorrhoea	Absence of menses
Last menstrual period (LMP)	Date of first day of bleeding
K7–10/28–32	Menstrual cycle length 28 to 32 days with 7 to 10 days of bleeding
Menopause	The last menstruation
Oligomenorrhoea	Infrequent menstruation
Menorrhagia	Regular heavy menses
Intermenstrual bleeding (IMB)	Bleeding between menses
Postcoital bleeding (PCB)	Bleeding after intercouse
Dysmenorrhoea	Pain associated with menstruation

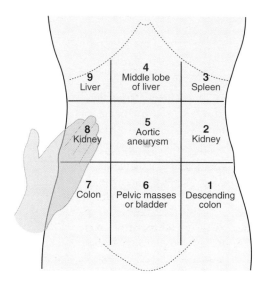

Fig. 1 **Abdominal palpation of the nine areas of the abdomen.**

Past obstetric history

The level of detail required of the past obstetric history is dependent on the presenting gynaecological complaint with more details being relevant in someone complaining of recurrent spontaneous miscarriage or infertility than in an older patient complaining of urinary symptoms or prolapse. It is usual to record the number of pregnancies and the outcome, the mode of delivery, the weight of the heaviest baby and any complicating factors during or after the pregnancies.

Contraception

Record the method used, satisfaction with the method, any side effects or problem with compliance and the consistency of use of the method.

Examination

After performing a general systems examination, breast and abdominal examination precede the pelvic examination.

Breast examination

Using the palmar aspect of the fingers palpate for lumps in the breast using circular motions starting over the nipple and radiating outwards, finishing with palpation of the axilla and supraclavicular areas for palpable lymph nodes.

Abdominal palpation

The nine areas of the abdomen are examined (Fig. 1), the right-handed examiner usually commencing in the left iliac

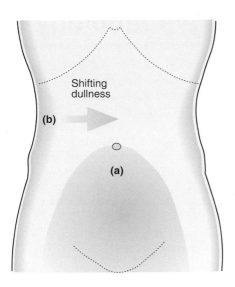

(a) Dullness on percussion over fibroid uterus or ovarian cyst is noted centrally

(b) Dullness on percussion in the flanks is associated with ascites. The level rises as the patient rolls to her side

Fig. 2 **Difference in percussion findings in cysts/fibroids versus ascites.**

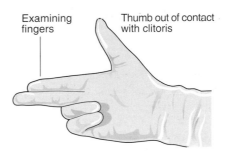

Fig. 3 **The correct hand position for vaginal examination.**

fossa progressing up towards the spleen, down the centre of the abdomen towards the pelvis and up the right hand side of the abdomen towards the liver. Superficial then deep palpation should be performed looking for tenderness and masses, which would be delineated by percussion.

If tenderness is present, peritonism is then sought – rebound tenderness or guarding. A check of hernial orifices and femoral pulses is usual and, if ascites is thought to be present, it may be confirmed with a check for 'shifting dullness' (Fig. 2). Auscultation for bowel sounds completes the examination.

Pelvic mass
A mass arising from the pelvis will have free lateral and upper borders but the examining hand cannot go between the symphysis pubis and the lower border of the mass. To determine whether the mass is cystic or solid use a ballotting motion. The regularity, mobility, firmness and tenderness are assessed during the examination. Percussion would elicit central dullness over a large ovarian cyst or fibroid uterus; the dullness would be in the flanks if the abdominal distension is due to ascites.

Pelvic examination
The vulva should be inspected for any lesions as indicated from the history. The oestrogen status of the patient can be determined by the degree of atrophy of tissues and white plaques (leucoplakia) or ulcerated areas may be noted. The labia are parted with the left hand, inspecting the introitus and noting any discharge and its nature. The external urethral meatus is observed, noting urethral caruncles and urinary incontinence.

Speculum examination
A Cuscoe bivalve speculum is introduced with a 90 degree rotation allowing comfortable insertion. The use of lubricants (KY jelly) does not disturb the taking of a smear. Once the speculum has achieved its full length the jaws are fully opened revealing the cervix, noting any discharge or ectopy (see p. 134). A cervical smear and bacteriological swabs are obtained as required.

A Sims' speculum examination may be performed in cases of prolapse or urinary symptomatology (see p. 154).

Bimanual examination
Two fingers of the gloved hand are introduced into the vagina keeping the thumb off-centre to avoid the clitoris, which is tender to palpation (Fig. 3). With the fingers in the posterior fornix, the other hand is placed on the lower abdomen and is the working hand during the pelvic examination. Downward pressure on the abdominal hand should trap the uterus between the hands allowing a determination of its size, regularity, whether it is ante- or retroverted, presence of tenderness and the mobility of the uterus.

Palpation for the adnexa commences at the anterior superior iliac spine on each side, using downward pressure to trap the adnexa between the examining hands. The ovary is small and firm, often described as like a walnut, thus only in slim patients would you expect to feel a normal ovary, but masses should be palpable and tenderness would be elicited.

To check for cervical excitation pain the cervix is pushed to the right, checking right adnexa and then to the left, checking for pain on the left side. This puts the parametrium on each side in turn on the stretch and, indirectly, tests for inflammation and tissue oedema.

Gynaecological assessment

- The patient history starts with the presenting complaint.

- This is followed by menstrual history, any pains, urinary symptoms and details of past history.

- Physical examination begins with general systems, followed by breasts, abdomen then pelvis.

Developmental and paediatric gynaecology

(See also Puberty and its abnormalities, p. 90, and Amenorrhoea, p. 112.)

Those with an XY karyotype require both testosterone and Müllerian inhibiting factor to develop normal genitalia. Testosterone masculinizes the otherwise female external genitalia and stimulates the mesonephric (Wolffian) system to develop. Müllerian inhibitory factor inhibits the paramesonephric (Müllerian) system, which would otherwise form female internal genitalia.

Intersex disorders and ambiguous genitalia

Early multidisciplinary sub-specialist involvement is essential, particularly surrounding the issues of genital surgery and gender assignment. There will be initial parental shock at the diagnosis, with possible subsequent depression, doubts of gender, concerns over fertility, issues of sexuality, cultural problems and a sense of worthlessness. Peer support from those with similar problems is essential.

XY but look female (male pseudohermaphroditism)

Testicular feminization syndrome (androgen insensitivity). This is an X-linked recessive disorder caused by an absence of androgen receptors. Although testosterone is present, it has no effect on the external genitalia and these individuals appear female. Müllerian inhibitory factor is also still present and therefore no internal genitalia form. Presentation is usually after puberty with amenorrhoea in the presence of normal breast development, scanty pubic and axillary hair, a blind-ending vagina, absent uterus and female habitus and psychosexual orientation. Gonadectomy is essential because of the risk of malignant change.

There is a small phallus, some degree of hypospadias, a bifid scrotum and a blind vaginal pouch.

5α-reductase deficiency. There is an autosomal recessive target enzyme defect of 5α-reductase. This converts testosterone to dihydrotestosterone in the target organs, and is therefore important for male development. At puberty considerable, but still incomplete, virilization occurs with male body habitus, psychosexual orientation and gender conversion.

XX but look male (female pseudohermaphroditism)

Congenital adrenal hyperplasia (accounts for 70% of ambiguous genitalia). There is an autosomal recessive

enzyme defect in aldosterone synthesis that leads to reduced aldosterone production and an increase in androgen production (Fig. 1a). In the commonest form, 21-hydroxylase deficiency, two-thirds have a salt-losing crisis, often within the first 4 weeks of life, which requires long-term mineralocorticoid replacement. There are ambiguous genitalia (Fig. 1b), which may require a reduction clitoroplasty, although there is an argument against such a procedure as future sexual sensation may be reduced.

Exogenous administration of androgens (e.g. danazol). This may lead to virilization of a female fetus.

Other rare abnormalities

These may occur with XO, XX or XY chimerism. True hermaphroditism (i.e. the presence of male and female gonadal tissue) is also rare.

Abnormal genital tract development

Vagina (Fig. 2)
There may be horizontal septae, vertical septae or the vagina may be absent.

Horizontal septae. There may be cryptomenorrhoea with cyclical pain and a haematocolpos. If obstruction is caused simply by the hymen (blood looks blue behind it) then a cruciate incision, usually under anaesthesia, is all that is required. If the septum looks pink rather than blue the situation is potentially more serious and should be referred to a specialist surgeon. If the septum is in the low or midportion of the vagina, total excision and resuturing is necessary. If the septum is high, a combined abdominal and vaginal approach may be required. Pregnancy rates are excellent with low septae, but only around 25% for those higher in the vagina.

Vertical septae. These may be associated with abnormal uterine development. Although presentation may be with dyspareunia or infertility, they may occasionally present in advanced labour. They can be surgically removed.

Vaginal atresia. This is associated with an absent, or only a rudimentary, uterus and is known as the Rokitansky syndrome. Presentation is at puberty with amenorrhoea (or

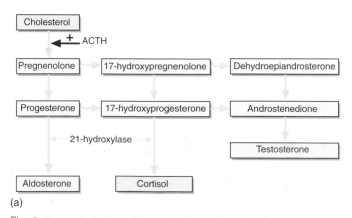

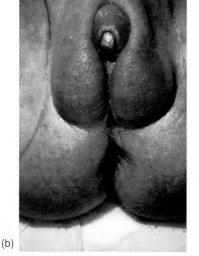

Fig. 1 **Congenital adrenal hyperplasia. (a)** Steroid pathway.
(b) Ambiguous genitalia.

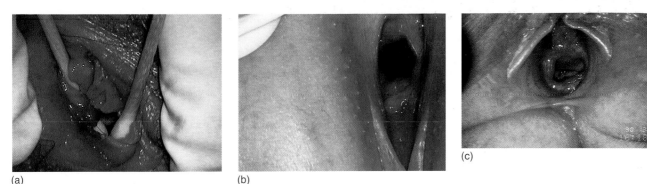

(a)   (b)

(c)

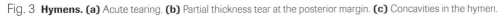

Fig. 3 **Hymens. (a)** Acute tearing. **(b)** Partial thickness tear at the posterior margin. **(c)** Concavities in the hymen.

cryptomenorrhoea) in the presence of normal secondary sexual characteristics. It is possible to create a vagina with regular use of vaginal dilators, or by one of a variety of surgical techniques. Surrogacy is an option for childbearing.

Uterus (Fig. 2)

Abnormal uterine shapes are usually asymptomatic but may present with primary infertility, recurrent pregnancy loss or menstrual dysfunction (oligomenorrhoea, dysmenorrhoea or menorrhagia). In pregnancy, there may be miscarriage (p. 92), preterm labour or an abnormal fetal lie.

Unicornuate uterus. With this there is a higher miscarriage rate and risk of preterm labour.

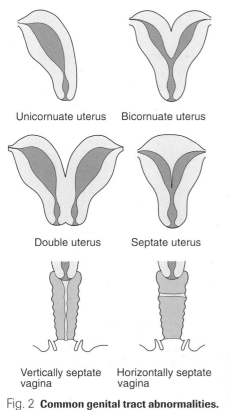

Unicornuate uterus   Bicornuate uterus

Double uterus   Septate uterus

Vertically septate vagina   Horizontally septate vagina

Fig. 2 **Common genital tract abnormalities.**

Bicornuate uterus. This may often carry a pregnancy to an adequately advanced gestation, and the chance of this probably increases with subsequent pregnancies. A 'Strassman' procedure will correct the defect, but the benefits for pregnancy are unproven. A bicornuate uterus may be asymmetrical with one side hypoplastic. Pregnancy in the hypoplastic horn carries a risk of rupture.

Septate uterus. If appropriate to remove the septum, a hysteroscopic approach is probably the most appropriate.

Prepubertal problems

Sexual abuse

This is the involvement of dependent sexually immature children and adolescents in sexual activity they do not truly comprehend, and to which they are unable to give informed consent, and which violates social taboos or family roles. The abuser is usually male and well known to the child and family. It may present acutely, following injury or allegation, or may be suggested by precociousness and other behavioural disorders.

There are numerous pitfalls to the clinical examination, and a depth of experience is required for an examination to stand up in court. Early senior multidisciplinary help is essential in this highly emotive area where incorrect interpretation of the signs may have major consequences. A colposcopic examination is helpful and photographic records are extremely useful.

The history should be carefully taken and documented, and the social work team involved if appropriate. Swabs (which may include swabs for DNA analysis) should be taken with a 'secure chain of evidence' in case they are required for a later legal action. Particular attention should be paid to bleeding, bruising or any other area of injury, particularly lacerations at the posterior fourchette and perineal abrasions.

A normal hymen has a number of different shapes (annular, crescentic, fimbriated, septate, sleeve- or funnel-shaped). Notches and clefts can be highly suggestive of penetrating injury, but may be normal if associated with an intravaginal ridge above them; they are very rare in the posterior segment in non-abused girls (Fig. 3). Straddle injuries very rarely affect the hymen, and there is much more likely to be bruising anterior to the vagina or laterally (e.g. labia majora). It is also rare for tampon use to cause hymenal injury (although it may increase the diameter slightly), and there are no reported cases of congenital absence of the hymen. A normal pre-pubertal hymen does not exclude abuse.

Puberty and its abnormalities

Puberty is the time during which there is development of secondary sexual characteristics and attainment of sexual maturity. There is some form of hypothalamic trigger which leads to pulsatile release of luteinizing hormone (LH) and follicle-stimulating hormone (FSH) between 5 and 10 years of age, with ovarian release of oestrogen usually from the age of 8. This oestrogen mediates the pubertal changes. The sequence starts with a somatic growth spurt followed by breast development, then development of pubic hair followed by axillary hair and finally the menarche (first period) (Fig. 1).

Normal puberty

Growth spurt

The somatic growth spurt is the first notable change due to oestrogen stimulation. After the menarche somatic growth will continue for approximately 2 years until fusion of the epiphyses, after which no further growth is possible. Precocious puberty may lead to premature epiphyseal closure and the child may fail to attain its full height potential.

Breast development (thelarche)

This is the next stage in pubertal development with four stages of breast development (Fig. 2). The breast bud is followed by breast and areola enlargement. The nipple and areola then enlarge further and the final stage is development of the adult breast.

Hair growth

Pubic hair precedes axillary hair development and also shows four stages. Initially there is sparse hair on the labia; this then grows centrally and advances onto the mons pubis. The next stage is for the hair to spread laterally a little, with the full adult triangular distribution as the final stage.

Menarche

The first menstrual period is the final stage in pubertal development, and occurs in 95% of girls between the ages of 11 and 15 years. The average age of the menarche in the UK is

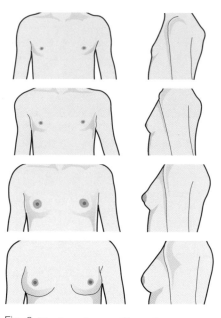

Fig. 2 **The four stages of breast development.**

13 years, a fall in the age of menarche being noted in children in developed countries. This is thought to be a reflection of improved nutritional status – some researchers believing that a critical body weight must be reached before menarche is achieved. This theory has some merit as it is noted that moderately obese girls have an earlier menarche than those of more normal weight. Conversely, girls with anorexia or adhering to an intensive exercise programme may show delay in the age of menarche.

Abnormalities of puberty

Precocious puberty

Signs of pubertal development before the age of 8 are accepted as precocious puberty which in three-quarters of females has an idiopathic aetiology. However, before allocating a child to this category, it is important to rule out treatable causes (Table 1).

The idiopathic group includes girls with constitutional sexual precocity due to premature maturation of the hypothalamic–pituitary–ovarian axis.

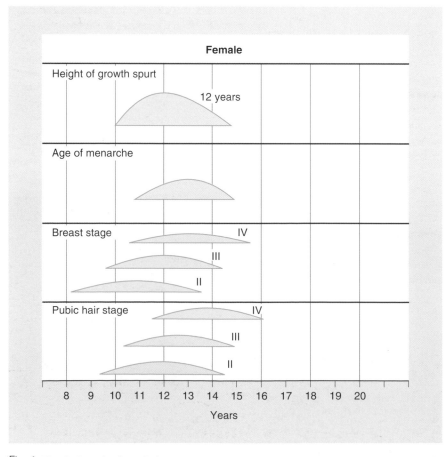

Fig. 1 **The timing of pubertal changes.**

Table 1 **Causes of precocious puberty**	
Cause	**Percentage**
Idiopathic	74%
Ovarian hormone production	11%
Intracranial pathology	7%
McCune–Albright syndrome	5%
Adrenal problem	2%
Ectopic gonadotrophin production	Less than 1%

This tends to run in families and tends to occur around the cut-off age of 8 years. Intracranial pathology includes cranial trauma, encephalitis, cysts or tumours – the mechanism by which they produce precocious puberty being uncertain. Ovarian hormone production is usually associated with an ovarian cyst which should be diagnosable by ultrasound scanning, but is often present as a palpable mass in the abdomen. The McCune–Albright syndrome (polyostotic fibrous dysplasia) presents with cystic bone lesions which easily fracture, café-au-lait patches and sexual precocity. The cause is uncertain.

Referral to a paediatric endocrinologist ensures everything is addressed.

Delayed puberty

Delayed puberty (Table 2) is rare with only 1% of females not having had menarche by the age of 18. If there are no secondary sexual characteristics by the age of 14 delay is diagnosed and investigation is appropriate. The largest group are those with ovarian failure, more than half of whom have chromosomal anomalies.

In girls with hypergonadotropic hypogonadism the ovarian failure may be associated with an abnormal karyotype, particularly Turner's syndrome. In those with a normal karyotype it may be that there is gonadal dysgenesis (the external genitalia are usually of infantile female type) or the resistant ovary syndrome with normal appearance of external genitalia (where the ovary fails to respond to the increased levels of LH and FSH) but where there can be spontaneous ovulation and obviously pregnancy can thus occur, though prognosis with respect to future pregnancy in these cases should be guarded.

With hypogonadotropic hypogonadism (low levels of LH and FSH) the delay may be constitutional – particularly when short compared to her family but appropriate for the stage of puberty and bone age – or due to a chronic medical condition or anorexia nervosa.

In the eugonadotropic group (normal LH and FSH) congenital absence of the uterus (Rokitansky syndrome) or vaginal developmental obstruction should be considered.

Treatment of delayed puberty

Initial management
First exclude pregnancy.

Table 2 **Causes of delayed puberty**		
Cause	Percentage	Underlying cause
Hypergonadotropic hypogonadism	43%	Gonadal dysgenesis, e.g. Turner's syndrome
Hypogonadotropic hypogonadism	31%	Constitutional, chronic medical illness, anorexia
Eugonadism	26%	Abnormal genitalia, e.g. absent uterus, vaginal septum

Ask about chronic illnesses, anorexia, excessive physical exercise or family history of delayed puberty. Heart problems may be found with chromosomal disorders, urinary or bowel disorders with anatomical disorders of the genital tract, hernia repairs may suggest gonadal disorder and slow general development is associated with hypothyroidism. Examination should include measurement of height, weight and visual fields; check for secondary sexual characteristics, virilization and hirsutism. Vaginal examination is inappropriate unless the girl is sexually active. Check for stigmata of Turner's syndrome (short stature, webbed neck, and wide carrying angle).

Investigations include sending serum for LH and FSH (low with constitutional delay), testosterone (increased in polycystic ovarian syndrome), free T4, TSH (increased in primary hypothyroidism) and prolactin (ideally measured under non-stressed conditions). Karyotype is needed if a chromosomal problem is suspected; if an XY chromosomal pattern is found, it is usual to suggest gonadectomy due to the 25% risk of tumour in the gonad. X-ray for bone age would confirm constitutional delay. Assessment of 17-hydroxyprogesterone when congenital adrenal hyperplasia is suspected, pelvic ultrasound to assess pelvic anatomy and skull X-ray if prolactin is raised are appropriate.

Causes and further management
Normal secondary sexual characteristics but with primary amenorrhoea. This is most commonly caused by an imperforate hymen and is characterized by cyclical pain and a haematocolpos (see p. 88). A progesterone challenge test will identify constitutional menstrual delay, i.e. will result in bleeding only with an adequate estradiol level and normal genital tract. Give 5 days of oral progesterone and there should be a withdrawal bleed within 10–14 days of stopping.

Poor or absent secondary sexual characteristics. These comprise:

1. Constitutional delay. The diagnosis is likely in a healthy adolescent who is short for the family but appropriate for the stage of puberty and bone age. There is often a family history and it may be associated with chronic systemic disease (rare, but consider hypothyroidism and malabsorption). If the bone age on X-ray is less than the chronological age than it is reasonable to adopt a conservative approach. Anorexia nervosa should also be considered.

2. Ovarian dysfunction. This may be due to gonadal agenesis with Turner's syndrome or Turner's mosaic. Treatment is specialized as oestrogen treatment may predispose to short stature by premature epiphyseal closure. Therapy is with low-dose ethinylestradiol initially, increasing over the next 18 months. A progestogen is then added for 5 days every 4 weeks. The dose of oestrogen is increased if response is adequate and the contraceptive pill substituted.

3. Hypothalamopituitary disorders. Hypogonadotropic hypogonadism is usually associated with pituitary tumours and other pituitary deficiencies. In Kallmann syndrome there is a congenital deficiency of luteinizing hormone-releasing hormone (LHRH) and absent olfactory sensation. Hypothyroidism is likely to cause pubertal delay.

Puberty and its abnormalities

- For puberty to occur there must be oestrogen production from the ovaries.
- Thelarche and sexual hair growth follow the somatic growth spurt. Menarche is the final stage of puberty.
- Precocious puberty is associated with failure to achieve full adult height so must be treated.
- Delayed puberty is only found in 1%.

Miscarriage

Spontaneous miscarriage

- Spontaneous miscarriage is the loss of a pregnancy before 24 weeks' gestation. It is most common in the first trimester and is said to occur in ≈ 25% of all pregnancies.
- The word 'abortion' has connotations of induced abortion and should not be used for miscarriage. The term 'blighted ovum' used to describe an anembryonic pregnancy should be discarded.
- Extreme care must be taken not to advise uterine evacuation if there is any possibility of viability.
- It should not be assumed that the pregnancy is non-viable simply because the gestation does not agree with the expected dates.
- There should also be a low threshold of suspicion for ectopic pregnancy.
- Approximately 50% of miscarriages occurring early in the first trimester are associated with chromosomal abnormality (trisomy, monosomy, polyploidy), although this becomes less with increasing gestation.

Presentation

There is usually a history of bleeding per vagina and lower abdominal pain, although an empty gestational sac (or fetal pole with absent fetal heartbeat) may be an asymptomatic finding at booking scan ('missed'). Miscarriage is 'inevitable' if some products of conception (*not clots*) are passed. Rarely, products of one twin may be passed, with the other twin being viable, justifying an ultrasound scan in every case. The miscarriage is said to be 'threatened' if the pregnancy is still viable, and 'incomplete' if there is residual tissue within the cavity (Fig. 1).

Management

This is based on USS findings.

Viable intrauterine pregnancy. The prognosis is good and the parents can be offered reasonable reassurance.

Empty gestational sac. A true gestational sac usually has a double decidual ring, unlike a pseudosac which is suggestive of ectopic pregnancy. If there is an empty gestational sac greater than 25 mm maximum diameter, the pregnancy is very likely to be non-viable (Fig. 2).

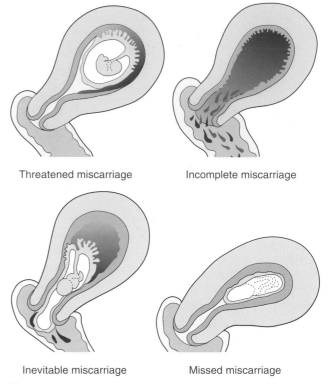

Threatened miscarriage   Incomplete miscarriage

Inevitable miscarriage   Missed miscarriage

Fig. 1 **Different types of miscarriage.**

Pseudosac. See Ectopic pregnancy, page 98, and Figure 3.

Fetal pole with no fetal heartbeat (FH). An FH is usually seen on transvaginal (TV) scan if the fetal pole is > 2–3 mm in diameter, but will always be seen by 6 mm diameter (Fig. 4). A similar cut-off of 15 mm diameter is appropriate for a transabdominal (TA) scan. If in doubt, rescanning should be arranged in 7–10 days.

Empty uterus. Either there has been a complete miscarriage (tissue may have been passed), or the pregnancy is very early (e.g. < 5 weeks), or there is an ectopic pregnancy. Ectopic pregnancy must be excluded. An intrauterine sac will usually be seen on TV scan if the human chorionic gonadotrophin (hCG) is > 1000 IU (> 6500 IU for a TA scan) and its absence

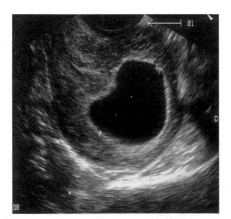

Fig. 2 **35-mm empty gestational sac.** If the mean sac diameter is greater than 25 mm, the pregnancy is almost certainly non-viable.

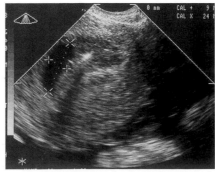

Fig. 3 **Pseudosac, with intrauterine contraceptive device (IUCD) in situ,** in a patient with a 6-week, right-sided tubal ectopic pregnancy.

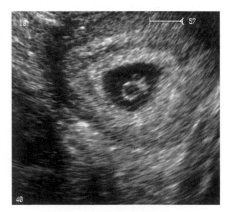

Fig. 4 **4-mm fetal pole with no fetal heartbeat on transvaginal scan.** Viability is unlikely but the patient should be rescanned in 7–10 days.

raises the possibility of an ectopic pregnancy. Serum levels of hCG should double in 48 hours if the pregnancy is viable and intrauterine; less suggests an ectopic pregnancy (although by using this method in isolation, 15% of intrauterine pregnancies would be diagnosed as ectopics and 13% of ectopics as intrauterine). If the level doubles and the patient remains well, the ultrasound scan should be repeated in 1 week to ensure that the pregnancy is ongoing. If less than doubling, steady, or only slightly reduced, a laparoscopy should be considered to exclude ectopic pregnancy.

Retained products. Evacuation of retained products of conception (ERPOC) has become the established management for miscarriage with retained products. For those with heavy bleeding this remains appropriate, although it is occasionally possible to remove retained products from the cervical os at speculum examination and save the need for further intervention. While ERPOC may still be offered to those with little bleeding, there is evidence that if the diameter of retained products is small (e.g. < 40 mm), ERPOC may not be necessary. An additional option is also available to give mifepristone and misoprostol for a 'medical' evacuation of retained products (see p. 94).

Adnexal mass or ectopic. Possible adnexal findings with an ectopic pregnancy are of a sac (30%), a sac containing a yolk sac (15%) and a sac with a fetal pole and FH (15%). The absence of adnexal findings on USS therefore *does not exclude an ectopic pregnancy.*

After the miscarriage

There has been a bereavement and the parents have lost 'a baby'. They should be reassured that they did nothing which might have caused the miscarriage and given time to grieve. There is no medical indication to wait before trying again, but they may require contraception to allow time to grieve. There is often further upset around the date the baby would have been born.

Septic abortion

This is rare unless after illegal terminations with inadequate asepsis, and therefore more common in countries with anti-abortion policies.

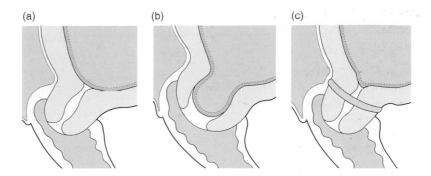

Fig. 5 **Cervical incompetence. (a)** Normal cervix. **(b)** Incomplete cervix. **(c)** Cerclage with a non-absorbable suture.

There is usually raised temperature > 38°C, tachycardia, malaise, abdominal pain, marked tenderness and purulent vaginal loss. Endotoxic shock may develop and there is a significant mortality. The usual infecting organisms are Gram-negative bacteria, streptococci (haemolytic and anaerobic) and other anaerobes (e.g. *Bacteroides*).

Recurrent spontaneous miscarriage

This is the consecutive loss of three or more fetuses weighing < 500 g (incidence 0.5–1%). Those who have had three consecutive miscarriages still have a 70% chance of a normal outcome in their next pregnancy.

Investigation

- Karyotype from both parents.
- Maternal blood for lupus anticoagulant and anticardiolipin antibodies.
- Possible hysterosalpingogram and/or pelvic ultrasound examination (uterus and ovaries) to look for uterine abnormalities (see p. 89).

Causes and management

Antiphospholipid syndrome (≈ 15%). Miscarriage is more likely to occur in the presence of lupus anticoagulant and raised anticardiolipin antibodies.

Chromosomal abnormality (≈ 5%). This is usually a balanced reciprocal or

Robertsonian translocation, and the finding of such an abnormality should prompt genetic referral.

Cervical incompetence. This is a cause of mid-trimester miscarriage, and cervical cerclage should probably only be considered when the miscarriage has been preceded by spontaneous rupture of membranes or painless cervical dilatation (Fig. 5). Use of such a suture probably provides a small improvement in the prognosis in the next pregnancy, but at the risk of infection developing after insertion. Transabdominal cerclage has also been used but is not without risk and should be considered a sub-specialist procedure.

Thrombophilic defects. Retrospective studies have indicated an increased incidence of thrombophilic defects in those with recurrent miscarriage (activated protein C resistance, antithrombin III, protein C and protein S deficiency ± hyperhomocystinaemia). Evidence for the efficacy of treatment in this group is lacking.

Anatomical uterine abnormality (see also p. 89).

It is very difficult to estimate the significance of anatomical abnormalities and great caution is required before undertaking significant surgical procedures.

Miscarriage

- Extreme care must be taken not to advise uterine evacuation if there is any possibility of viability.

- A positive pregnancy test and an empty uterus should be considered as an ectopic pregnancy until proven otherwise. The absence of adnexal findings does not exclude an ectopic pregnancy.

- Those with recurrent spontaneous miscarriage associated with lupus anticoagulant or raised anticardiolipin antibodies should be given aspirin and heparin in the next pregnancy.

Induced abortion (termination of pregnancy)

Termination of unwanted pregnancies, or abortion, has been carried out for thousands of years. Both Aristotle and Hippocrates favoured its selective use, and yet its provision in a legal, medically supervised and safe framework is still one of the most contentious issues in medicine. Strictly speaking, the term 'termination' is used here to refer to any pregnancy induced at < 24 weeks' gestation (UK) or with a fetal weight of < 500 g, but as neonatal survival has been achieved below these parameters, the definitions are debatable. The term 'abortion' here refers to induced abortion, and the expression 'miscarriage' is reserved for spontaneous loss.

Ethics

Many people have an opinion, often strongly held, about abortion (Table 1). Those who are pro-abortion argue they are 'pro-choice' and believe in the right of individuals to make their own decisions. They focus on the potential problems of bringing an unwanted baby into the world, and of the surrounding social difficulties the child might face. Those who are anti-abortion, 'pro-life', argue that the fetus is more than just part of the mother, but a life in itself and should be protected as such, even to the extent of limiting the mother's own actions.

Worldwide, unsafe abortion is a major public health issue. At least 20 million women undergo unsafe abortion each year and some 67 000 women die as a result, with many others suffering chronic morbidities and disabilities. Unsafe abortions may be induced by the woman herself, by non-medical persons or by health workers in unhygienic conditions. Such abortions may be induced by insertion of a solid object (usually root, twig or catheter) into the uterus, an improperly performed dilatation and curettage procedure, ingestion of harmful substances, or exertion of external force. The complications of sepsis,

Table 2 The five sections of the UK Abortion Act

A	To save the mother's life
B	To prevent grave permanent injury to the mother's physical or mental health
C	If < 24 weeks, to avoid injury to the physical or mental health of the mother
D	If < 24 weeks, to avoid injury to the physical or mental health of the existing child(ren)
E	If the child is likely to be severely physically or mentally handicapped

haemorrhage, genital and abdominal trauma, perforated uterus or poisoning may be fatal if left untreated. Death may also result from secondary complications such as gas gangrene and acute renal failure. The mortality from an appropriately conducted abortion, however, is minimal, and the morbidity small. In the United States, for example, the death rate for abortion is now 0.6 per 100 000 procedures, compared to perhaps several hundred times this rate for an unsafe abortion. The abortion rate is also much higher in those countries with limited access to contraception. Where abortion is permitted by the law, the large majority of abortions (typically > 90%) take place before the end of the 12th week of pregnancy.

Abortion is legal in the UK under the Abortion Act 1967 amended by the Human Fertilisation and Embryology Act 1991 (Table 2). Two doctors are required to sign a form, and if a doctor does not wish to sign he or she has a duty to refer to another doctor who would. There is also a duty to treat complications in an emergency situation.

In practice, Section 'C' can be interpreted in such a way as to support termination of pregnancy, as it could be argued that continuing an unwanted pregnancy might be injurious to the mother's mental health. The risk of psychiatric morbidity is significantly greater after delivery of a baby than after a termination. Furthermore, women

with an unwanted pregnancy may display evidence of an anxiety state or reactive depression. Categories A, B and E do not specify a gestation limit and category E only allows termination of a major potentially serious anomaly. If abortion is required to save a women's life in emergency circumstances, one doctor may act alone.

Counselling for Section 'C' terminations

Counselling needs to explore many areas. It is often helpful to start by acknowledging that this is a difficult situation, e.g. 'This must have been a very difficult week or two for you', and then follow with an open question: 'Tell me what has been happening.' It is important to find out the patient's own views and to ensure that she is not being forced against her will. If a parent is present, it is often useful to see the patient alone for at least part of the time.

It is also important to find out whether the baby's father knows, how he and the baby's mother get on together, who else knows and what they all feel. The counsellor should try to explore how they might cope afterwards, or how they would feel if they went ahead with the pregnancy. They should also consider whether there are plans to have children in the future, whether they have considered adoption and what the plans for contraception are afterwards.

The woman should be aware that there is a possibility, albeit rare, that infection following termination of pregnancy (TOP) may lead to tubal occlusion and second-degree infertility. There is also a small procedure failure rate, and either a clinical follow-up or pregnancy test 2–6 weeks post-termination is important (note: the pregnancy test may remain positive for up to 4 weeks despite successful TOP). It is important to either screen for and treat infections (including chlamydia), or treat all prophylactically, e.g. with oral metronidazole and azithromycin.

Method

In general, the complication rate is lower the earlier the procedure is carried out. The risk of major complications from termination at 15 weeks' gestation is double the risk from termination at 8 weeks' gestation.

Table 1 Induced abortion

Advantages	Disadvantages
■ Reduces illegal abortions and their complications (particularly sepsis and uterine perforation)	■ Moral, ethical and religious objections
■ Allows an opportunity to screen for sexually transmitted diseases (STDs), discuss contraception and support the patient through difficult circumstances	■ May be inappropriately looked upon as a form of contraception
■ Reduces the births of unwanted children	

It is important to confirm that the woman is pregnant and to establish the gestation either clinically or by USS. Blood should be sent for grouping and testing for antibodies, and anti-D should be given post-termination to Rhesus-negative women. Options (if available) should be explained and the woman given the choice as outlined below:

- less than 9 weeks: suction evacuation or medical termination
- 9–12 weeks: suction termination only
- more than 12 weeks: medical termination only.

(Note: some experienced practitioners will consider surgical dilatation and evacuation up to 18 weeks' gestation.)

The pros and cons of medical vs surgical termination at less than 9 weeks' gestation are as follows:

- Medical TOP avoids a general anaesthetic.
- There is probably little to choose in terms of the infection risk, pain, post-procedure bleeding and subsequent fertility.
- Those that choose either method are usually satisfied with their choice.
- Medical termination may be more effective at earlier gestations, and surgical better closer to 9 weeks.

Surgical termination (Fig. 1)

Prostaglandin pessaries 4 hours prior to the operation are useful to soften the cervix and minimize trauma from the dilatation, particularly if the woman is a primigravida or at a gestation of > 10 weeks. Surgery is usually carried out under general anaesthetic (local anaesthesia is occasionally an option) and cervical dilators are used to dilate the cervical os. A rigid or flexible suction curette is then used to remove the pregnancy. It is important to check and document that definite products of conception are seen to be coming away at the time of surgery.

Medical termination

First trimester

Mifepristone is given orally and the patient admitted to hospital 36–48 hours later for a prostaglandin pessary. Eighty

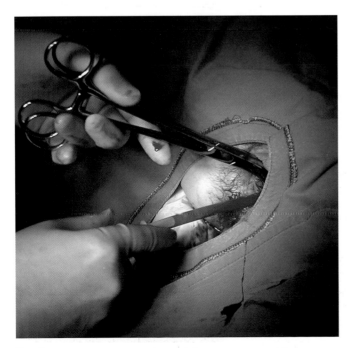

Fig. 1 **Surgical TOP is performed in the same way as this evacuation of retained products of conception.**

per cent will pass products of conception in the following 4 hours and this should be confirmed by clinical inspection and speculum examination before discharge. Ninety-four per cent will abort spontaneously and most will bleed for a total of 10 days. Follow-up should be arranged for 2 weeks to ensure that bleeding has settled and to confirm complete abortion by bimanual examination. If in doubt, an ultrasound scan is useful. Retained products can almost always be managed conservatively unless bleeding is particularly heavy. Less than 5% require uterine evacuation.

Second trimester

Mifepristone is given orally and the patient admitted to hospital 36–48 hours later for a prostaglandin pessary. She is then fasted until abortion occurs, and an intravenous infusion is set up if more than 6 hours pass. Further prostaglandin pessaries are inserted 6-hourly to a maximum of 24 hours (nearly all will abort by 24 hours, average 8 hours). During this time analgesia, emotional and sympathetic support are required. It is important to ensure that the placenta appears complete and that the uterus is well contracted on bimanual examination. Approximately 6% will require a uterine evacuation.

Risks of termination

Although early termination of pregnancy is a relatively safe procedure, there are risks which, generally, increase with advancing gestation. The first possibility is of failure to terminate the pregnancy, which is greater at the earlier stage when the gestational sac is smallest. With suction termination, there is a risk of uterine perforation with damage to the abdominal viscera, and possible longer-term consequences of cervical trauma which might lead to cervical incompetence. Postoperative pelvic infection may occur with either method and may lead to tubal occlusion. With pregnancy termination overall, however, there seems to be little statistical impact on the outcome of subsequent pregnancies.

Follow-up

After termination, anti-D should be given to those who are Rhesus-negative and the results of any infection screens should be assessed. Follow-up can be in either the hospital or community setting, and it is important to ensure that it is organized. This is to check that the TOP is complete, that contraception has been arranged and to discuss the emotional aspects.

Psychological problems after termination

Most women feel tearful and emotional a few days after termination of pregnancy, but there is good evidence that most feel psychologically much better 3 months later when compared with their feelings before the procedure. There is no evidence that termination causes serious psychiatric morbidity, although relapse of existing psychiatric problems can occur. On the other hand, the incidence of depression, suicide and child abuse is higher in women who have continued with the pregnancy because termination was refused.

> ### Induced abortion
> - Unsafe abortion is a major worldwide public health issue.
> - There is strong 'pro-life' and 'pro-choice' support.
> - Termination can be either medical or surgical.

Trophoblastic disorders

Trophoblast is naturally invasive, but the invasion normally ceases after placentation has occurred. Gestational trophoblastic disorders represent an abnormal proliferation of trophoblastic tissue, leading to often massive placental overgrowth, occasional invasion and rarely even metastases. Malignant change can also occur with transformation to choriocarcinoma. Trophoblastic disorders occur in approximately 1 : 1000 UK pregnancies. Large differences in incidence between different racial groups have been reported (e.g. 1 : 85 in Indonesia, 1 : 1700 in USA) but are not confirmed by all authors. All secrete human chorionic gonadotrophin (hCG), making it a very useful tool to monitor treatment and screen for recurrence. In the UK, management of post-uterine evacuation is confined to one of the three centres: Charing Cross, London; Ninewells, Dundee; Weston Park, Sheffield.

Hydatidiform mole

This is the commonest type of gestational trophoblastic disease.

Partial hydatidiform mole

This is triploid with one set of maternal and two sets of paternal chromosomes, usually 69 XXY (Fig. 1). There may

initially be a fetus, but it often dies early in the first trimester. Although 1% invade ('invasive mole') and a few of these can develop metastases, they virtually never become choriocarcinoma. Only 0.5% require treatment following uterine evacuation.

Complete hydatidiform mole

This is the 'classical' molar pregnancy. It is androgenetically diploid; in other words, although there are the normal number of chromosomes, all are paternally derived and the female nuclear DNA is inactivated (Fig. 1). In 90% there is duplication of one haploid sperm (XX) and the rest are from two spermatozoa, i.e. dispermic (and usually XY). There is never an embryo and the patient usually presents at 8–24 weeks' gestation with vaginal bleeding (± the passing of grape-like tissue). The uterus may be soft, doughy and large for dates. There may also be pre-eclampsia, hyperemesis, cardiac failure and thyrotoxicosis, probably related to the very high levels of hCG (hCG and thyroid-stimulating hormone share a common structure and α subunit). Ultrasound is said to show a 'snowstorm appearance' but this describes the older B-scan pictures. On a real-time scan it more correctly looks as if the cavity is

filled with relatively homogeneous solid tissue with a vesicular appearance (Fig. 2). There may also be multiple luteal cysts on the ovaries from stimulation by the very high hCG levels. Ten per cent invade through the uterus ('invasive mole' – Fig. 3) and can metastasize to

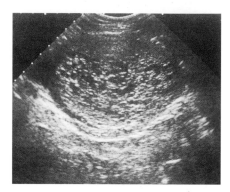

Fig. 2 **Ultrasound scan of hydatidiform mole.**

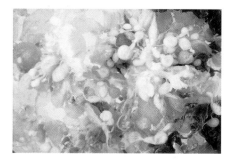

Fig. 3 **Invasive mole.**

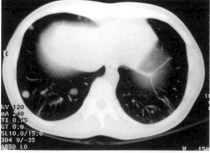

Fig. 4 **CT scan of pulmonary metastases with choriocarcinoma.**

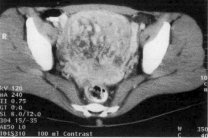

Fig. 5 **CT scan of pelvis in the same patient showing a large vascular mass.**

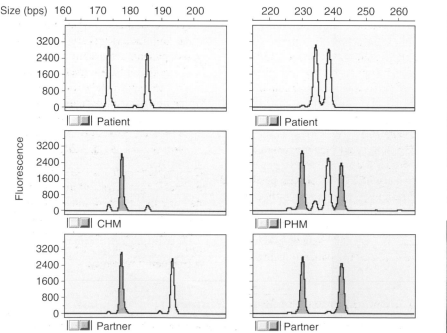

Fig. 1 **Fluorescently labelled products of conception.** In the complete hydatidiform mole (CHM; left) the genetic material is of paternal origin following duplication of one haploid sperm. On the right, the partial hydatidiform mole (PHM) is triploid with two different sets of paternal chromosomes and one maternal haploid set. bps, base pair size.

lung, vagina, liver, brain and the gastrointestinal tract (Figs 4 and 5). These may occasionally regress spontaneously. Approximately 15% of complete moles require chemotherapy after uterine evacuation. The incidence of choriocarcinoma is 3%.

Gestational choriocarcinoma

Gestational choriocarcinoma contains both syncytiotrophoblast and cytotrophoblast and is histologically different from a hydatidiform mole (absence of villi). It may arise from a hydatidiform mole (50%) or follow a live birth, stillbirth, miscarriage or ectopic pregnancy de novo. It contains maternal and paternal chromosomes, unlike choriocarcinoma of ovarian origin.

Placental site trophoblastic tumour

This contains largely cytotrophoblast (therefore it has lower hCG) and occurs almost exclusively following a normal pregnancy. It is much rarer than gestational choriocarcinoma and presents with amenorrhoea or irregular bleeding.

Clinical presentation

Partial and complete mole

Molar pregnancy becomes clinically apparent because of its pathophysiological features.   Most molar pregnancies will miscarry spontaneously and the commonest clinical presentation, therefore, is pain and vaginal bleeding. It may also be asymptomatic and discovered at a routine early pregnancy ultrasound scan. The uterus is often large for dates. Excessive production of hCG may be one of the reasons why a molar pregnancy may present with hyperemesis gravidarum or even (very rarely) with extremely early-onset pre-eclampsia.

Gestational choriocarcinoma

An invasive mole is usually identified because of persistent hCG levels or ongoing bleeding after surgical evacuation of the uterus. Choriocarcinoma may present either because of the primary intrauterine lesion, in which case the pathology after surgical evacuation will confirm the diagnosis, or because of a metastasis. Metastases may be to:

- the lung, causing haemoptysis
- the brain, leading to neurological abnormalities

Score	0	1	2	4
Age	<39	>39		
Previous pregnancy	Mole	Miscarriage	Term pregnancy	
Interval from previous pregnancy (months)	4	4–6	7–12	>12
hCG	<1000	1000–10 000	10 000–100 000	>100 000
Parental blood group		O or A	B or AB	
Size of tumour		3–5 cm	>5 cm	
Metastasis site		Spleen, kidney	GI tract, liver	Brain
Metastases number		1–4	4–8	>8
Previous chemotherapy			Single drug	≥ 2 drugs

Table 1 **Prognostic factors in gestational trophoblastic disease.** Differing forms of chemotherapy are used for differing risk groups: low risk is < 4, medium 4–8 and high > 8

- the GI tract, causing chronic blood loss or melaena
- the liver, leading to jaundice
- the kidney, causing haematuria.

Initial management

If gestational trophoblastic disease is suspected, then an ultrasound scan and chest X-ray should be arranged. Blood should be sent for measurement of hCG, thyroid function tests and cross-matching prior to undertaking the uterine evacuation. The risk of bleeding with or without perforation is significant but uterine evacuation for a complete mole is superior to both medical evacuation of the uterus (may lead to increased risk of dissemination) and hysterectomy. Medical evacuation may be appropriate for a partial mole, particularly if a larger fetus is present, but should be followed with a surgical evacuation of any retained products of conception. It is recommended that oxytocics be avoided until after the uterine evacuation, and used preoperatively only if they are necessary to control severe haemorrhage, as uterine contractions may precipitate distant spread. Mifepristone and prostaglandin analogues should also be avoided unless clinically essential.

Management after uterine evacuation

- The patient should be registered with a regional centre.
- Urinary hCG levels should be checked fortnightly until undetectable, then monthly for 6 months and 3-monthly for the second year. This may be best achieved by the patient posting

specimens directly to the regional centre. Following a complete mole, the patient must wait at least 6 months from the hCG returning to 0 (or for 1 year following chemotherapy) before trying for a further pregnancy to minimize the risks of recurrence. Condoms or an intrauterine contraceptive device may be used. The combined oral contraceptive can only be taken when the hCG has returned to zero, although some advocate waiting an extra 6 months beyond this time, again to minimize recurrence risk.

- Chemotherapy may be required if the hCG rises progressively following the uterine evacuation, or is > 20 000 U at 4 weeks, or if the pathology is reported as choriocarcinoma. Of those patients who develop persistent trophoblastic disease, approximately 80% are low risk and 20% high risk on the scoring system shown in Table 1. Of the low-risk group, 80% respond to low-dose methotrexate but 20% need additional chemotherapy because of methotrexate resistance. All low-risk patients are cured. High-risk patients are usually given chemotherapy over several cycles. Chemotherapy is always given if the diagnosis is choriocarcinoma, or if there are metastases to liver, brain and gastrointestinal (GI) tract (80% of high-risk patients are cured).

Of long-term survivors, 85% have normal pregnancies, but if a patient has had one hydatidiform mole, the risk of a second mole is 2% and a third 20%. Follow-up with checking of hCG levels must be undertaken after any subsequent pregnancy.

Trophoblastic disorders

- Gestational trophoblastic disorders represent an abnormal proliferation of trophoblastic tissue.
- It is important to track urinary hCG after uterine evacuation to ensure that there is no residual tissue and that there is no invasion.
- There is an increased recurrence risk in subsequent pregnancies.

Ectopic pregnancy

An ectopic pregnancy is one which implants outside the uterine cavity. It occurs in about 1 in 200 pregnancies in the United Kingdom, 1 in 30 in the West Indies and in the United States is found twice as commonly in the non-white as in the white population. The incidence has been rising slightly, but the death rate of about 1 per 1000 ectopic pregnancies has been falling due to earlier diagnosis and treatment in western societies.

Aetiology

The mechanism by which the fertilized ovum reaches the uterine cavity is dependent upon motility of the tube, the movement of the cilia of the fallopian tubes, and currents set up within the tubes. These all contribute to the sperm making passage upward to meet the egg which is coming down the fallopian tube. Three or four days after fertilization the fertilized ovum implants within the uterine cavity. This implantation will occur at the appropriate time wherever the zygote happens to be at that stage. The associations and possible causes of ectopic pregnancy are thus thought to operate by changing the motility of the tube or damaging the cilia and disturbing the normal progression of the fertilized ovum.

Any past history of pelvic infection or ruptured appendix which will cause peritubular adhesions or pelvic inflammatory disease causing damage to the internal structure of the tube may predispose to ectopic implantation. Tubal surgery, even using microsurgical techniques, is unlikely to reconstruct the tube to its native form and thus predisposition to ectopic pregnancy remains. Reversal of sterilization is the tubal surgery with the lowest incidence of ectopic pregnancy. With other indications for tubal surgery the incidence of ectopic pregnancy is dependent upon the original damage to the tube. Where there has been conservative surgery for an ectopic pregnancy the chance for a future ectopic pregnancy is dependent upon the pre-existing tubal disease.

The presence of an intrauterine contraceptive device is associated with a higher rate of ectopic pregnancy, thought to be due to the ability of the device to prevent intrauterine but not ectopic gestation. The presence of the device may also alter tubal motility which is the mechanism that has been proposed for ectopic pregnancy seen in association with progestogen-only oral contraception (see p. 108). About half of all ectopic pregnancies are idiopathic.

Site of ectopic pregnancy

The commonest site for an ectopic pregnancy is along the fallopian tube (Fig. 1), though ovarian pregnancy, abdominal pregnancy and cervical pregnancy are all reported (Fig. 2). Ovarian and abdominal pregnancies may be primary implantations on those sites or may follow a tubal abortion which re-implants.

Presentation

The patient may present with sudden onset of symptoms or a more gradual course. The classical, though rare, acute presentation is of sudden collapse in a previously well young woman after a period of amenorrhoea with possibly some brown vaginal loss. There may be a history of fainting or shoulder tip pain and acute abdominal pain. The patient is likely to be shocked and requiring resuscitation. Abdominal

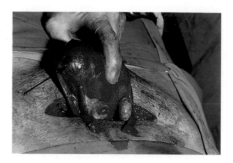

Fig. 1 **A cornual ectopic (rare).** This is dangerous as it ruptures early and bleeds heavily.

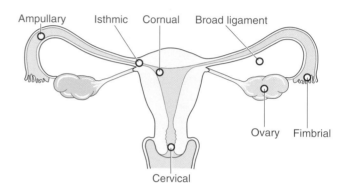

Fig. 2 **Sites of ectopic pregnancies.**

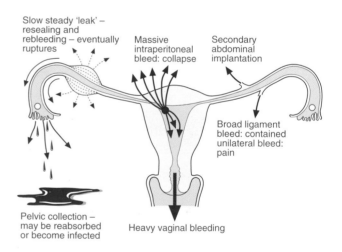

Fig. 3 **Sequelae of ectopic pregnancies.**

palpation reveals a rigid abdomen and immediate laparotomy is necessary to control the haemorrhage. Haemoperitoneum with rupture of the fallopian tube would be noted (Fig. 3).

The subacute presentation is much more common and diagnosis depends on a high index of suspicion. The patient may complain of lower abdominal pain which may be central or localized to the side of the ectopic gestation. The period of amenorrhoea is commonly between 6 and 8 weeks with the history that the patient is trying to conceive or not using contraception. She may have frank red vaginal bleeding, but more commonly would have brown vaginal loss. Vaginal bleeding occurs as the decidua sloughs after the demise of the fetus.

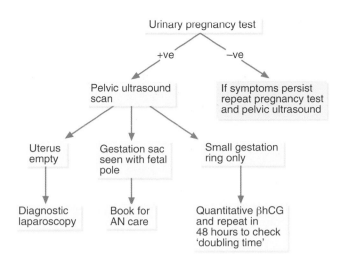

Fig. 4 **Investigations in cases of suspected subacute ectopic pregnancy.**

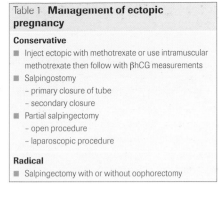

Clinical examination may reveal peritonism with guarding and rebound on abdominal palpation, but often the findings are more vague with only tenderness in the lower abdomen. Prior to pelvic examination, if ectopic pregnancy is expected it is wise to site an intravenous line as rupture of the ectopic may occur during the examination. Gentle pelvic examination may reveal cervical excitation pain, because the tube is distorted by the enlarging ectopic pregnancy. It may be possible to feel a mass in the adnexal region in about 20%. The uterus would be bulky due to the normal early pregnancy changes.

Since assays have been available for the detection of the sub-unit of human chorionic gonadotrophin (hCG) it has been possible to detect this in the serum of a pregnant patient between 7 and 10 days after ovulation has occurred. Thus diagnosis of pregnancy can occur before the patient has missed her period. In a normally-sited pregnancy the doubling time for hCG levels is approximately 48 hours, so serial measurements of hCG may help in the diagnosis of an ectopic pregnancy (Fig. 4). The detection of urinary hCG is the standard pregnancy test and with a positive pregnancy test an intrauterine gestation sac would be seen from 5 weeks onwards.

Ultrasound examination earlier than this may reveal an empty uterus with a positive pregnancy test. Failure to detect a sac should raise the possibility of ectopic gestation. The thickening of the endometrium for the implantation of the fertilized ovum may lead to an ultrasound picture known as a 'pseudo-sac', which should be distinguishable from a normal gestation sac. An hCG discriminatory zone is described whereby a titre of 1000–1500 IU/ml is associated with the presence of an intrauterine sac on transvaginal ultrasound (6000–6500 IU/l for transabdominal scan). This may help to increase the accuracy of the diagnosis.

Management (Table 1)

The initial management of the acute patient involves correction of shock with rapid fluid replacement, cross-matching of blood, check on the haemoglobin and immediate recourse to laparotomy to stem the source of the haemorrhage. In the more usual subacute presentation a laparoscopy is performed to make the definitive diagnosis and to plan the type of treatment that would be appropriate. The laparoscopic treatment of ectopic pregnancy offers a quicker recovery associated with an improved rate of subsequent intrauterine pregnancy compared to treatment by laparotomy. There is also a lesser risk of recurrent ectopic but a higher rate of persisting trophoblastic tissue during laparoscopic management.

The surgery may be laparoscopic or may require laparotomy. Laparotomy would be indicated where access to the tube was limited by adhesions or in a patient with haemorrhagic shock, but ectopic pregnancies are commonly managed laparoscopically. The tube may be removed (salpingectomy) or conserved (salpingostomy). Salpingectomy is associated with a lower rate of persisting trophoblast and subsequent repeat ectopic, whilst having a similar intrauterine pregnancy rate to salpingostomy. The advent of laparoscopy has reduced laparotomy rates during ectopic pregnancy by at least 40% and as conservative management down the laparoscope proceeds many fewer laparotomies need be performed.

The ultimate conservative management would be to cause tubal abortion by ensuring death of the ectopic tissue – attempts have been made to inject the ectopic with methotrexate or with high-dose potassium, a risky procedure due to the possibility of intravascular injection and harm to the mother. Follow-up with hCG levels to ensure non-continuation of the trophoblastic tissue is essential.

The future

Most patients will wish to discuss the recurrence risk for ectopic pregnancy – this being highly dependent upon the reason for the current ectopic pregnancy. The usually quoted risk of ectopic pregnancy after surgery is approximately 5–15%, depending on whether management is laparoscopic or open. Some patients will not wish further conception after an ectopic pregnancy but of those who do, approximately 50% achieve a live birth.

Ectopic pregnancy

- Ectopic pregnancy is a diagnosis easily missed unless a high index of suspicion is maintained.

- The fallopian tube is the commonest site for ectopic implantation.

- Slow rise in hCG levels may indicate an ectopic pregnancy.

- On ultrasound examination beware the pseudo-sac and look for free peritonal fluid or an adnexal mass.

- There is decreased fertility after ectopic pregnancy.

Pelvic inflammatory disease

There is a broad spectrum of disease included under the term pelvic inflammatory disease (PID), ranging from an acute, life-threatening presentation to a more chronic but disabling disorder. In many instances it may be that the disorder is completely asymptomatic, which means that the incidence is usually under-reported.

The term covers ascending infection of the genital tract and usually includes an endometritis and salpingitis – though parametritis, salpingo-oophoritis, pelvic peritonitis and pelvic abscess may all be found (Fig. 1). It is a disease of the reproductive years so most patients are young (75% of cases are under 25 years) and are sexually active (90% of infections are sexually acquired). Pelvic infection may follow childbirth or instrumentation (insertion of intrauterine contraceptive device, hysterosalpingography) of the uterus in 10%. The reported incidence varies geographically (Table 1).

Acute PID

Presentation and diagnosis

The clinical presentation may be very varied but low, bilateral pelvic pain with associated fever is suggestive of the

Table 1	Incidence of pelvic inflammatory disease
Country	**Incidence**
USA	10%
Sweden	0.27%
Africa	15–20% incidence of gonorrhoea
Uganda	6–19% PID

Table 2	Diagnosis of pelvic inflammatory disease
All three of:	**And at least one of:**
■ Abdominal tenderness	■ Temperature > 38°C
■ Cervical excitation	■ WBC > 10 × 10⁹/l
■ Adnexal tenderness	■ ESR > 15 mm/hour

diagnosis. It is important to question about the time of the last menstrual period and use of contraception as the differential diagnosis includes ectopic pregnancy, threatened abortion, menstrual pain (dysmenorrhoea) and endometriosis. Vaginal discharge may be profuse, purulent and offensive, blood-stained or minimal. Onset of symptoms is likely to have been over a few days with possibly deep dyspareunia and general malaise.

If the diagnosis is based on Table 2, then laparoscopic findings will be 70% with salpingitis, 30% with adhesions and 6% with tubal occlusion.

PID may be caused by a variety of organisms. As they are known to have ascended from the lower genital tract this may explain why swabs taken from the high vagina or endocervix are frequently unhelpful in isolating the cause of symptoms. The natural history of the disease is incompletely understood, though the relationship with sexually transmitted disease raises the possibility of damaged mucosal surfaces being more prone to ascending infection. Proposals as to how organisms ascend the genital tract include being swept upwards during retrograde menstruation, which might explain why the onset of PID is often associated with menstruation.

The two organisms most commonly associated with PID (60% of cases) are *Chlamydia trachomatis* and *Neisseria gonorrhoeae*. They have changed in prevalence over the past 30 years – *Chlamydia* increasing whilst gonorrhoea is less prevalent. Chlamydiae are obligate intracellular parasites and appear to be able to influence the host's immune response in ways beneficial to their survival. It may be the immune response to the chlamydiae which determines the extent of tubal damage. The necessary investigations in suspected cases are:

- FBC (full blood count) – looking for a raised white blood cell count as response to infection
- ESR > 15 mm/hour
- temperature – raised in response to infection
- triple swabs – from high vagina, endocervix, urethra
- diagnostic laparoscopy – may be considered for a definitive diagnosis, investigation of a pelvic mass, or failure to respond to treatment.

Related factors

Sexual history. An increased risk of PID has been noted in association with a young age at first sexual intercourse, a high frequency of sexual intercourse and multiple sexual partners.

Contraception. Use of the oral contraceptive has a lower risk of PID, possibly due to the changes in the cervical mucus making this impenetrable to ascending organisms. On the other hand, there is an increased chance of PID in association with the

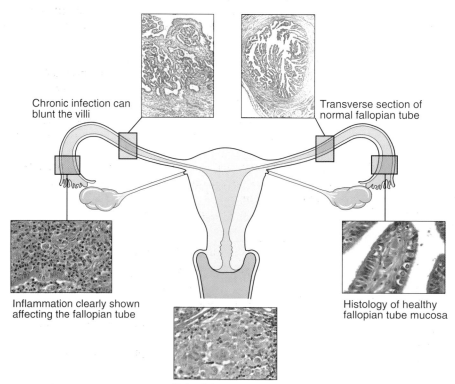

Chronic infection can blunt the villi

Transverse section of normal fallopian tube

Inflammation clearly shown affecting the fallopian tube

Histology of healthy fallopian tube mucosa

Tuberculosis infection of the fallopian tube – a rare cause of infertility

Fig. 1 **Changes to fallopian tubes resulting from pelvic inflammatory disease.**

use of the intrauterine contraceptive device (IUCD). This may be due to the introduction of organisms at the time of coil insertion or the presence of the thread leading from the endometrial cavity down to the vagina – which may allow organisms to ascend.

Smoking. Smoking is also noted to be associated with an increased risk of PID.

Treatment of acute PID

This illness is polymicrobial in nature and thus requires the use of broad-spectrum antibiotics. With 60% of cases due to *Chlamydia trachomatis* or *Neisseria gonorrhoeae* it seems prudent to base treatment around coverage of these organisms. A single oral dose of azithromycin and a course of metronidazole should be given. In the unwell patient the addition of cefuroxime or gentamicin will be necessary. In those with excessive vomiting, intravenous fluids will also be helpful.

Treatment regimes should include treatment of the sexual partner(s) as more than 50% will have evidence of genital tract infection. Contact tracing is thus important and it may be wise to call on the services of the genitourinary medicine team who have this facility set up already.

If after 48 hours of antibiotic therapy there is no improvement in the patient's condition, laparoscopy can be considered to exclude the possibility of a developing pelvic abscess, which would require surgical incision and drainage. Recurrent episodes of acute PID are associated with increasing chance of tubal blockage – after one episode 17%, two episodes 35% and three episodes 70%.

Chronic PID

This follows inadequately treated acute PID or may follow cases where low-grade symptoms mean the patient did not seek help. It can also occur even with good treatment of the first infection in the presence of tubal damage or reinfection with *Streptococcus*, *Staphylococcus*, anaerobes or *Actinomyces*. Inflammation leads to fibrosis and adhesions develop between pelvic organs with, in severe cases, obliteration of the pelvis with a matted mass of bowel loops above the pelvic organs.

The tubes may be distended with pus (pyosalpinx) or fluid (hydrosalpinx, Fig. 2). They become distorted and form a characteristic retort shape round the ovary. The function of the tube in transporting eggs and sperm is disrupted, leading to infertility. The management of pain may require frequent hospital admissions. Treatment of the infectious cause is often unsatisfactory as scarring means an inadequate blood supply with poor delivery of antibiotics to the affected area. Surgical clearance of the pelvis may be the final step in a long line of treatments – there is a 10-fold increase in hysterectomy rates following PID and 7–10-fold increased rate of ectopic pregnancy.

Presentation and diagnosis

Pelvic pain may be associated with menstruation (secondary dysmenorrhoea), deep dyspareunia, or be present constantly with disruption of lifestyle. Heavier menstrual loss is seen which may be due to increased blood flow to the uterus associated with infection or may result from interference with the function of the spiral arterioles which normally control volume of blood loss.
Vaginal discharge is usually minimal in chronic cases but may be increased and offensive.

Infertility may be noted in a patient who has had numerous

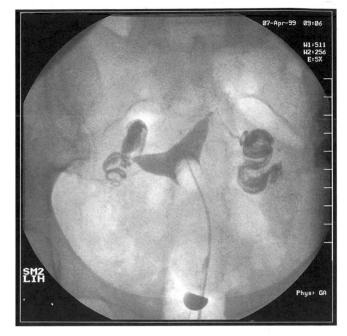

Fig. 2 **Bilateral hydrosalpinges on hysterosalpingography.**

treatments for PID or the findings at laparoscopy during fertility investigations may be consistent with a diagnosis of PID. If investigation of infertility includes hysterosalpingography (Fig. 2) there may be a flare-up in cases due to chronic PID.

The definitive test is laparoscopy when pelvic adhesions may be seen. Culture of organisms from fluid obtained from the pouch of Douglas is more likely to direct antibiotic prescribing correctly but is frequently unhelpful.

Treatment

Analgesia in increasing strengths may be necessary to control pain. Antidepressant medication may potentiate the effect of analgesics, and short-wave diathermy may have a role. If a desire for fertility is not a consideration then removal of infected tissue may be the only way to get pain relief. This may involve total abdominal hysterectomy with bilateral salpingo-oophorectomy as leaving the ovaries behind at hysterectomy results in continuing pain in a number of patients. Resolution of symptoms is usual after the menopause though it may be unrealistic to expect the patient to wait until this stage.

If menstrual problems predominate and are not amenable to non-steroidal anti-inflammatory therapy or antifibrinolytics then hysterectomy may be necessary.

For treatment of infertility see page 132.

Pelvic inflammatory disease

- Early and vigorous treatment of acute PID should decrease the incidence of secondary complications.

- Triple swabs are frequently negative.

- Antibiotics should be broad-spectrum and cover *N. gonorrhoeae*, *C. trachomatis* and anaerobes.

- Infections are usually sexually transmitted and contact tracing is an essential part of therapy.

- Chronic pain management may require hysterectomy with bilateral salpingo-oophorectomy

Genital infections

Introduction

The World Health Organization (WHO) estimated that, in 1995, there were over 333 million cases of curable sexually transmitted infections (STIs) in adults aged 15 to 49 throughout the world. Many of the STIs can cause long-term morbidity, particularly in females. Untreated, some infections can lead to infertility or cause miscarriage, premature birth, or infection of the newborn. Prompt diagnosis and appropriate management are crucial in reducing these complications. This may be difficult as some infections, for example, for example *Chlamydia trachomatis*, are often asymptomatic until complications arise.

Certain demographic features increase the likelihood of someone having an STI. There are:

- age under 25 years
- lack of barrier contraception use
- being single, separated or divorced
- having an occupation involving staying away from home.

Women undergoing termination of pregnancy and those with an infection such as genital warts are at increased risk of STIs. In reality, these factors are surrogate markers of sexual activity and rates of partner change, as it is these factors mainly that determine the risk of transmission and acquisition of an STI. To be able accurately to assess someone's risk of having an STI, therefore, it is necessary to take a good sexual history.

History

A good history should be taken in a relaxed, communicative and non-judgmental way with reassurances about confidentiality. Choice of words, appropriate facial expressions and appropriate body language by the questioner are extremely important. There is never a 'routine' way to take a history, but the questions will need to cover:

- Symptoms
  - vaginal discharge – is it offensive (vaginosis) or does it cause irritation (candida)?
  - dysuria – suggestive of gonorrhoea or chlamydial infection
  - genital ulcers – timing, prodromal symptoms (e.g. before herpes), painful (also genital herpes)
  - abdominal pain or dyspareunia – suggestive of pelvic inflammatory disease (PID) (see p. 100)
- The place and time of recent sexual contacts
- Whether the contact was penile–vaginal, or anal, or oral
- Sexual orientation and whether the contacts were with a man or a woman
- Foreign travel and sexual contact
- Contraceptive precautions, and the requirement for postcoital contraception
- Risk factors for HIV, especially:
  - unprotected sexual activity with others at high risk for HIV, or in areas of the world where HIV is endemic
  - injected drug misuse by the patient or partner
- A gynaecological history to exclude the possibility of pregnancy and to check cervical smear test results.

Physical examination

The skin and mouth should be examined and the abdomen palpated looking especially for tenderness (PID) or for evidence of lymphadenopathy. The external genitalia should be examined for skin lesions, particularly genital warts, genital herpes and ulceration. The commonest cause of genital ulceration in the UK is herpes; syphilis is rare. The urethra should be inspected for inflammation urethritis. Where appropriate, the anal area needs to be inspected.

On speculum examination, the posterior fornix should be inspected for discharge, and the cervix examined for discharge, ulceration, bleeding, polyps, tumours or the threads of an intrauterine contraceptive device. A bimanual pelvic examination should also be performed to detect tenderness of the cervix or adenexa.

Swabs should be taken from the urethra, vagina and endocervix. Although chlamydia is readily identified from appropriate endocervical swabs, the ligand chain reaction (LCR) or the polymerase chain reaction (PCR) testing of urine is also an extremely sensitive test. Immediate microscopy of vaginal swabs can detect yeasts, *Trichomonas vaginalis* and 'clue cells' – vaginal epithelial cells covered with large numbers of Gram-positive and Gram-variable bacilli, characteristic of *Gardnerella vaginalis*. Measurement of vaginal pH may be useful. It is normally ≤ 4.5 but will be > 4.5 in bacterial vaginosis and trichomonal infection.

(See also HIV infection, p. 16.)

With the possible exception of PID, genital infections are best managed in an STD clinic with facilities for counselling, contact tracing and on-site Gram staining and microscopy.

Actinomycosis

Actinomyces are Gram-positive bacteria which only rarely cause salpingitis (often unilateral, more often on the right), chronic tubo-ovarian abscesses and fistulae. Actinomycosis may occur secondary to appendicitis or with use of an intrauterine contraceptive device (IUCD). It is not sexually transmitted and is treated with long-term high-dose oral or parenteral penicillin.

Bacterial vaginosis

This is very common and occurs when lactobacilli are replaced by anaerobes, particularly *Bacteroides* species (Fig. 1). It is not sexually transmitted and many women are asymptomatic, but it can cause an offensive green or grey discharge (the pH is raised to ≈ 5.5 and bacterial metabolites produce volatile amines with a 'fishy' odour), particularly after intercourse. On

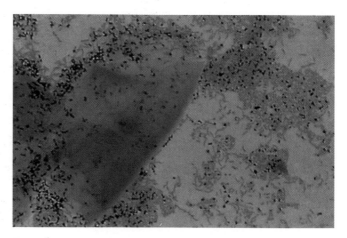

Fig. 1 **Gram-stained smear of bacterial vaginosis.**

wet microscopy, there are 'clue' cells (see above). If symptomatic, it is treated with oral or vaginal metronidazole or with vaginal clindamycin cream (if the woman is pregnant, ampicillin may be more appropriate). There is no benefit in treating the partner or in using condoms.

Bacteroides spp.

These are commensals but may cause a vaginal discharge (see 'Bacterial vaginosis', above) or complicate pre-existing PID (leading to chronic infection). They are not sexually transmitted. Treatment is with metronidazole or with clindamycin cream.

Candida or thrush (*Candida albicans*)

This presents with a whitish discharge and pruritus and is not sexually transmitted (Fig. 2). The vulva and vagina may be fissured and painful. It occurs more commonly in the sexually active, the pregnant, the immunocompromised, the diabetic and after antibiotic treatment. The combined oral contraceptive (COC) probably makes no difference. Microscopy reveals yeasts and pseudohyphae, and a high vaginal swab may be cultured on Sabouraud's medium. Treatment is with clotrimazole (e.g. Canesten) pessaries and cream. Oral fluconazole (Diflucan) given immediately is also effective, but may have systemic side effects, and should not be used in pregnancy. If proven infection is recurrent, there is no benefit from treating the partner.

Prophylactic treatment, however, may be of benefit, e.g. if the patient's symptoms are particularly troublesome premenstrually, a single pessary may be inserted midcycle. Alternatively, a weekly pessary may be used. Natural yoghurt on a tampon for 3 nights, acetic acid jelly, wiping the anus front to back, and cotton underwear may also be of help.

Chlamydia

This is the commonest bacterial sexually transmitted infection in the UK (0.5–15% depending on the sample selected), and is a much commoner cause of infection than the gonococcus (*Neisseria gonorrhoeae*). In the female it is often asymptomatic, but may cause PID, bartholinitis, spontaneous abortion, premature labour, neonatal conjunctivitis (5–14 days postnatally, Fig. 3) and neonatal pneumonia. PID with associated perihepatitis is known as the Fitz-Hugh–Curtis syndrome (Fig. 4). Reiter's syndrome (arthritis, mucosal ulceration and conjunctival

symptoms) is very rare in women. In the male, *C. trachomatis* infection may cause urethral discharge, dysuria, epididymo-orchitis and Reiter's syndrome. Diagnosis in the female is by endocervical swabs, urethral swabs or first-void urine sent in a specific transport medium for investigation via the LCR or the PCR. Uncomplicated infection may be treated with an immediate oral dose of azithromycin or with doxycycline for 7–10 days or erythromycin for 7–10 days. Increased doses plus the addition of metronidazole are employed for complicated infection. Contact tracing is important and individuals should avoid unprotected intercourse for 2 weeks.

The main concern with chlamydial PID is its association with tubal damage and infertility. As infections may be subclinical, it has been suggested that at-risk groups should be screened – particularly as this can now be achieved simply through LCR/PCR testing of urine. Those at greatest risk are those aged < 25 years, particularly those with

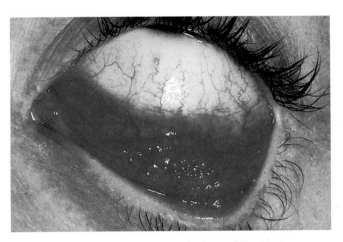

Fig. 3 **Chlamydial conjunctivitis occurs in 50% of neonates born to an infected mother.**

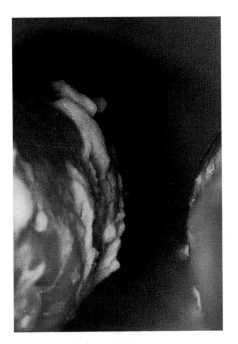

Fig. 2 **Candidal vaginitis.**

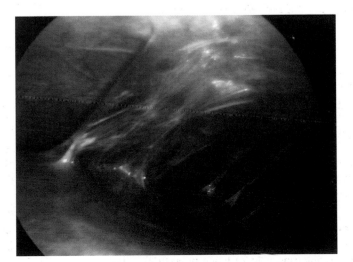

Fig. 4 **Fitz-Hugh–Curtis syndrome.**

two or more sexual partners in the preceding year or who are presenting with a request for termination of a pregnancy. It has also been argued that all women under 25 years old should be regularly screened.

Genital warts (Fig. 5)

These are usually caused by human papilloma virus (HPV) types 6 and 11, though types 16 and 18 are occasionally implicated. Most patients with genital HPV have no visible warts but the virus can be transmitted to sexual partners who may then develop visible lesions. Twenty-five per cent of those with warts have other demonstrable STIs. Podophyllin paint can be applied weekly to the non-pregnant patient by medical staff, with advice to wash the solution off 6 hours later. Self-treatment is also available with podophyllotoxin solution – this is applied twice a day for 3 days, and the treatment repeated on a weekly cycle for four cycles. For patients with multiple or large warts, treatment with cryotherapy using liquid nitrogen, or laser treatment, or diathermy under general anaesthetic is appropriate. Annual cervical screening is not required but those with visible cervical warts or abnormal cytology should be colposcoped.

Gonorrhoea (*Neisseria gonorrhoeae*)

The incubation period is 2–5 days for men. The vast majority of women are asymptomatic but infection may cause PID (often at the time of menstruation),

urethritis, polyarthralgia, miscarriage, premature labour and neonatal ophthalmia (2–7 days postnatally). Most men have symptoms of urethritis and penile discharge (Fig. 6). Swabs should be taken from the urethra and cervix and placed in Amies transport medium. A Gram stain of an endocervical swab shows Gram-negative intracellular diplococci in only 50% so that definitive diagnosis is by culture on NYC (New York City) medium. Treatment is with ampicillin orally stat. together with probenecid. Ciprofloxacin orally stat. is used in penicillin allergy and for infections acquired in regions where resistance is common.

Herpes (herpes simplex virus, HSV)

This infection classically occurs secondary to the sexually transmitted Type II virus, but infection with Type I from cold sores is increasingly common. The incubation is 2–14 days with itch and dysuria prominent early symptoms. The vulva becomes ulcerated (Fig. 7) and exquisitely painful and, in the first attack (which may last 3–4 weeks), there may be systemic flu-like symptoms with or without secondary bacterial infection. Autoinoculation to fingers and eyes can occur and there may be a sacral radiculopathy giving a self-limiting paraesthesia to the buttocks and thighs. Only very rarely is there an associated meningitis or encephalitis. Strong oral or intramuscular analgesia and advice to micturate while in the bath may be of help (lidocaine (lignocaine) gel is

painful to apply and may lead to hypersensitivity reactions). Aciclovir orally shortens the duration of symptoms and lessens infectivity (famciclovir and valiciclovir are alternatives). Recurrent infections are shorter (lasting 5–10 days) and usually less severe. Ninety-five per cent of Type II and 5% of Type I infections recur in the first year. Aciclovir cream should be used at the start of subsequent infections. Prophylactic oral aciclovir should be reserved for those with frequent incapacitating infections (e.g. > 10/year) and should be continued for at least 12 months. There is no necessity for annual cervical cytology. (See p. 15 for 'infections in pregnancy'.)

Syphilis (*Treponema pallidum*) (Table 1)

A primary chancre (raised, round, indurated usually painless ulcer; Fig. 8) resolves in 3–8 weeks and may be followed by secondary fever, headaches, bone and joint pain, generalized rash, flat papules known as condylomata lata and generalized painless lymphadenopathy. Following the latent phase, there may be tertiary gummas (Fig. 9) or quaternary neurological and cardiovascular disease. Congenital syphilis may lead to intrauterine death or midtrimester loss. Survivors may be premature, have intrauterine growth restriction, and failure to thrive as well as bone, joint, liver and kidney disease. The diagnosis is made serologically, with most laboratories using the Venereal Disease Research Laboratory

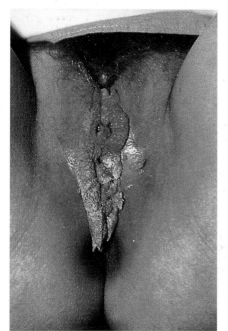

Fig. 5 **Extensive vulval warts.**

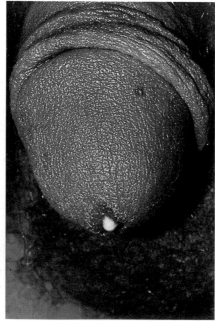

Fig. 6 **Gonococcal urethritis in a male – most women are asymptomatic.**

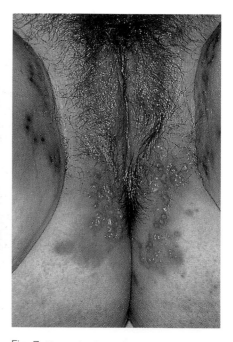

Fig. 7 **Herpetic ulceration of the vulva.**

Table 1 **Syphilis**

Stage	Timing	Features
Primary	Usually 14–28 days from contact	Chancre
Secondary	Approx. 6 weeks after chancre	Rash, condylomata lata, lymphadenopathy
Tertiary	More than 10 years after infection	Gumma in skin, mucous membranes, long bones
Quatenary	Late	Cardiovascular and neurosyphilis

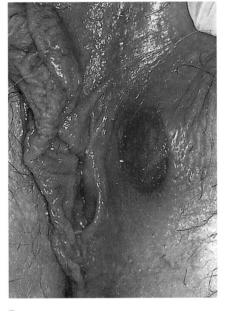

Fig. 8 **Vulval chancre.**

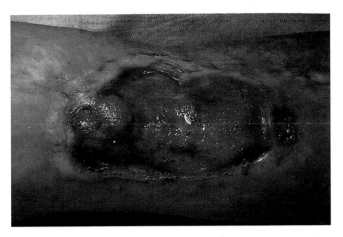

Fig. 9 **Gumma of the leg.** 'Punched-out' ulcers classically occur in the leg, scalp and sternoclavicular area.

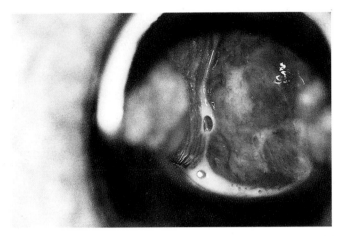

Fig. 10 **Trichomonal vaginitis.** Note that the classical 'frothy yellow' discharge is found in only a third of cases.

(VDRL), *T. pallidum* haemagglutination (TPHA) and fluorescent treponemal antibody (FTA) tests. Many laboratories now screen with an anti-treponemal IgG enzyme-linked immunosorbent assay (ELISA) that is highly sensitive but does give false-positive results. True positives are confirmed by the more traditional tests. Treatment is with procaine benzylpenicillin (procaine penicillin) i.m. for 10–21 days depending on the stage of the disease.

Trichomonas vaginalis

This is usually sexually transmitted. There is a foul-smelling, purulent vaginal discharge with accompanying symptoms of dysuria and vulval soreness (Fig. 10). Diagnosis is by identification of the flagellate organism on a wet film. Treatment is with metronidazole as for bacterial vaginosis.

Vaginal discharge

History

Physiological vaginal discharge changes throughout the reproductive life, increasing as the oestrogen level increases (e.g. at puberty, in pregnancy or with the COC). An itchy discharge suggests *Candida*, an offensive one a foreign body, *Trichomonas vaginalis* or bacterial vaginosis. Ask whether there is pain or fever (PID causes abdominal pain, HSV causes vulval pain). A sexual history should also be obtained.

Management

Perform a speculum examination to see whether the discharge is vaginal or cervical.

- If the history is one of pruritus vulvae, the patient is well and the discharge is white, prescribe antifungal preparations (swabs for culture are optional). See 'Candida' above.
- The treatment of bacterial vaginosis is described above.
- If there is no response to the above, or there are concerns about STIs, or there is an endocervical discharge, swabs should be taken for *N. gonorrhoeae* and *C. trachomatis* (or first-pass urine for PCR/LCR if available) and a fresh wet smear examined for *Trichomonas vaginalis*.
- If there has been no response to the above measures and there are no identifiable organisms, it is worth formally calling a halt to investigations and reviewing the original history. Discussion about the changing nature of a physiological discharge and reassurance about the absence of infection is often reassuring. Treating a cervical ectropion to cure vaginal discharge is frequently unrewarding. Topical or systemic oestrogen treatment for recurrent vaginal infections may be of help in atrophic vaginitis (e.g. postmenopausally or in those on depot progestogens).

Genital infections

- *Chlamydia* and gonococcal infections are often asymptomatic in the female, but may cause tubal damage and infertility.
- Active herpes simplex virus infection may lead to serious neonatal infection.
- Contact tracing is very important.

Oestrogen-dependent hormonal contraception

The combined oral contraceptive pill is still the commonest form of contraception used in the UK, and is highly effective, with a failure rate of 0.1 per 100 woman-years (i.e. if 100 women took the pill for 1 year, one woman would conceive).

The combined oral contraceptive pill (the 'pill')

The pill is a combination of synthetic oestrogen and progestogen (synthetic progesterone). The main oestrogen is ethinylestradiol, although mestranol is used in two products. The progestogens are all C19 nor-testosterone derivatives, apart from cyproterone acetate (used in Dianette) which is a pregnane-type anti-androgen. The majority of pills contain second generation progestogens.

More recent pills contain third generation progestogens. The latter display higher binding affinity for progesterone than for androgen receptors, and therefore produce fewer side effects, e.g. acne, weight gain and premenstrual tension. They have better carbohydrate and lipid metabolism profiles and, despite recent controversy, probably have no increased risk of venous thromboembolism compared to their second generation counterparts.

Most contraceptive pill packets (Fig. 1) contain 21 tablets, allowing 7 pill-free days for the withdrawal bleed. 'Everyday' packs including seven dummy pills are available. This may enhance compliance in certain groups, e.g. adolescents.

- The monophasic pills contain the same dose of oestrogen and progestogen in all 21 tablets.
- Biphasic pills maintain the same dose of oestrogen, but vary the progestogen so that there is a lower dose in the first half as compared to the second half of the cycle.

Table 1 Benefits of combined pill use		
Menstrual related	**Protective effect for**	**General**
■ Regular cycles	■ Ovarian cysts	■ Reduction in acne
■ Reduction of blood loss	■ Ovarian cancer	■ Reduction in hirsutism
■ Less anaemia	■ Endometriosis	(in certain circumstances)
■ Reduction of dysmenorrhoea	■ Endometrial cancer	■ Reduction in anxiety
■ Control of premenstrual syndrome	■ Benign breast disease	(reliable contraception)
	■ Pelvic inflammatory disease	■ Seizure control improves with a steady
	■ ? Rheumatoid arthritis	hormonal environment

- In triphasic contraceptive tablets the dose of oestrogen varies slightly to mimic the mid-cycle surge and there are three phases of progestogen doses.

When prescribing the oral contraceptive pill consider:

- benefits (Table 1)
- disadvantages (Table 2)
- risk factors or contraindications to pill prescribing
- any concurrent therapy that might interact with the pill
- whether or not the individual will be a reliable pill taker
- whether or not she might exhibit oestrogen or progestogen sensitivity.

Absolute and relative contraindications

The ideal pill user is fit, thin, and a non-smoker with no personal or family history of venous thromboembolism. This ideal category may be allowed to continue to take a low-dose third generation progestogen pill until the menopause. Contraindications include the following:

- cigarette smokers – advised to stop the pill at age 35
- previously existing hypertension, obesity and diabetes mellitus (in the presence of other risk factors, diabetes is a contraindication, especially if there is evidence of microvascular disease, or if there is retinopathy or nephropathy)
- as sickle cell disease is associated

with thrombotic episodes the pill is contraindicated in homozygotes (heterozygous carriers may use the pill)

- coronary artery disease, cardiomyopathy and pulmonary hypertension are all absolute contraindicators to the pill due to an increased risk of myocardial infarction
- inflammatory diseases are relative contraindications (ulcerative colitis and Crohn's disease)
- focal, crescendo and severe migraine requiring ergot treatment are contraindications because the vasoconstriction associated may add to the thrombotic risk of the pill. Some women, however, have so-called menstrual migraines and these improve if the cycles are ablated by running three packets of the pill together before having a withdrawal bleed, i.e. tricycling.

Breast disease and the pill

Controversy surrounds the issue of breast disease. The use of the contraceptive pill appears to reduce the incidence of benign breast disease (Table 1). The incidence of breast cancer is slightly higher in women who began taking the pill before the age of 20. Against this the benefits of the pill must be considered.

Practical prescribing

The current advice is to start the contraceptive pill on the first day of a period. This provides immediate contraception. It is important to link taking the pill with an everyday activity to reduce the likelihood of the pill being forgotten As there are seven pill-free days each packet is always started on the same day of the week. New patient guidelines have been issued for cases of missed pills (Table 3).

Drug interactions

Although anticonvulsants can reduce the contraceptive effect of the pill (Table 4), seizure control is improved

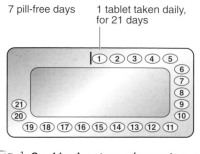

7 pill-free days   1 tablet taken daily, for 21 days

Fig. 1 **Combined oestrogen/progestogen pill.**

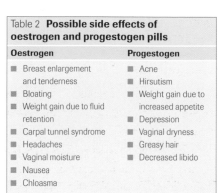

Table 2 Possible side effects of oestrogen and progestogen pills	
Oestrogen	**Progestogen**
■ Breast enlargement and tenderness	■ Acne
	■ Hirsutism
■ Bloating	■ Weight gain due to increased appetite
■ Weight gain due to fluid retention	■ Depression
■ Carpal tunnel syndrome	■ Vaginal dryness
■ Headaches	■ Greasy hair
■ Vaginal moisture	■ Decreased libido
■ Nausea	
■ Chloasma	

Table 3 Advice to be given to women who miss the combined contraceptive pill

Omission	Advice
For single pill omissions of less than 12 hours	Take the pill immediately and further pills as usual
For one, or more, pill omissions, more than 12 hours late:	
– in week 1 of pill packet	■ Take the pill immediately ■ Continue the packet as usual ■ If intercourse has not occurred for 7 days – use sheath in addition for 6 days ■ If intercourse has occurred – see a doctor (consider emergency contraception)
– in week 2 of pill packet	■ Take the last pill immediately ■ Continue with the packet as usual ■ If four, or more, pills are missed – use sheath for 7 days as well
– in week 3 of pill packet	■ Take the pill immediately ■ Continue with the packet as usual ■ At the end of the packet continue with the next packet *without* a break. (breakthrough bleeding may occur)

After Korver. T et al. 1995. Br J. Obstet. Gynaecol. 102: 601–7.

Table 4 Drug interactions with the combined contraceptive pill

Drug category	Example	Drug effect	Notes
Drug interactions that may lead to contraceptive failure			
■ Broad-spectrum antibiotics	Ampicillin, tetracycline, cephalosporins (? erythromycins)	Disturb bowel flora and affect absorption	–
■ Rifampicin	–	Potent enzyme inducer (even brief exposure can interfere with contraceptive cover for 1 month)	Used to treat tuberculosis, but more commonly encountered as prophylaxis following meningococcus exposure
■ Antifungal agents	Griseofulvin (? oral imidazoles, fluconazole, ketoconazole, itraconazole)		Anecdotal reports of pill failure with oral imidazoles
■ Anticonvulsants	Barbiturates, phenytoin, primidone, carbamazepine	Enzyme-inducing agents	The *newer* anticonvulsants are *safe* to use with the pill – sodium valproate, clonazepam, vigabatrin
The contraceptive pill may interfere with drug action:			
■ Antihypertensives	Ace-inhibitors, beta blockers	Oestrogen antagonizes hypotensive effect	–
■ Anticoagulants		Effects antagonized	–
■ Antidepressants		Effects antagonized	–
■ Oral hypoglycaemics		Effects antagonized	–
■ Diuretics		Effects antagonized	–

with a steady hormonal environment. Monophasics are recommended in epileptics. A stronger pill is normally prescribed, often tricycling three packets (to minimize risks from the pill-free week). The pill itself may interact with pre-existing medication.

Surgery and the pill
The pill should be stopped at least 4 weeks before major surgery, and before minor surgery where immobilization follows. For emergency (i.e. unplanned) surgery the pill should be stopped and heparin prophylaxis provided. The pill should be recommenced 2 weeks after full mobilization.

Breast feeding
The pill is contraindicated in breast feeding as it inhibits breast milk production. Women who plan to bottle feed their baby may start the pill 3 weeks after delivery. The relative thromboembolic risk is high in the immediate postpartum period. Most postpartum regimens would advise waiting until the sixth postnatal week (see p. 65).

Emergency contraception
There is still a problem with the under-utilization of emergency contraception due to a lack of awareness. The much used misnomer 'the morning after pill' is confusing:

■ progestogen-only emergency contraception (Levonelle-2) – can be used for up to 72 hours post unprotected intercourse
■ the intrauterine device (a copper coil) – may be fitted up to 5 days after unprotected intercourse.

The Levonelle-2 pill is very effective, preventing four out of five potential pregnancies with few side effects.

Adolescent contraception
Many adolescents are mentally and emotionally unprepared for early sexual experience. There is a risk of unwanted pregnancy, sexually transmitted diseases, pelvic inflammatory disease, and cervical dyskaryosis.

It is important that any service for young people is user-friendly, confidential, approachable and offers a full range of options. The pill is the most popular choice, but other methods including the sheath are frequently used – the latter because it is easy to obtain.

Controversy surrounds treating under 16-year-olds. Since 1985 in the UK there are strict guidelines covering these circumstances, including that the girl fully understands the doctor's advice *and* that the doctor tries to persuade her to inform her parents or guardian – but obviously will respect her confidentiality if she decides she does not wish to do so.

Oestrogen–dependent hormonal contraception

■ The contraceptive pill is the most widely prescribed contraception available with a safety rate of approximately 0.1 per 100 woman-years
■ The major side effects include venous thromboembolism, arterial thrombosis, hypertension and subarachnoid haemorrhage.
■ Antibiotics, antifungal agents, antiepileptics and rifampicin can reduce the pill's contraceptive effect.
■ Progestogen-only emergency contraception may be used for up to 72 hours after unprotected intercourse.
■ Adolescents must be treated as a special category in an approachable and confidential manner.

Progestogen-dependent hormonal contraception

It is in this area that contraception has made the most advances in recent years. Oral, depot and intrauterine treatment modalities are now available with the length of activity ranging from 24 hours to 5 years, allowing the clinician to pick the contraception that is most suitable to the individual woman's needs.

Progestogen-only pill (POP)

The progestogen-only pill contains norethisterone, levonorgestrel or norgestrel. There are three possible modes of action:

- cervical mucus changes
- ovulation either prevented or interrupted (in 60% of cases)
- some antinidatory action on the endometrium (producing an atrophic endometrium).

Some women bleed regularly, 30–50% have irregular bleeding, and the rest become amenorrhoeic. Prolonged amenorrhoea, e.g. for up to 5 years, especially in a woman who smokes, should prompt an assessment of bone mineral density. Being oestrogen free, the POP may be used in certain medical conditions where the combined pill is contraindicated (Table 1).

However, it should still not be prescribed in pregnancy, undiagnosed abnormal vaginal bleeding, severe arterial and ischaemic heart disease and previous ectopic pregnancies. The incidence of ovarian cysts is more common in POP usage. Older users appear to be more at risk.

The failure rate with the POP varies with age. It can be as high as 3.1 per 100 woman-years in women aged 25–29 and drop to 0.3 per 100 woman-years for women over 40 years of age. It is therefore more suitable contraception for the older woman

Table 1 Clinical situations where POP may be useful

- Older women, especially smokers, over the age of 35 years
- Breast-feeding women
- Women who suffer side effects with the combined contraceptive pill (COC)
- Medical conditions which are contraindicated to COC usage, e.g. sickle cell disease, past history of venous thromboembolism
- Migraine sufferers

than for the young teenager. Body mass index also exerts an effect on the failure rate and in the very overweight two tablets per day are advised.

Missed or late pills constitute the biggest cause of POP contraceptive failure, as it *must* be taken within 3 hours of the same time each day. If taken late, other precautions should be taken for the following 7 days.

Pills are usually started on day 1 or 2 of the cycle. Postpartum contraception is usually started on day 21.

Depot progestogen injections

Long-term depot progestogen provides contraception by suppressing ovulation as well as exerting effects on the endometrium and cervical mucus. The injections are highly effective convenient contraceptives which are particularly useful for women who are unable to remember to take the oral contraceptive methods.

The depot progestogens have been widely used in developing countries, and the World Health Organization has a vast body of literature on their efficacy and safety. Depo-Provera, lasting 12 weeks, has been used the longest and more extensively worldwide. Noristerat is active for 8 weeks and frequently used in Germany. They are somewhat under-utilized, however, in the United Kingdom, where they are licensed as 'second choice contraceptive methods, to be used only after counselling'.

Overdue injections pose a risk of contraceptive failure. It is generally thought that 7 days of latitude exist. Longer delays should be followed by emergency contraceptive advice.

Table 2 Disadvantages of the depot progestogen injections

Menstrual cycle disturbance	Initial irregular bleeding
	Eventual amenorrhoea
Weight gain	Often 4–5 lbs
	Commoner in slimmer women
Fertility	Slower return to fertility than with oral methods
	Usually returns by 5 months after last injection
	This may be a deciding factor in some women
Osteoporosis	Conflicting evidence, certainly no noticeable increase in osteoporotic fractures in long-term users
	However, generally, not recommended for women > 45 years
	Amenorrhoea induced by depot could mask the onset of the menopause
General symptoms	Tiredness
	Low mood
	Low libido
	Mastalgia

Although a very safe method of contraception, certain disadvantages have been identified (Table 2).

The Fem-ring

The progestogen-only ring looks similar to a vaginal ring pessary and is 5–6 cm in diameter (Fig. 1).

The Fem-ring releases 20 mg levonorgestrel locally each day, absorbed through the vaginal mucosa. The ring is effective for 3 months.

The main contraceptive activity is to thicken the cervical mucus. There is a failure rate of 3–4 per 100 woman-years. Studies have demonstrated a 7% expulsion rate, mainly related to pelvic wall laxity. Continuation rates are between 50 and 75%. Irregular bleeding has been the most-cited problem. Asymptomatic erythematous vaginal wall patches have been noted.

The Fem-ring offers certain advantages over Depo-Provera, the alternative 3-monthly progestogen contraception:

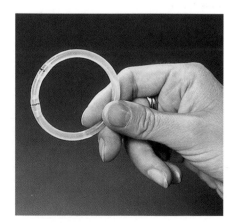

Fig. 1 **The Fem-ring.**

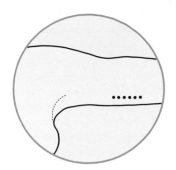

Fig. 2 **Site of insertion.**

- Reversibility
- Much smaller risk of amenorrhoea
- No concern regarding osteoporosis
- No problem with delay in return to fertility.

Progestogen implants

Implanon is the newest progestogen implant pellet (Fig. 2). It is a biodegradable, single flexible rod 4 cm long × 2 mm in diameter. It contains 68 mg etonogestrel, an active metabolite of desogestrel. It is licensed for 3 years and has the same mode of action as Norplant. Being biodegradable, the rod does not require removal. Follow-up is advised 3 months after insertion and every 3–6 months thereafter.

Implants have a low pregnancy rate of 0.2 per 100 continuing users for the first year, with an accumulative pregnancy rate of 3.9 per 100 users over 5 years. On removal or degradation, the contraceptive effect ceases almost immediately.

The majority of women (60–80%) will experience some change in bleeding pattern during the first year. Menstrual irregularities tend to settle with time. Occasionally women complain of headaches, mastalgia, dizziness or hair growth (5–10%).

The levonorgestrel intrauterine system

The levonorgestrel intrauterine system (LNG-IUS), otherwise known as the Mirena coil (Fig. 3), is a major breakthrough in contraception. Not only does it provide reversible contraception, but it is a highly effective device with failure rates lower than those seen with the combined oral contraceptive pill and even sterilization. The failure rate is reported as 1 per 500 woman-years of use. The Mirena is licensed for 5 years' contraceptive cover.

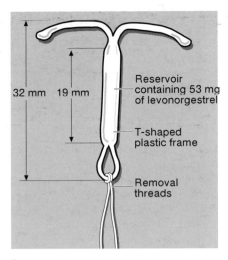

Fig. 3 **The Mirena coil (LNG-IUS).**

There are added benefits to the Mirena coil since the direct action of progestogen on the endometrium is to produce atrophic change:

- menstrual blood loss is dramatically reduced in 70% of cases over the first year (now licensed in the UK for treatment of menorrhagia)
- dysmenorrhoea is greatly reduced
- uterine fibroids are less likely to grow and may indeed shrink
- pelvic infection is uncommon. The LNG-IUS may exert a protective effect
- endometrial hyperplasia and atypia are prevented and in established cases the histology appears to reverse
- there is the potential that the Mirena could provide the progestogen component of a hormone replacement therapy (HRT) regimen in conjunction with systemic oestrogen by providing endometrial protection 'at source' (awaiting licence).

The expulsion rate is low (2–5%), but is most likely to occur in the first few weeks after fitment, if at all.

Difficulties with the Mirena coil

5–10% of women are progestogen sensitive and may exhibit some systemic side effects.

Initially erratic bleeding or spotting may occur for up to 3–4 months in approximately 30% of cases. Very occasionally the problem persists. In most cases the woman will settle into light, regular cycles. Twenty per cent of women become amenorrhoeic by the end of the year, and must be counselled accordingly.

Although expensive, if the cost is divided by its duration of action, i.e. 5 years, then the cost per month is not greatly different from that of other forms of contraception.

The stem is wider than those of most other coils. In consequence some women will require cervical dilatation to allow correct placement of the device with appropriate analgesia.

The Mirena coil is subject to the limitations of fitting any intrauterine device (see p. 111, Table 1). If the uterus is particularly enlarged, or the uterine cavity distorted, by fibroids, then the effect on contraception and menstrual loss may be inadequate.

Contraindications to the use of the Mirena coil are few; the same as those for any other uterine device. Women should be checked 6 weeks following insertion and should be encouraged to check their own threads by vaginal examination after each period.

Progestogen-dependent hormonal contraception

- There are now a considerable number of progestogen-only contraceptive methods available.
- The progestogen-only pill may be used in situations where the combined contraceptive pill is considered unsafe, but must be taken within 3 hours of the same time each day.
- Women rendered amenorrhoeic by the POP may have a marginally increased risk of osteoporosis.
- Depot injections are safe but can produce irregular bleeding, weight gain and a slower return to fertility than oral methods.
- The Fem-ring provides 3 months' contraceptive cover and is more easily reversible than the Depo-Provera injection.
- Implanon is a biodegradable implant lasting 3 years.
- The Mirena coil is effective for 5 years, has both a low failure and expulsion rate and markedly reduces menstrual blood flow and dysmenorrhoea.
- Some women will require analgesia to allow insertion of the Mirena coil.

Non-hormonal methods of contraception

Some women do not want to commit themselves to a hormonal method of contraception. Advances have been made in the types of diaphragm and cap available, with the introduction of the new female condom, and in different types of copper-bearing coil.

Natural methods of family planning

Natural family planning has a high failure rate but is suitable for committed couples in stable relationships who may wish to extend their family. It requires abstinence from penetrative intercourse at the most vulnerable time of the cycle. There are several options available, all of which exploit different methods to identify the fertile period of the cycle. Some women with religious and moral objections to artificial forms of contraception would find this method ideal.

Barrier methods of contraception

The male condom

Most condoms are manufactured from latex, with spermicides incorporated into the lubricant. Hypoallergenic varieties are available. Latex can perish in hot, humid climates and can be damaged by a variety of compounds, including sun tan oils and some vaginal antifungal agents, that lead to loss of tensile strength and potential rupture of the sheath.

The condom is a popular choice amongst young people as it is easily obtainable, but users must be instructed regarding safe application.

There has been a resurgence of interest in the condom recently. Barrier methods protect against STDs including HIV. Evidence exists that adolescent girls are less likely to develop cervical dysplasia (see p. 134). This has led to the introduction of the 'double Dutch' approach to contraception, where teenagers are encouraged to use the combined oral contraceptive pill, which offers the most efficient method of contraception, in conjunction with the condom, which offers the protection of a barrier method.

The female condom (Femidom)

The Femidom was introduced as a barrier method that would be under the woman's control. It is a lubricated polyurethane sleeve sealed at one end (Fig. 1). The Femidom is available over the counter, should be fitted before sexual activity and can remain in place well after ejaculation has occurred. It has been reported that men find that the Femidom allows for more sensation than the male condom.

The diaphragm

Diaphragms stay in place because of the tension of the metal spring in the rim. Therefore the correct choice of size is essential and they should be fitted by a trained clinician. The woman must be taught how to insert and remove the diaphragm and should return for a follow-up appointment to check that she has the correct technique. The diaphragm may be inserted several hours before intercourse. Spermicidal cream or gel should be applied to both sides of the diaphragm as well as around the rim. Extra spermicide should be applied if more than 2 hours have elapsed from the insertion of the diaphragm to when coitus occurs. The diaphragm should not be removed for a minimum of 6 hours after intercourse.

The diaphragm cannot be relied upon in the same way as the condom to protect against sexually transmitted disease.

Caps

Contraceptive caps are occlusive. They rely on suction because of the close application to the vaginal vault or cervix and because of this, they are not susceptible to the vaginal wall expansion that occurs during arousal and orgasm. They do, therefore, prevent sexually transmitted diseases. Unlike diaphragms, they can be left in place for several days, but 24 hours is the recommended length of time. Prolonged use can give rise to offensive discharge.

Chemical methods

Spermicidal agents

Spermicides are generally advised for use as supplements to other methods. They have a mild bactericidal action. The active agent for most products is nonoxynol-9. Spermicides can be manufactured as foam, pessary, cream or gel. Use of spermicides as a sole method of contraception is advisable only in couples with very low fertility, i.e. perimenopausal or oligospermia.

The contraceptive sponge

This is a soft doughnut-shaped device that needs to be lubricated with water and inserted high into the vagina before intercourse takes place. The sponge is a delivery system for spermicide but also acts as a barrier and absorbs the ejaculate. It can be inserted into the vagina up to 24 hours before intercourse and must remain in place for at least 6 hours afterwards. A ribbon attached to the sponge allows removal.

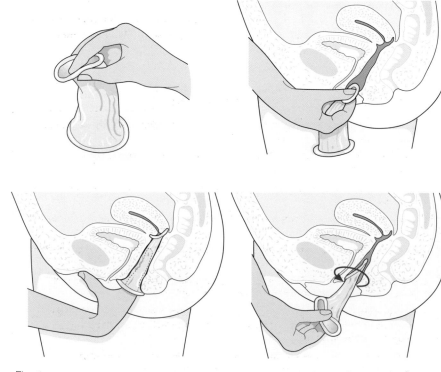

Fig. 1 **The Femidom device.**

Intrauterine contraceptive methods

All coils are copper bearing except the Mirena IUS. The Nova T and the Nova Gard contain both silver and copper. These coils are licensed for 5 years' contraceptive use and have a failure rate of 1–2 per 100 woman-years. A Multiload Cu 250 is licensed for 3 years. There are two third generation copper devices, the Multiload Cu 375 and the Gynae T 380 slimline. The former is licensed for 5 years and the latter for 8 years; both have a failure rate as low as 0.5 per 100 woman-years. Should pregnancy occur, the miscarriage rate is increased.

Problems can be encountered when the coil is fitted (Table 1) which should only be done by a certified practitioner. Fitting in women with a regular cycle can be done from the end of the period up until day 19 of the cycle. Removal should be preceded by either 7 days' abstinence or the use of other contraceptive precautions. Ideally, devices should not be removed after day 19 of a 28-day cycle.

Areas of concern

The copper-bearing coils often produce menorrhagia and dysmenorrhoea. The coil is relatively contraindicated in a history of previous ectopic pregnancy, subfertility, immunosuppression and where infection would be of grave concern, e.g. previous tubal surgery, bacterial endocarditis and the presence of prosthetic heart valves. Fibroids are not a contraindication unless the uterine cavity is distorted.

Previous cervical surgery resulting in stenosis may make insertion difficult and the coil should not be fitted during active pelvic infection.

Actinomyces israelii is more common in women with an IUD.

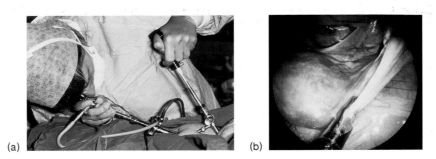

Fig. 2 **Female sterilization. (a)** Operation to apply clips to tubes. **(b)** Clip on tube.

Sterilization

Sterilization offers a permanent method of contraception once the decision has been made that the couple's family is complete. Appropriate counselling is needed, and if there is any ambivalence alternatives should be considered.

Male sterilization

Vasectomy offers several advantages:

- It can be performed under local anaesthetic.
- Significant operative morbidity and mortality are virtually non-existent.
- It is an easy procedure to perform.
- It is certainly cheaper than female sterilization as it does not require such sophisticated operative equipment.
- It usually involves less disruption to family life than female sterilization.
- No inpatient stay is needed.

The man can return to work after 1–3 days depending on whether he is an office or manual worker.

Seminal analysis should be performed at 12 and 16 weeks. Two negative semen analyses are required to confirm that the procedure has been effective. Complications are rare, but scrotal haematomas, wound infection or epididymitis may occur. Sexual activity may be resumed as soon as there is no further discomfort.

Female sterilization

This is a more invasive technique and carries the risks of any laparoscopic procedure. Originally the tubes were diathermied but this increased the risk of postoperative pelvic pain and sometimes caused ovarian dysfunction. Currently, the application of tubal clips is the most common technique (Fig. 2).

The current failure rate stands at 1.5 per 1000. There may be certain situations where a mini laparotomy will be required, e.g. if there are multiple adhesions that block access to the tubes or if the tubes are too thick for the application of the clips with guaranteed occlusion.

Women can be advised that they may return to work within 5–7 days, that tubal ligation is effective at once and that there is no need to continue contraception following the procedure if it is performed immediately postmenstrually. Sterilization does not affect menstruation, but does increase the incidence of tubal pregnancy.

Table 1 **Risks associated with the fitment of an IUD**	
Expulsion	Most often occurs in the first few weeks after fitting
Perforation	Most commonly occurs with inexperienced fitters and when the uterus is retroverted
Pain	Lidocaine (lignocaine) gel may be inserted intracervically Paracervical block Oral analgesia (NSAIDs) or Voltarol suppositories, given prior to fitting
Prolonged vasovagal bradycardia	Have atropine available
Bronchospasm	Have intubation equipment, oxygen and adrenaline (epinephrine) available
Small risk of infection	

Non-hormonal methods of contraception

- There are many approaches to the natural method of family planning. It has a high failure rate and requires considerable commitment
- The sheath is easy to obtain but is often not used correctly by young people. It does have the advantage of reducing sexually transmitted disease.
- The 'double Dutch' technique utilizes the contraceptive pill for safe contraception and the sheath to prevent STDs.
- The diaphragm is easy to use and does not need to be inserted immediately prior to intercourse. It is not particularly effective in preventing STDs.
- The cap is occlusive and is therefore a good barrier method to infection; it can be left in place for several days.
- Spermicidal agents and the contraceptive sponge have higher failure rates and should not be used alone except in perimenopausal women with reduced fertility.
- There are several different types of copper-bearing IUD. They carry a slight risk of infection. The coil should be fitted by a trained certified practitioner and there should always be equipment on hand for the emergency situation.
- Sterilization should be considered as final. Female sterilization carries the risks of any laparoscopy. Male sterilization is under-utilized, and is cheap and safe.

Amenorrhoea

Amenorrhoea can be considered under two categories – physiological (including prepuberty, pregnancy-related and postmenopausal) and pathological (primary and secondary). Disorders which can lead to amenorrhoea are shown in Table 1.

Physiological

Puberty occurs between the age of 10 and 16 years, so amenorrhoea before this is normal and only requires investigation if at age 16 no menstrual loss has been noted. Puberty is associated with a somatic growth spurt, breast budding and pubic hair growth. Menarche (the first period) is within 2 years of breast development. Any obvious causes for not reaching puberty have often been sorted out in childhood so with otherwise normal development it may be expected that menses will arrive. Menarche often follows a familial pattern – if the girl's mother had a late menarche it may be anticipated that this will occur in the patient.

Pregnancy should always be excluded before any investigation for amenorrhoea commences. The postpartum period will be associated with absence of menstrual loss for a variable phase, particularly in association with breast feeding.

The menopause is the last menstrual period and can only be recognized in retrospect, being diagnosed after amenorrhoea for a year. This signifies the end of the reproductive phase of a woman's life and bleeding after this is abnormal, unless she is taking cyclical hormone replacement therapy.

Pathological

Primary amenorrhoea is defined as the failure of any menstrual loss by the age of 16 years. This requires systematic investigation if the correct diagnosis is to be reached and to ensure appropriate management. If secondary sexual characteristics fail to develop it is appropriate to investigate earlier (age 14).

Secondary amenorrhoea is arbitrarily defined as a 6-month absence of menses without any physiological reason.

Investigation of amenorrhoea

Normal secondary sexual development should not preclude chromosomal analysis as Turner's mosaic and testicular feminization are associated with normal secondary sexual characteristics. Measurement of follicle stimulating hormone (FSH), luteinizing hormone (LH), thyroid stimulating hormone (TSH), prolactin, estradiol and testosterone will clarify most other problems. A progestogen challenge test determines whether the endometrium has been exposed to oestrogen and is a more physiological method than measuring estradiol levels. Raised prolactin levels indicate the possibility of a pituitary adenoma, which should be further investigated with appropriate imaging.

Investigations and their interpretation

Blood tests

LH – low level implies no stimulation from the hypothalamus; higher than usual levels may be found in polycystic ovarian syndrome (PCOS), or very high levels suggest ovarian failure.

FSH – low if no stimulation from the hypothalamus; high levels found with ovarian failure.

TSH – raised with hypothyroidism, an easily treatable cause of amenorrhoea.

Prolactin – raised implies a pituitary adenoma; arrange a CT scan.

Testosterone – levels at upper end of female range found in PCOS, levels in male range suggest ectopic production.

Estradiol – low levels need to be interpreted with LH/FSH values as they can be due to no stimulation from the hypothalamus or pituitary, or may suggest ovarian failure.

Progestogen challenge test

Administer a progestogen for 5 days and within 3 days of stopping there will be a withdrawal bleed. This implies that the endometrium has been primed with oestrogen, that the uterus is present and that there is no outflow tract obstruction.

Ultrasound

Ultrasound scanning shows the pelvic organs. Absent uterus may be due to Müllerian failure or testicular feminization (see p. 88). A fluid-filled uterus and vagina implies cryptomenorrhoea (see p. 89). Ovaries showing a dense stroma and more than 10 follicles per field are classical of PCOS (see p. 114).

CT scan of pituitary

Prolactinomas are classified as microadenomas (< 1 cm in diameter) or macroadenomas (Fig. 1).

Management of amenorrhoea

Abnormalities causing amenorrhoea are usually divided into anatomical areas to facilitate both the investigation of the problem and management, which follows logically from the diagnosis.

Asherman's syndrome is caused by scarring of the endometrial cavity and synechiae are seen at hysteroscopy. It may follow over-vigorous surgical curettage or endometrial infection including tuberculosis. After breaking down these adhesions, a coil may be inserted to allow endometrial regrowth.

'*Imperforate hymen*' represents one form of failure of complete canalization of the vagina (see p. 88).

Gonadal dysgenesis occurs with streak gonads and is characterized by an infantile female phenotype from low levels of oestrogen. A karyotype is required to exclude any Y chromosome material necessitating

Table 1 **Disorders leading to amenorrhoea**		
Site of disorder	**Diagnosis**	**Investigations**
Hypothalamus	Hypothalamic hypogonadism (rare)	FSH, LH and estradiol – all low
	Weight-related amenorrhoea (common)	FSH, LH and estradiol – low
Pituitary	Pituitary adenoma (common)	Prolactin – raised, FSH, LH and estradiol – low
	Sheehan's syndrome (rare)	LH, FSH and estradiol – low
Endocrine – thyroid	Hypothyroidism (rare)	TSH – raised, T4 – low or normal
Ovary	Gonadal dysgenesis (rare)	FSH, LH – high, estradiol – low
	Polycystic ovarian syndrome (common)	LH – high, FSH – normal, androgens – high normal
	Premature ovarian failure (rare)	FSH, LH – high, estradiol – low
Müllerian tract	Absence of uterus (rare)	Ultrasound and progesterone challenge
Genital tract	Imperforate hymen (common)	Ultrasound and examination
	Asherman's syndrome or endometrial fibrosis (rare)	HSG and AAFB testing

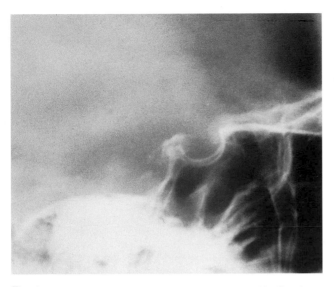

Fig. 1 **CT scan of enlarged pituitary fossa with double-flooring effect.**

gonadectomy. Development of secondary sexual characteristics requires slow introduction of oestrogens. The patient will require long-term hormone replacement therapy and will not become pregnant without oocyte donation.

Testicular feminization presents with amenorrhoea in a phenotypically female patient who has absent uterus and gonads that are testes (see p. 88).

Turner's syndrome (Fig. 2) will usually have been detected sooner but mosaic forms may present at puberty. Short stature, webbed neck, increased carrying angle at the elbow and sexual infantilism is found in XO females, but with Turner's mosaic any combination of normal and abnormal may result. The streak ovaries found in this syndrome are responsible for the low oestrogen levels and lack of sexual development. A karyotype will confirm the diagnosis and management will be dependent on factors such as coexisting cardiac lesions.

In PCOS (*polycystic ovarian syndrome*) fertility can usually be induced with clomifene. Treatment with combined oral contraceptive therapy will result in regular artificial bleeds (see p. 114).

Pituitary adenomas produce high levels of prolactin and may present with amenorrhoea and galactorrhoea. However, in only a third of patients with raised prolactin will there be galactorrhoea and a third of patients with galactorrhoea will have normal menses. The high prolactin level inhibits pulsatile release of gonadotrophin releasing hormone (GnRH) from the hypothalamus but therapy with a dopamine agonist (e.g. bromocriptine, cabergoline) will lower the levels of prolactin in microadenomas enabling ovulation to occur. These block the prolactin receptors and negative feedback reduces prolactin secretion.

Trans-sphenoidal neurosurgery achieves complete resolution of hyperprolactinaemia with resumption of cyclic menses in about 40% of patients with macroadenomas and 80% of patients with microadenomas, but may be associated with cerebrospinal fluid leaks, meningitis or diabetes insipidus which is usually transient. The choice between surgical and medical treatment is not clear-cut but can be simplified – dopamine agonist therapy is used to shrink macroadenomas then reduced to a low maintenance dose which will need to be continued long term. This therapy may be used to shrink the tumour prior to surgery. Some patients will prefer surgery to avoid long-term therapy but long-term dopamine agonists will cause fibrosis, making surgical removal difficult.

Agonist therapy is the treatment of choice in microadenomas but treatment is directed to management of infertility or treating breast discomfort. If the patient with a microadenoma only requires treatment for amenorrhoea and has no wish for fertility, then oestrogen therapy may be preferable.

Sheehan's syndrome is panhypopituitarism and is usually associated with a massive postpartum haemorrhage with concomitant hypotension and inadequate fluid replacement. It is rare. The pituitary blood supply is via end arteries and a dramatic fall in blood pressure may result in necrosis of the gland. After determining which hormonal deficiencies exist replacement therapy will be necessary.

Hypothalamic amenorrhoea accounts for most cases of hypogonadotrophic amenorrhoea and is diagnosed by exclusion of pituitary lesions. Stress, low weight or strenuous exercise are the usual causes and patients will have low gonadotrophins, normal prolactin and will fail to respond to a progestogen challenge. Treatment depends on the patient's requirements – if pregnancy is desired then ovulation induction is appropriate but hormone replacement therapy is the better management of amenorrhoea due to low oestrogen. Stress management may need to be addressed.

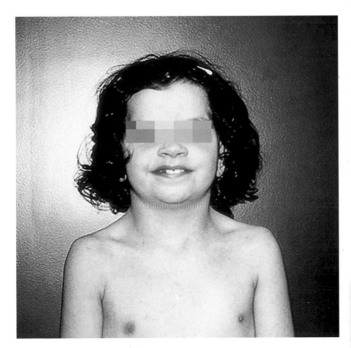

Fig. 2 **Turner's syndrome.**

Amenorrhoea

- Exclude pregnancy before any investigation of amenorrhoea.
- Only use investigations that will confirm or refute a suspected diagnosis; it is inappropriate to do all tests on all patients.
- Follow a logical plan of investigation and the diagnosis will become clear.

Polycystic ovarian syndrome

Polycystic ovarian syndrome (PCOS) is so prevalent as to be a variation of normal – the polycystic appearance has been reported in 20–25% of ultrasound scans in a random population (Fig. 1). The classically enlarged ovaries are due to numerous unruptured follicles which surround a stroma that appears dense and gives a pearl necklace scan picture. The syndrome was first described by Stein and Leventhal in 1935 with obesity, hirsutism, oligomenorrhoea and infertility associated with enlarged ovaries seen at laparotomy. Now we recognize both polycystic ovaries seen on ultrasound scan and the above features with biochemical abnormalities – raised luteinizing hormone (LH) levels and low normal follicle stimulating hormone (FSH), giving a reversal of the LH : FSH ratio, and raised androgen levels – within the normal female range but associated with a higher free androgen index due to lower sex hormone binding globulin (SHBG) (Fig. 2).

Both insulin resistance and hyperinsulinaemia are found in anovulatory patients with PCOS, being more evident in the obese patient. Hyperandrogenaemia is associated with the obesity and hence with higher levels of serum insulin. The hyperandrogenaemia and insulin resistance are associated with a characteristic atherogenic lipid picture. Long term there is an increased risk of cardiovascular disease, non-insulin-dependent diabetes mellitus (NIDDM), endometrial hyperplasia and endometrial and breast carcinoma, though there is no proven link with ovarian tumours.

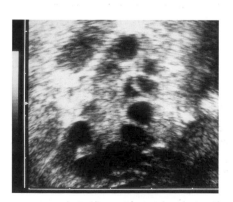

Fig. 1 **Polycystic ovary showing dense stroma and multiple follicles/cysts.**

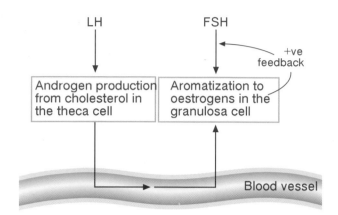

Fig. 2 **Ovarian follicular steroidogenesis.**

The range of presentations is wide, varying from the classical scan picture noted in an asymptomatic patient to the patient with all the symptoms noted below.

Symptoms
- Acne – found in patients whose sebaceous glands respond to the higher free-circulating testosterone
- Hirsutism – in these patients the response to the higher free testosterone is production of terminal hair in a male pattern
- Obesity – the reason for this is unclear but it is responsible for the suppression of SHBG production by the liver, giving higher free levels of testosterone
- Oligomenorrhoea – ovarian dysfunction with irregular ovulation leads to menstrual upset; there is also excessive production of androgens from the ovarian stroma
- Infertility – due to irregular ovulation.

Hirsutism
The extra hair growth that affects some women (Fig. 3) is due to the influence of testosterone on hair follicles in the areas pictured. Lanugo hair is converted to terminal hair in a one-way process. Fine, light, short hair is replaced by thicker, darker, longer hair. Once hirsutism has developed it is thus only possible to ensure no further conversion of lanugo to terminal hair and use oestrogens to make the hair finer, paler and less firmly attached. The genetic influence on hair growth is worth discussing, e.g. the Japanese have less androgen-sensitive hair follicles and thus seldom respond to raised androgen levels by

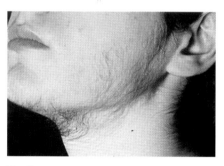

Fig. 3 **Hirsutism.** In this case affecting jawline, upper lip and sideburns. Other areas that may be affected include anterior abdominal wall, inner aspect of upper thighs, circumareolar and upper back.

developing hirsutism. Africans, Asians and Caucasians may become hirsute. In some, the androgen sensitivity affects the sebaceous glands and excess oil production may result in acne with a similar distribution to that illustrated for hair growth.

The active form of testosterone is that which circulates unbound to plasma proteins. Usually 1% is in this form but this is raised in patients with polycystic ovarian syndrome. Oestrogen therapy will raise the level of SHBG and mop up excess testosterone. Weight loss removes the inhibition of SHBG production by the liver.

Seventy per cent of anovulatory females will develop hirsutism.

Investigations
These will be directed towards the possible cause of the problem but need only be few and mainly need to exclude any tumour:

- check LH, FSH and the LH : FSH ratio
- a progestogen challenge test – see page 112

- prolactin – raised levels suggest pituitary adenoma as a cause of amenorrhoea
- thyroid levels – altered values may be associated with menstrual upset
- testosterone – levels in the male range may be found with androgen-secreting tumours
- ultrasound scan may show characteristic appearances with a dense ovarian stroma, more than 10 follicles in a cross-sectional view, increased ovarian volume and thickening of the ovarian capsule.

Treatment

As PCOS is found in a large proportion of the female population, treatment is only required for the patient's symptoms.

Amenorrhoea

Either induce ovulation which will result in regular menstruation (see below), or protect the endometrium against the effects of unopposed oestrogen stimulation by:

- using the oral contraceptive pill which will result in regular menses
- giving progestogens three or four times per year to induce endometrial shedding.

Infertility

These patients pose problems as they are more likely to respond to clomifene therapy with multiple ovulation (in 10%) and are at greater risk of ovarian hyperstimulation syndrome. The importance of monitoring these patients while using ovulation-inducing agents cannot be over-stressed (see p. 133). There is an 80% chance of ovulation using clomifene. In patients resistant to ovulation-induction therapies, the high androgen level within the ovary is thought to be detrimental and may be lowered with a resulting normalization of hormone levels, even if temporarily, by laser drilling of the ovary. Formerly wedge resection of the ovary was used, which would result in removal of some ovarian stroma and a consequent lowering of androgen levels. This would also result in periovarian adhesion formation and so is no longer used.

Metformin has been shown to improve reproductive performance and reduce insulin resistance independent of weight loss.

Hirsutism

The aim is to reduce androgen levels by either turning off ovarian production of androgen or mopping up the free androgen by raising the SHBG level using oestrogen and weight loss (Fig. 4). The oral contraceptive pill can usefully achieve a decreased production of testosterone and raise the SHBG level. Setting out what can be achieved is important so that the patient does not become disheartened.

There are many cosmetic approaches to dealing with the existing hair – plucking, shaving, waxing, electrolysis, laser treatment and using hair removal creams. These will be necessary in conjunction with therapy to prevent further new hair growth such as the antiandrogen cyproterone acetate (CPA) – usually given in combination with oestrogen (as an oral contraceptive pill) to ensure menstrual cycle control. Better results may be achieved initially by giving a larger dose of CPA daily with ethinylestradiol used for the first 10 days of each month. Once new hair growth has been

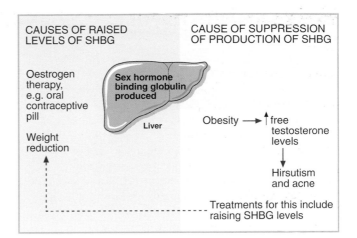

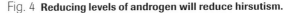

Fig. 4 **Reducing levels of androgen will reduce hirsutism.**

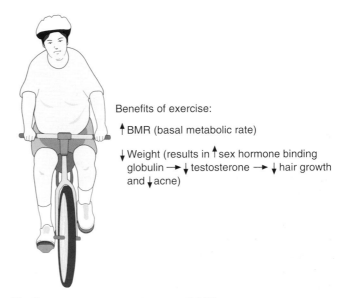

Fig. 5 **The benefits of weight loss in PCOS.**

controlled then it may be appropriate to consider permanent removal of established hair by electrolysis.

Obesity

Weight reduction has many benefits for the patient but usually proves very difficult. Once considerably overweight, patients become less active and their basal metabolic rate (BMR) is reduced, thus they require less calories to maintain their body weight. The resulting frustration for them can mean they become very disheartened with attempts to lose weight – a full explanation before commencing a weight loss programme may avert this problem (Fig. 5).

Polycystic ovarian syndrome

- PCOS affects such a large proportion of the female population as to be a variation of normal.
- There are five main presenting symptoms, though many females may have no symptoms and will be found to have the polycystic appearance on ultrasound scan of their ovaries.
- Treatment is symptomatic as polycystic ovaries are not the primary disorder but a manifestation of a systemic metabolic condition.

Day care surgery

Day surgery has been defined by the UK National Health Service Executive as 'an operational procedure performed on a particular patient who is admitted on a non-residential basis'. In gynaecology 60–70% of cases are now dealt with as outpatient or day care procedures.

Outpatient procedures include colposcopy and cervical treatment modalities (see p. 135), hysteroscopy and endometrial sampling techniques (see p. 125), videocystography (see p. 154), flexible cystoscopy and, in some centres, suction termination of pregnancy (see p. 95) Periurethral injections of bulking agents can also be performed under local anaesthetic in suitable cases.

Day care procedures requiring a light general or spinal anaesthetic routinely include suction termination of pregnancy, laparoscopic sterilization, cystoscopy, diagnostic laparoscopy, laparoscopy with dye insufflation, ovarian drilling, endometrial ablation, transvaginal tape (TVT) and periurethral injections (PUIs) (see p. 155). Cases unsuitable for outpatient procedures (e.g. certain cervical cone biopsies and hysteroscopies with dilatation and curettage) are performed as day cases with a light general anaesthetic.

The setting

The ideal day surgery unit (Fig. 1) should be completely self-contained with its own operating theatre, ward and staff, a consultant director and an experienced nurse manager. Purpose-built units are often built onto the back of existing hospitals to facilitate intercommunication with the main theatre suite and intensive care facilities should complications occur. In other situations they are built as freestanding units, containing several operating theatres, consulting rooms and a medical day unit.

Ambulatory care and diagnostic (ACAD) centre (Figs 2 and 3) developments are substantially larger and include radiology suites, endoscopy units, lecture theatres and outpatient consulting rooms allowing for diagnostic imaging and interventional radiology (e.g. arterial embolectomies) on site. All units should be light, bright and welcoming with good access for the staff and patients. Some hospitals still nurse day surgery patients on general gynaecology wards, converting a 4–6-bedded bay for this purpose. The patients are then cycled through the main theatre suite. Children are usually admitted via the paediatric wards.

Changing surgical practice

Reasons for the increase in gynaecological day surgery are:

- advances in anaesthesia and pain control, particularly the introduction of propofol, which permits sedation and anaesthesia to be tailored to the patient and the procedure
- advances in surgical techniques, especially in endoscopic and laser surgery
- fiscal considerations – day surgery is cost effective if inpatient throughput and bed occupancy are reduced
- patient considerations (Table 1).

Most units run audit programmes where patient satisfaction, efficiency and safety are constantly evaluated.

Preoperative evaluation

For day surgery to be successful and safe there must be adequate preoperative assessment and strict patient selection criteria (Table 2). Problems may potentially arise if there is a long time interval between the outpatient clinic visit and the admission date for surgery, as the presenting complaint may have altered or the general medical condition deteriorated. Most units, therefore, have introduced preoperative assessment sessions where clerking is performed by either

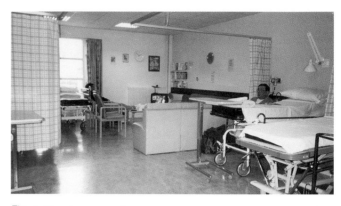

Fig. 1 **The day care unit.**

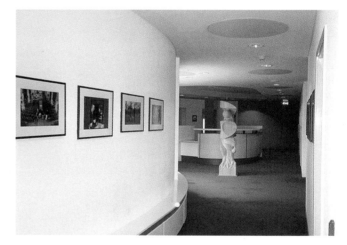

Fig. 2 **Ambulatory care and diagnostic centre.**

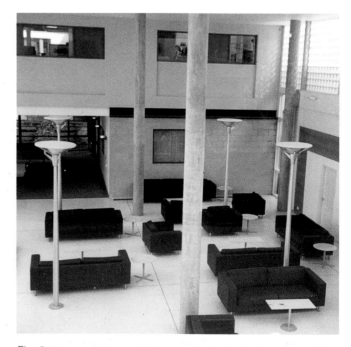

Fig. 3 **Entrance foyer, ambulatory care and diagnostic centre**

Table 1	**Advantages of day care surgery**

- Minimal disruption to patient's personal life
- Earlier return to work or school
- Patients prefer day surgery
- Psychological benefits, especially for children
- Shorter waiting lists for admission
- Reduced incidence of hospital-acquired infection
- Reduced incidence of respiratory complications
- Reduced frequency of medical errors
- Large numbers of patients may be treated
- Cost effective

Table 2	**Preoperative selection guidelines for day care surgical admissions**

Surgical
- Operations lasting less then 1 hour
- Minor and intermediate procedures
- Exclude procedures where severe postoperative pain is likely
- Exclude procedures where significant postoperative bleeding is likely
- Exclude procedures where significant disability is likely, e.g. bilateral varicose veins, bilateral herniae, bilateral Keller's

Social
- Must live within 15 miles or 1 hour's drive of the hospital
- Must not go home by public transport
- Must have responsible fit adult escort home.
- Must be supervised by responsible fit adult for at least 24 hours

Medical
- Patient's age > 6 months and < 70 years
- Obesity – BMI > 30 not accepted to day unit
- ASA class 1 and 2 only
  - ASA 1: a normal healthy individual
  - ASA 2: a patient with mild systemic disease which does not interfere with normal life including mild medical conditions which are well controlled on treatment, e.g. mild hypertension, asthma, osteoarthritis or epilepsy, and also non-insulin-dependent diabetes.

Antiepileptics and antihypertensives should be taken on the day of surgery

Oral hypoglycaemic agents should not be taken on the day of surgery

The American Society of Anesthesiologists (ASA) classification ranks patients in classes 1 to 5. Class 1 is essentially a fit normal individual with only localized pathology requiring treatment. Class 5 is moribund with poor chance of survival.

junior medical staff or trained day care nurse practitioners. Many units have designed specific history proformas to aid clerking and have devised protocols for the assessment and pre-clerking process (Fig. 4).

Investigations are kept to a minimum and are performed at the outpatient appointment with results available on the day of surgery. All patients for therapeutic termination of pregnancy will have their Rhesus status and blood group checked. Patients of West Indian, African and Mediterranean origin will have their sickle cell status tested. In some centres the preoperative anaesthetic assessment is performed in specific outpatient assessment clinics. More usually patients are seen in the day unit on the day of surgery.

The role of the nurse practitioner

The day surgery unit (DSU) nurse represents a new development in the emerging role of the nurse practitioner. Some units will use the assessment nurse solely for information-giving and counselling and have designed excellent patient information leaflets. In other centres the assessment nurse has an independent and well-defined role. Patients will be referred directly from the outpatient clinic and the preoperative clerking will be undertaken by the DSU nurse, who will refer to medical staff only if the selection criteria are not met or there are medical concerns. These nurses will perform phlebotomy and undertake electrocardiograms if required. In America, anaesthetic nurse practitioners are now trained and certified to deliver straightforward general anaesthetics. This concept is being evaluated in the UK.

Postoperative surgical findings are usually discussed with the patient by the medical team but the DSU practitioners will reinforce information and will certainly be involved with counselling regarding contraceptive

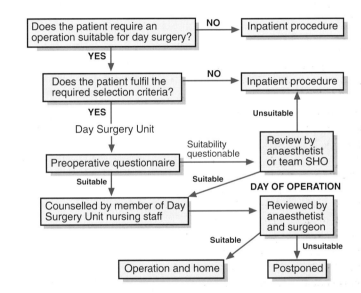

Fig. 4 **Day care patient selection and preparation process.**

issues, hormone replacement therapy or other outpatient prescriptions. They will organize the outpatient follow-up visit, the documentation of the day care episode and the general practitioner (GP) discharge summary. Courses have now been developed between the British Association of Day Surgery (BADS) and the English National Board of Nursing (ENB) to enable training and certification of specialist nurses in this area.

As, in the UK, the model for health-care provision increasingly emphasizes primary care and community settings for services, the day care unit could become an attractive interface between the primary and acute sectors with the possibility of the GP coming in to perform minor operations on his/her own patient.

Day care surgery

- 60–70% of gynaecological surgery is now performed as outpatient or day care procedures.
- Day care surgery is financially effective and has reduced the waiting time for surgery.
- Units are run with strict guidelines and protocols.
- Preoperative assessment is often performed by specialist day unit nurse practitioners.

Uterine fibroids

Correctly known as leiomyomas, fibroids are benign tumours of uterine smooth muscle interlaced with connective tissue which develop within the wall of the uterus causing distortion, and disturbance of menstrual and reproductive function.

Approximately 20% of women of reproductive age have fibroids, commonly presenting later in reproductive years with menstrual problems. Presentation may be earlier following infertility investigations. In Afro-Caribbeans up to 50% of women may have fibroids.

Aetiology

The actual cause of fibroids is unknown although it is appreciated that raised oestrogen levels are associated with increased growth of fibroids. This might explain the association between obesity and the presence of fibroids, as there is peripheral conversion of androgens to oestrogens in adipose tissue. Hormone replacement therapy (HRT) can be given to women with fibroids without adverse effect as the hormone levels achieved from standard HRT are much lower than in pregnancy when fibroids do grow.

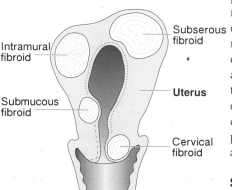

Fig. 1 **Types of fibroids.**

Pathology

Fibroids may be found singly within the uterus, but are more commonly multiple and may vary in size from seedling fibroids to enormous tumours filling the whole pelvic cavity and extending into the abdominal cavity. They often start intramurally (Fig. 1) but as they grow become more predominantly submucosal or subserosal (Table 1). The cut surface has a characteristic whorled appearance where the interlacing of the muscle and fibrous tissue can be clearly seen (Fig. 2). After the menopause fibroids are noted to shrink and regress, presumably due to the withdrawal of oestrogen support. Fibroids can go through a variety of degenerative processes (Table 2).

Presentation

Menorrhagia

Menorrhagia is the common presenting symptom of fibroids and is thought to arise due to the increased surface area of the endometrium which bleeds at the time of menstruation. It may also be due to pressure from the fibroid on venous drainage increasing blood flow. A disturbance of the balance of E and F prostaglandins noted within the menstrual effluent raises the question of whether a disturbance in the metabolism of prostaglandins is a contributory factor or possibly even an aetiological factor. Another theory is that ulceration of endometrium overlying a submucous fibroid may cause haemorrhage. Large fibroids can present with pressure symptoms on adjacent organs (Table 3).

Subfertility

This is a well recognized association, although whether the presence of the

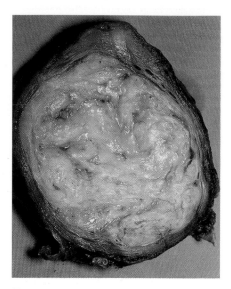

Fig. 2 **Cut surface of a fibroid showing fibrous tissue and whorled appearance.**

fibroids decreases successful implantation resulting in subfertility, or whether it is the lack of pregnancy that predisposes to fibroid growth in later reproductive years is uncertain. In patients with recurrent abortion, fibroids may be responsible due to the mechanical distortion of the endometrial cavity disturbing implantation. Pedunculated fibroids within the uterus may block the cornual region, decreasing fertility.

Investigations

Pelvic examination usually reveals an irregularly enlarged uterus of firm consistency and the presence of fibroids may be confirmed by ultrasound (Fig. 3). Ultrasound will clearly show intramural and submucous fibroids but distinguishing subserous fibroids from the ovary may not be easy.

Submucous and intramural fibroids will show as a filling defect on a hysterosalpingogram. A hysterosalpingogram should be considered for those with infertility to assess tubal function and cavity structure. The presence of fibroids does not necessarily imply a causal relationship to subfertility – they may be coincidental.

Management

Medical

Medical management is appropriate for patients with menorrhagia and small fibroids or for those with subfertility where fibroid size requires some shrinkage. Anti-prostaglandins

Table 1	**Fibroids are predominantly submucosal or subserosal**
Site	**Findings**
Submucosal	These lie under the endometrial lining of the uterus and may cause distortion of the uterine cavity leading to menorrhagia, subfertility and late miscarriage
	If polypoid they may grow from the endometrial lining and appear to develop a stalk. They may then be extruded by the uterus through the cervix causing cramping uterine pain and often heavy bleeding
Subserosal	Predominantly under the outer peritoneal coat of the uterus and may cause distortion of the pelvic anatomy. They grow between the leaves of the broad ligament, down towards the cervix and can make surgery complicated
	Fibroids under the serosal surface of the uterus may grow out on a stalk-like projection – parasitic fibroid, which takes blood supply from elsewhere (commonly the omentum) and becomes detached from the uterus

Table 2	**Fibroid degeneration**
Hyaline degeneration	This occurs due to a process of atrophy with loss of the muscular component and hyaline degeneration within the fibrous tissue element
Cystic degeneration	The centre of the fibroid becomes ischaemic and degenerates, becoming cystic
Calcification	Degeneration may proceed to calcification at a later stage, and therefore tends to be found in older patients. In an extreme form it may be found as 'womb stones', the uterus containing a collection of stony masses
Torsion	Pedunculated fibroids may undergo torsion with pain and haemorrhage into themselves. Rarely this subsequently becomes infected but more commonly would go on to cystic degeneration and possibly calcification
Red degeneration	This is the classic degeneration of a fibroid during pregnancy associated with rapid uterine growth. The cut surface would appear red but the fibroid should not be surgically removed during pregnancy due to a very high risk of haemorrhage. Can be extremely painful requiring analgesia and bed rest
Sarcomatous change	Very rare (< 0.1%) but should be considered if the fibroid is growing rapidly (see p. 139)

Table 3	**Effects of large fibroids on adjacent organs**
Organ	**Symptoms**
Bladder	Frequency, urgency and nocturia
Rectum	Diarrhoea or constipation
Uterus	Cramping abdominal pain due to attempts at extrusion of fibroid polyp
Acute abdominal pain	Torsion or degeneration of fibroid

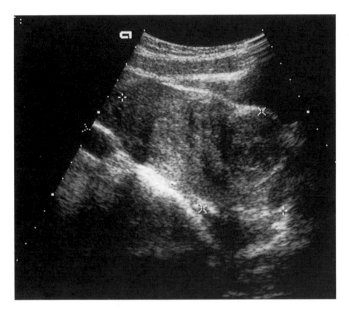

Fig. 3 **Appearance of fibroid uterus on an ultrasound scan.**

incision. Any incision should be placed on the anterior surface of the uterus if possible to avoid adhesions involving the fallopian tubes. It is usual to avoid entering the uterine cavity at operation to avoid intrauterine adhesions which may compromise future fertility or necessitate caesarean section in a future pregnancy due to the presence of a full thickness scar.

Endoscopic removal of fibroids is a possibility but is more commonly used in the treatment of menorrhagia than of subfertility because of the resultant scarring within the uterine cavity. Submucous fibroids may be resected hysteroscopically (Fig. 4) and subserous fibroids approached laparoscopically with removal by morcellation.

Embolization of the blood supply to the fibroid will result in shrinkage but this can be associated with considerable pain.

might be the first approach in menorrhagia and are associated with an 80% reduction in blood loss. Gonadotrophin releasing hormone (GnRH) analogues will cause shrinkage of fibroids, which may be appropriate short term either in the management of subfertility or prior to surgical removal of large fibroids – limiting blood loss at the time of operation and decreasing morbidity. Long-term use is limited by the loss of bone mineral and fibroids will return to the previous size after cessation of treatment.

Surgical

Hysterectomy is the definitive surgical approach for fibroids. A myomectomy is associated with greater morbidity than hysterectomy – so unless fertility needs to be conserved it is not the operation of choice. The patient should be consented for hysterectomy as well as myomectomy as the procedure may prove to be associated with excessive blood loss. Prior shrinkage with GnRH analogues may improve surgical access and lessen bleeding. Multiple incisions on the uterus may be necessary but to limit adhesion formation postoperatively, as many fibroids as possible are removed through a single

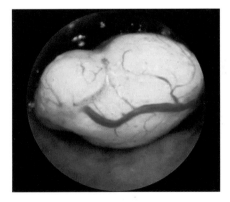

Fig. 4 **A hysteroscopic view shows a fibroid polyp within the uterine cavity.**

Uterine fibroids

- Leiomyomas are found in 20% of women of reproductive age
- Menorrhagia is the main presentation though pressure effects may also be a problem.
- Medical management for menorrhagia may tide a woman over to menopause when natural shrinkage occurs.
- Surgery involves either myomectomy or hysterectomy.

Physiology of menstruation

The physiology of menstruation is closely linked to factors controlling ovulation. If ovulation is regular, so is the menstrual cycle.

The ovulation process

Follicles of all stages of development are found within ovarian stroma. Folliculogenesis takes place in several steps – recruitment and intermediate follicular development. Most follicles are primordial and only a few are recruited into the 'growing' pool, the group designated to develop. This cohort of growing follicles undergoes a process of development and differentiation spanning 85 days, i.e. three ovarian cycles. The recruitment process is probably independent of pituitary control and may depend on paracrine factors. Growing follicles induce changes in surrounding cells, which differentiate into granulosa and theca cells. Only a fraction of these follicles reach a stage of maturation where ovulation is possible, the rest become atretic.

Follicle stimulating hormone (FSH) pushes responsive follicles into the final stages of the growth phase. Luteinizing hormone (LH) binds to the theca cells, stimulating androgen production. FSH binds to granulosa cells activating the aromatase enzyme system, enabling the conversion of androgens to oestrogen (Fig. 1). One dominant follicle responds to the high oestrogen milieu and ripens.

The rising oestrogen level produces a negative feedback on the anterior pituitary to inhibit FSH secretion. FSH levels fall, preventing further follicles ripening, but the dominant follicle continues to grow. Once it reaches maturity, oestrogen levels are sufficient to induce a positive feedback, and a massive discharge of LH occurs. The LH surge, acting through prostaglandins, produces follicular rupture. LH then binds to granulosa cell receptors to stimulate progesterone secretion. The main product of the corpus luteum is progesterone. The lifespan of the corpus luteum is 12 to 14 days. As it degenerates, progesterone levels fall and menstruation occurs.

The secretion of FSH and LH is controlled by luteinizing hormone releasing hormone (LHRH), released by the hypothalamus (Fig. 2). The

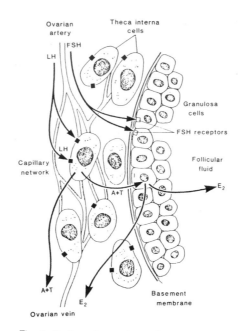

Fig. 1 **Action of gonadotrophins on the theca and granulosa cells of the ovary and the ripening follicle.**

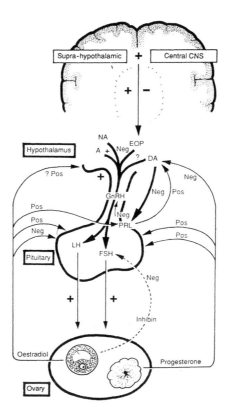

Fig. 2 **Feedback control mechanism in the hypothalamic–pituitary–ovarian axis.**

control of LHRH secretion is highly complex, depending on a number of inhibitory (dopamine) and excitatory (noradrenaline, prostaglandin) neurotransmitters, modulated by ovarian hormones. Ovarian steroids modulate the pattern of gonadotrophin

pulse secretion. The positive feedback of oestrogen and progesterone on gonadotrophin secretion may involve alteration of the sensitivity of the pituitary to LHRH action.

The normal menstrual cycle

Most cycles are between 24 and 32 days in length and the standard normal cycle is considered to be 28 days. Some irregularity occurs at both ends of the reproductive spectrum, i.e. at puberty and at the menopause. Once cycles are established, they are most regular between the ages of 20 and 40 years.

The mean menstrual blood loss in a healthy western woman is approximately 40 ml, 70% of which is lost within the first 48 hours. Within each individual the loss varies very little from one period to the next. There is a considerable variation, however, comparing one woman to another. The upper limit of normal menstruation is taken as 80 ml per menses. Reported menstrual loss can vary between a few ml to several hundred. Menstrual fluid loss contains mucus and endometrial tissue, as well as blood. Uterine contractility is usually greatest in the first 24 to 48 hours of the period. This possibly aids expulsion of degenerating endometrium. Contractility is variable and can produce only a mild discomfort or severe cramping pain (see p. 123).

Mechanisms of blood loss

The uterine wall consists of three layers: the serous coat, which is firmly adherent to the myometrium; the myometrium, which contains smooth muscle fibres and branches of blood vessels and nerves; and finally the endometrium, which consists principally of glandular and stromal cells. The blood supply is via the arcuate and radial arteries (Fig. 3). The radial arteries develop a corkscrew-like appearance as they approach the endometrial surface, at this point called spiral arterioles. These arterioles are sensitive to changing levels of sex hormones. A fall in progesterone results in constriction of the arterioles with ischaemia and shedding of the upper two-thirds of the endometrium. The end arterioles are lost with the glands and the stroma during menstrual shedding.

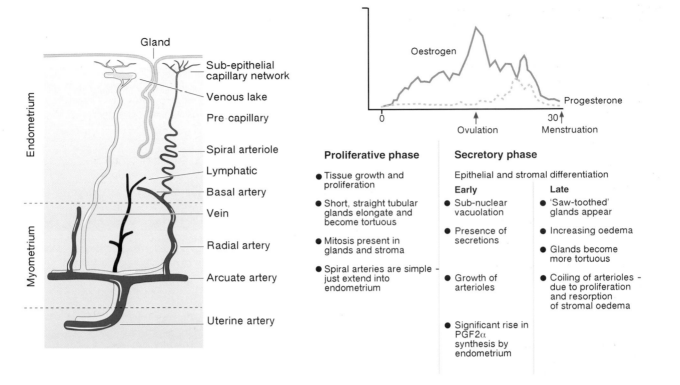

Fig. 3 **Blood supply to the uterus – cyclical changes in structure.**

Control of menstrual blood flow

The factors controlling blood loss include:

- myometrial contractility
- haemostatic plug formation
- vasoconstriction.

Myometrial activity is probably one of the lesser mechanisms since drugs which inhibit contractions, such as prostaglandin synthetase inhibitors, do not increase menstrual blood loss. Menstrual fluid and endometrium have marked fibrinolytic activity (hence antifibrinolytics can be useful in treatment) (see p. 124).

Vasoconstriction is probably the most important mechanism in controlling blood loss. Here the role of prostaglandins is central. Prostaglandin F2 alpha is a potent vasoconstrictor, whereas prostaglandin E2 and prostacyclin lead to vasodilatation. Prostacyclin is a potent inhibitor of platelet aggregation. Inhibitors of prostaglandin synthesis will therefore decrease blood flow to some extent (also dysmenorrhoea secondary to myometrial contractility; see p. 123).

Excessive bleeding may be related to an alteration in the ratio between the vasoconstrictor prostaglandin F2 alpha and the vasodilator prostaglandin E2. There may also be enhanced synthesis of prostacyclin from the myometrium in women with heavier periods, which, by inhibiting platelet aggregation, reduces haemostatic plug formation. As yet we do not understand the cause of the increased synthesis of these vasodilator substances.

Period pains (dysmenorrhoea)

There are several possible aetiological mechanisms causing period pains. Both prostaglandin F2 alpha and E2 are found in higher concentrations in the menstrual fluid of those with dysmenorrhoea. Prostaglandin F2 alpha is a potent oxytoxic and vasoconstrictor and administration to the uterus leads to dysmenorrhoea-like pain. The role of prostaglandin E2 is less clear, but it may work by increasing the sensitivity of nerve endings. An increase in uterine contractility can be demonstrated in women with dysmenorrhoea compared to controls by measuring the intrauterine pressure. This contractility may be associated with a decrease in endometrial blood flow.

Leukotrienes are also produced by the endometrium and increase myometrial contractility. Receptor sites are present in the myometrium. Vasopressin is also a stimulant of the non-pregnant uterus, and it is active at the onset of menstruation. The plasma concentration of vasopressin, which is known to stimulate prostaglandin release, is higher in those suffering with dysmenorrhoea.

Physiology of menstruation

- LHRH controls the secretion of both FSH and LH from the anterior pituitary.
- Ovarian hormones modulate the proportions of gonadotrophic secretion.
- The control of LHRH secretion is highly complex and depends upon inhibitory and excitatory neurotransmitters, again modulated by ovarian hormones.
- The recruitment process promotes some ovarian follicles into the growing pool; this is probably independent of pituitary control.
- FSH controls maturation of the growing follicle, the LH surge produces follicular rupture to allow ovulation.
- Following ovulation a corpus luteal cyst is formed producing progesterone; with falling progesterone levels menstruation occurs.
- The usual menstrual blood loss is approximately 40 ml.
- The interaction between vasodilator and vasoconstrictor prostaglandins controls menstrual flow; an alteration in the ratio of these prostaglandins can produce excessive bleeding and/or pain.

Disorders of menstruation I

This chapter considers menstrual abnormalities – regular and irregular heavy bleeding and painful periods. Disorders of menstruation are common, comprising 21% of gynaecological referrals.

Menorrhagia

This is heavy, regular bleeding defined as a menstrual blood loss greater than 80 ml. Women differ in their subjective reporting – some will describe loss as heavy when it is within normal limits, others cope stoically with excessive flow. A careful assessment should be made enquiring as to the type of protection (pads or tampons) used, the number of changes needed per day, the amount of clots and frequency of accidents (e.g. soiling of clothes or bed linen). A menstrual chart can be helpful (Fig. 1). Menorrhagia can be caused by:

- idiopathic
- fibroids (Fig. 2)
- bleeding disorders

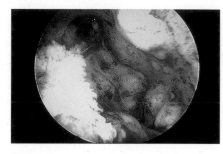

Fig. 2 **Multiple submucous fibroids.**

- intrauterine contraceptive devices (except the Mirena)
- pelvic infection (often heavy and painful menses).

Intermenstrual bleeding

This is bleeding occurring between menses. It may be physiological in origin, related to the sudden rise (and then fall) of oestrogen at ovulation. More often it is associated with cervical or endometrial polyps (Fig. 3), cervical erosions or, occasionally,

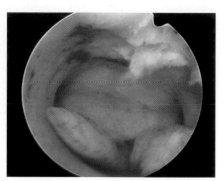

Fig. 3 **Hysteroscopic view of uterine cavity and endometrial polyps.**

Table 1 **Types of dysfunctional uterine bleeding**
Anovulatory
■ Impaired positive feedback, e.g. adolescents
■ Inadequate signal, e.g. polycystic ovaries and premenopause
Ovulatory
■ Inadequate luteal phase
■ Idiopathic

cervical carcinoma or stress. Postcoital bleeding may have similar causes.

Dysfunctional uterine bleeding

Dysfunctional uterine bleeding (DUB) is defined as heavy and often irregular bleeding, which occurs in the absence of any pelvic pathology, pregnancy or bleeding disorder. Both hypo- and hyperthyroidism can cause menstrual irregularity and should be excluded. Dysfunctional bleeding can be both anovulatory and ovulatory (Table 1).

Anovulatory dysfunctional bleeding

In the absence of ovulation, there is inadequate progestogenization of the endometrium, producing abnormalities in the production of prostanoids and steroid receptors. The unopposed oestrogen gives rise to persistent, proliferative or hyperplastic endometrium, resulting in irregular,

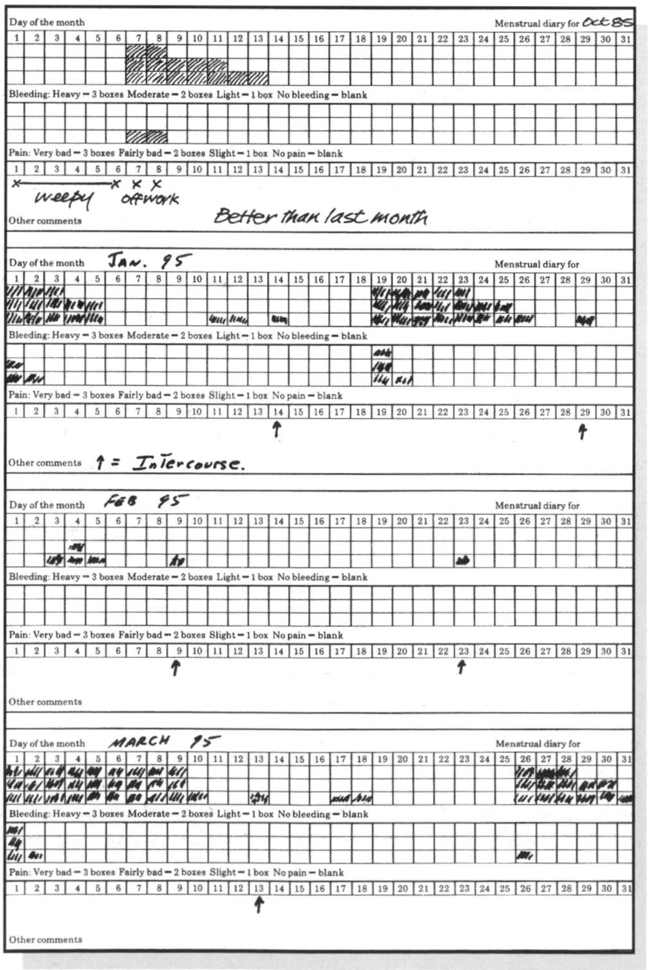

Fig. 1 **A typical example of a menstrual calendar.**

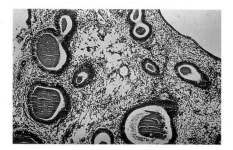

Fig. 4 **The 'Swiss cheese' appearance of the endometrium in metropathia haemorrhagica.**

painless bleeding. An extreme form of this (metropathia haemorrhagica), results in excessive bleeding after long intervals. The endometrium has a classic cystic appearance, often termed a 'Swiss cheese' pattern (Fig. 4).

Impaired positive feedback will cause anovulatory cycles by failing to produce the mid-cycle surge of luteinizing hormone that triggers ovulation. Failure of follicular development will occur in the perimenopausal age group, and in polycystic ovarian syndrome. If follicular development is insufficient there will be an inadequate oestrogen signal. Therefore a luteinizing hormone surge is not induced and ovulation does not occur.

Ovulatory dysfunctional bleeding

A shortened luteal phase arises from inadequate follicular development. Deficient luteal phase will cause irregular bleeding and may be associated with subfertility. The idiopathic category of ovulatory dysfunctional bleeding is probably related to intrinsic prostaglandin imbalance.

Dysmenorrhoea

Dysmenorrhoea can be either primary, with the onset of menarche, or secondary, developing later (Table 2). There may be cramping lower abdominal pains, which often radiate to the back, or down the inner aspect of the thigh. These may be accompanied by faintness or gastrointestinal symptoms, including loose stools or nausea.

Primary dysmenorrhoea

Menstrual symptoms vary widely amongst individuals, but some suffer more severely than others. Primary dysmenorrhoea occurs almost exclusively in ovulatory cycles.

Table 2 **Causes of dysmenorrhoea**	
Primary dysmenorrhoea	**Secondary dysmenorrhoea**
■ Prostaglandin production	■ Idiopathic
■ Increased myometrial contractility	■ Endometriosis
■ Decreased endometrial blood flow	■ Adenomyosis
■ Leukotrienes	■ Pelvic inflammatory disease
■ Vasopressin	■ Pelvic venous congestion
	■ Cervical stenosis
	■ Intrauterine device (IUD)

Table 3 **Treatment of primary dysmenorrhoea**

- ■ Analgesics
  - – e.g. paracetamol
- ■ Non-steroidal anti-inflammatory drugs (NSAIDs)
  - – mefenamic acid (Ponstan)
  - – ibuprofen
  - – naproxen
  - – diclofenac
  (NSAIDs work by direct inhibition of the cyclo-oxygenase system reducing prostaglandin production)
- ■ Combined oral contraceptive pill (COC) (suppresses ovulation)
- ■ Transdermal GTN

Treatment of primary dysmenorrhoea

Simple analgesia is often sufficient. Further treatment is based either on blocking prostaglandin formation with non-steroidal anti-inflammatory drugs (NSAIDs) or by suppressing ovulation (combined oral contraceptive pill) (Table 3). NSAIDs are best started just prior to the onset of menstruation, although timing this is only possible with regular predictable cycles. If symptoms remain debilitating, despite NSAIDs, the pill may be appropriate. This has the additional advantage of providing contraception. A 20 µg preparation may suffice, and recent concerns about the increased risk of venous thromboembolism in third generation progestogen pills seem unfounded. Third generation progestogen pills reduce side effects such as acne and weight gain which

make the pill unpopular amongst adolescents.

Reassurance is essential and it may be appropriate to substitute a transabdominal ultrasound for a vaginal examination in a young girl who is a virgin. Symptoms not uncommonly settle with time, and there is no association with later problems, particularly infertility.

Secondary dysmenorrhoea

This develops after menarche and there may be identifiable underlying pathology (see Table 2). Treatment is dependent on the cause. Investigation may include thorough examination, ultrasound scan and laparoscopy. Although psychological factors are quoted as being involved in both primary and secondary dysmenorrhoea, the evidence for physical factors is strong. Recurring, debilitating pain may well cause depression and anxiety, rather than depression initiating the pain.

Toxic shock syndrome

Toxic shock syndrome (TSS) is a rare condition occurring in women who forget to remove or regularly change tampons. It is caused by a *Staphylococcus aureus* exotoxin (toxic shock syndrome toxin-1). Influenza-like symptoms occur with high fever (39°C), diarrhoea, vomiting, rash, muscle aches and offensive vaginal discharge. Complications can be severe, including disseminated intravascular coagulation (DIC), renal, tubal or cortical necrosis, microthrombi, adult respiratory distress syndrome (ARDS) and tissue hypoxia. Mortality is in the order of 30 to 50%. Women should be advised to use the lowest absorbency tampon suitable for the flow, change 4- to 8-hourly and to wash their hands before and after insertion. Toxic shock syndrome can also be associated with cases of septic abortion.

Disorders of menstruation I

- ■ Disorders of menstruation are common; at some stage over 20% of women will complain of heavy periods.
- ■ Dysfunctional uterine bleeding is a diagnosis made by exclusion and can be either ovulatory or anovulatory.
- ■ Dysmenorrhoea may be primary or secondary – the latter requires full investigation.
- ■ Toxic shock syndrome (TSS) is caused by *Staphylococcus aureus* exotoxin – mortality is 30 to 50%, related to lost tampons and septic abortions.

Disorders of menstruation II

Management of dysfunctional uterine bleeding

Management should include an assessment of the situation, the pattern of bleeding and the degree of loss. Menorrhagia with a regular cycle is probably ovulatory and does not require endocrine investigation. Endometrial biopsy is not considered necessary in women under the age of 40 years.

Irregular periods warrant tests for follicle stimulating hormone, luteinizing hormone, prolactin, thyroid function and testosterone. A characteristic profile is found in cases of polycystic ovarian syndrome (see p. 115). Anovulatory menorrhagia is common in the older perimenopausal woman. Endometrial carcinoma can present as irregular bleeding in the mid to late 40s – if there is any suspicion, endometrial assessment is warranted (see p. 138).

Treatment for heavy bleeding

Medical

Treatment is initially by inhibition of prostaglandin synthesis (e.g. mefenamic acid) or an anti-fibrinolytic agent (e.g. tranexamic acid) (Table 1). The pill can also be used – it promotes anovulation by ovarian suppression, but provides short, regular controlled cycles. The levonorgestrel-impregnated intrauterine contraceptive device (Mirena) has changed the approach to the management of dysfunctional bleeding. It reduces blood loss in 70% of cases, and 20% of women will achieve amenorrhoea after 8 to 9 months of use. Initially, there is a 30% chance of irregular bleeding. It is not only effective, but also provides contraception. Cyclical progestogens and danazol have also been used.

Endoscopic

Hysteroscopy

This is the transvaginal approach to looking directly into the endocervical canal and the uterine cavity (Figs 1 and 2), with an endoscope introduced into the endocervical canal and advanced under direct vision until the uterine cavity is reached. Fibre-optically transmitted light provides illumination. The endocervical canal and uterine cavity are slightly distended with an appropriate medium to obtain a panoramic view of the uterine cavity. Saline or Hyskon (32% dextran-70 in 10% dextrose) are used as uterine distension media. Visualization can also be obtained with carbon dioxide, but vision is often obscured by gas bubbles. Complications related to dextran usage are very rare, but include anaphylaxis, pulmonary oedema, electrolyte imbalance (e.g. hyponatraemia and hypocalcaemia) and coagulation disorders. The incidence of complications is related to the volumes of Hyskon used, high distending pressures and long surgical procedures. Hysteroscopy itself has practically no complications. However, some blind manipulation may be required in sounding the uterine cavity

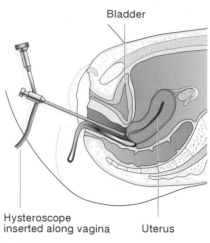

Fig. 1 **Hysteroscopy technique.**

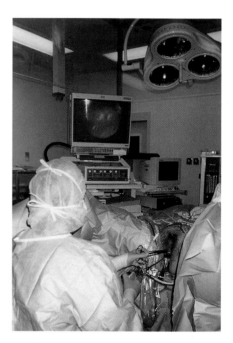

Fig. 2 **Performing hysteroscopy.**

or dilating the endocervical canal so that uterine perforation may occur, especially in the presence of severe cervical stenosis, acutely anteverted or retroverted uterus and the post-menopausal uterus. It is also associated with distortion of the uterine cavity secondary to myomas, occlusion secondary to adhesions and uterine anomalies or carcinomas.

Diagnostic hysteroscopy is performed with a small-calibre endoscope of 3–5 mm diameter (Fig. 3). The smaller scopes can be used without cervical dilatation as outpatient procedures.

Operative hysteroscopy requires a 7–8-mm diameter endoscope and therefore cervical dilatation. The operating hysteroscope can be used

Table 1 **Treatment options for heavy bleeding**		
Drug	**Regime**	**Notes**
Combined contraceptive pill	As for contraception	Useful if pain accompanies heavy, irregular bleeding and in the younger age groups. Also if there is a contraceptive need
NSAIDs	Ibuprofen 400 mg t.d.s. orally Naproxen 250 mg t.d.s. orally Mefenamic acid 500 mg t.d.s. orally	Act by inhibiting prostaglandin synthetase. More effective for pain control than blood loss, though will reduce this. Most effective if commenced 1–2 days before onset of menses. May cause side effects in patients with dyspepsia and asthma
Tranexamic acid	1 g t.d.s. orally during menses	An anti-fibrinolytic and inhibits plasminogen activators. Consistently effective in reducing flow, but will not regularize cycles. Can cause nausea, occasional vomiting and diarrhoea
Etamsylate	500 mg q.d.s. during menses	Reduces capillary fragility. Inhibits prostacyclin synthetase. Can cause nausea, headaches and rashes. Contraindicated with porphyria
Mirena IUD		Licensed now for 5 years in the UK. 20% of women become amenorrhoeic after 1 year. 70% successful in reduction of blood flow. 30% irregular bleeding/spotting initially
Progestogens	Duphaston 10–20 mg days 5–25 or days 14–28 Provera 10–20 mg as above Norethisterone 5 mg b.d. or t.d.s. as above	Still frequently prescribed. Poor bleeding control in clinical trials. Patients often report side effects of bloating, weight gain, premenstrual syndrome symptoms

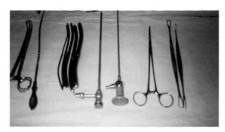

Fig. 3 **Hysteroscopic equipment.**

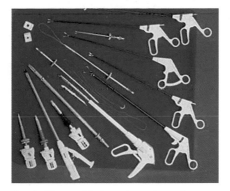

Fig. 4 **Disposable laparoscopic tools.**

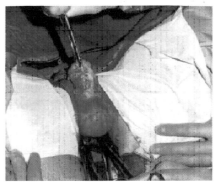

Fig. 5 **Vaginal hysterectomy.**

for division of uterine septa, severe intrauterine adhesions, tubal cannulation and some myomectomies for broad-based, sessile and large leiomyomas. Some authorities recommend simultaneous laparoscopy. Endometrial resection can be performed with laser ablation, roller-ball electrocoagulation or the hysteroscopic resectoscope. When current is applied, the resectoscope will easily cut through a leiomyoma to produce a shaving of the tissue; the tumour is progressively shaved down to the level of the endometrium. The haemostasis of cut vessels is performed one by one with coagulating current. The Nd-YAG lasers can also resect myomas. Carbon dioxide lasers have not proved effective. If perforation of the uterus occurs it is important to stop the procedure immediately and withdraw the instrument assessing where and how the perforation happened. Perforation with the larger operative instruments usually requires laparoscopy to assess the damage. Most perforations do not require active treatment unless bleeding persists.

In women who receive endometrial ablation techniques, 15–30% report dysmenorrhoea and some proceed to hysterectomy because of pain, despite achieving bleeding control. Cellular regeneration can occur following resection with return of bleeding, and even the potential for carcinomatous change.

Endometrial coagulation has been developed with an ultrasound-emitting probe or using heat.

Minimal Access Surgery

Laparoscopically assisted vaginal hysterectomy (LAVH) allows pedicles to be ligated and divided from above, whilst the uterus is removed, with morcelation if enlarged, from below.

This advancement has depended on better equipment, e.g. grasping forceps and cutting scissors (Fig. 4), improved imaging (fibreoptic telescopes, cameras and TV monitors) and an enhanced level of training.

Hysterectomy

The indications for hysterectomy have reduced following the introduction of tranexamic acid and the Mirena IUS as first-line treatment for dysfunctional bleeding, and minimal access and hysteroscopic techniques which allow resection of submucous fibroids. Hysterectomy, therefore, is reserved for either large fibroid masses that would be difficult to remove with the LAVH technique, which is time consuming, or for prolapse, when a vaginal hysterectomy would be preferred (Fig. 5). It is common practice to use GnRH analogues for 3 months prior to surgery in the case of very large fibroids to reduce the risk of interoperative bleeding (cf. myomectomies). It may also make the difference between entry via a paramedian incision or a Pfannenstiel incision. When counselling the patient preoperatively, a decision must be made whether to remove or conserve the ovaries which will depend on the

patient's age, whether she still has intrinsic ovarian function and, of course, her preference. A discussion should also take place as to whether the hysterectomy should be total or sub-total. Some authorities advocate conserving the cervix citing less risk to bladder and ureter, greater support to the vaginal vault with reduction in the risk of prolapse in later years and enhanced sexual function by preserving cervical orgasm. The counter-argument is the continuing need for cervical screening.

The vaginal hysterectomy is possible if there is primary- and, certainly, second-degree cervical descent present. Most ladies who have had previous pregnancies will have sufficient ligamental laxity to allow a vaginal approach which is preferable for the obese patient who is therefore able to mobilise more promptly without an abdominal scar reducing the risk of postoperative thromboembolism and wound sepsis.

All hysterectomy patients are advised that they will require 4–6 weeks' convalescence. The vaginal hysterectomy patient should be specifically counselled regarding pelvic floor exercises and the avoidance of lifting weights and straining to defecate which will weaken the pelvic floor healing process. The risks of surgery are those common to all major procedures – haemorrhage, infection and thrombosis – and prophylaxis is recommended.

Disorders of menstruation II

- Prostaglandin synthetase inhibitors decrease menstrual blood loss and myometrial contractility.
- Anti-fibrinolytics are useful as first-line management of dysfunctional bleeding.
- The Mirena progestogen-secreting coil plays a useful role in dysfunctional uterine bleeding, also providing contraceptive cover.
- Endometrial ablation can be used in women where medical treatment fails.

Acute and chronic pelvic pain

The elicitation of the history is very important in cases of pelvic pain as the patient may find it hard to express how the pain affects her. There may also be a lot of visual clues so watching the patient as she describes her illness is more important than writing down what is said! The nature of the pain, its site, radiation, relieving and aggravating factors should all be elicited.

Pain of visceral origin, conveyed along T10–L1 and associated with distension of organs or stretching of the overlying peritoneum, will be harder for the patient to pinpoint than pain of somatic origin (S2–4). Pelvic pain may be from the uterus, fallopian tube, ovary, bladder, ureter or bowel, so questions must cover all areas.

Acute pain

Pain may be due to ectopic pregnancy (see p. 98), miscarriage (see p. 92), ovarian cyst accident (see p. 140), pelvic infection (see p. 100), ureteric calculus, painful bladder conditions, appendicitis, diverticular disease or irritable bowel syndrome. Investigations of the cause of acute pelvic pain are listed in Table 1 and the management of acute pain is outlined in Figure 1.

Chronic pain

Chronic pelvic pain is a considerable problem in women of reproductive age and may account for as many as one-third of referrals in this group. Slightly more than half of diagnostic laparoscopies are carried out for investigation of chronic pelvic pain, often with a normal pelvis seen. An increased incidence of neurotic-type personality in these patients may be an effect of coping with pain long term rather than the cause of the problem.

Diagnosis (Table 2)

Assessment of pain may be facilitated by documentation (Fig. 2) which enables a clearer view of the timing of pain in relation to other events such as menstruation, bowel or bladder fullness and sexual intercourse.

Pelvic pain syndrome (PPS) is a disorder of the premenopausal woman. In PPS there would be tenderness on palpation over the ovary. The pain responds to postural change, in that lying flat eases the pain whereas standing, walking and bending all make the pain worse. The postcoital ache is characteristic in that, unlike that due to other pelvic pathologies, it continues after intercourse.

Irritable bowel syndrome (IBS), found twice as often in women compared to men, is commonly found in those presenting with pelvic pain. Pain may be localized to the left iliac fossa, there is an increase in flatus, increased rectal mucus and feelings of incomplete rectal emptying. From the long list of symptoms, three of the above noted will enable a diagnosis of IBS to be made.

Table 1	**Useful investigations in cases of acute pelvic pain**
Bimanual pelvic examination	To check for cervical excitation, size of uterus, state of os and presence of pelvic mass
Urine Dipstix	Protein may suggest infection
Immunological pregnancy test (IPT)	99.5% accuracy
Pelvic ultrasound scan	Gestational sac by 4.5 weeks, fetal pole by 5 weeks, fetal heart movement by 6 weeks
Quantitative beta hCG	48-hour doubling time is normal – less may indicate an ectopic pregnancy
Diagnostic laparoscopy	To investigate the acute abdomen

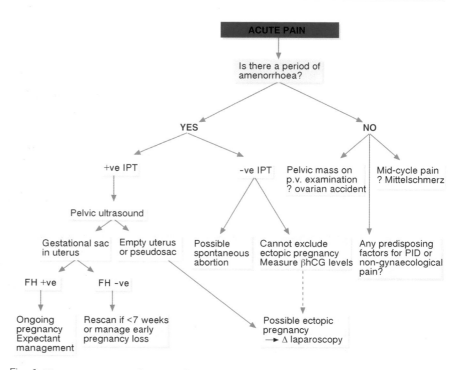

Fig. 1 **The management of acute pelvic pain.**

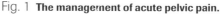

Table 2	**Diagnosis of the causes of acute pelvic pain**
Possible diagnosis	**Associated symptoms**
Chronic pelvic inflammatory disease (PID)	Vaginal discharge, pain worse during menses, sexually active
Endometriosis	Dysmenorrhoea, deep dyspareunia, pelvic ache
Pelvic pain syndrome (PPS)	Pain worse when standing or ambulant, deep dyspareunia and postcoital ache
Irritable bowel syndrome (IBS)	Alternating loose bowels and constipation, abdominal bloating, pain often in left iliac fossa
Nerve entrapment	Previous pelvic surgery, pain easy to pinpoint
Residual ovary syndrome	Previous hysterectomy, deep dyspareunia
Uterogenital prolapse	Dragging sensation, dull pelvic ache, vaginal bulge
Urethral syndrome	Urinary frequency and urgency, voiding difficulty
Interstitial cystitis	Urinary frequency and urgency, pain relief with voiding, haematuria
Idiopathic	Many other symptoms but other diagnoses excluded

PELVIC PAIN CLINIC QUESTIONNAIRE

For Office Use Only
Name of Interviewer
....
Date:......................

Please answer all the following questions by circling in pencil the correct answer(s) or putting an X on a line when indicated. Do not write in the right hand column. Bring the completed form when you come to this Clinic. Your answers are entirely confidential to the doctor/sis

Name:
Address:

Tel: ....
Name of G.P. ....
Occupation: ....

Pain

Main Complaints:

What are you complaining of:
If other(s), please desc
How long have you had the pa
Can you remember what start
Childbirth/after an op
Other cause(s):.........
What does the pain feel like?
Other:..................
How often do you get the pai
When you get an attack, how
Is the pain worse at some tim
Just before the period
Please indicate where the pai
If the pain is mainly on one si

Quality of Life

1. Number of times you have been to see a doctor for any reason in the last three months?

2. Number of 'pain killers' tablets and type you are using each day.

	No. used per day
Name of tablets -----------------	-----------------
Name of tablets -----------------	-----------------

Put an X on the lines to show the quality of life you think you have at present

3. How much was the pain affected with your daily activity in the last month (shopping, housework, etc)?

0 Not at all — 10 Totally

4. Do you do a full time job? *Yes / No*
If yes, how many days did you take off work in the last month? -----------

5. How much is the pain interferring with your social life (going out with your partner, seeing friends, etc)?

0 No effect — 10 No social life

6. How would you score your present enjoyment of life?

0 Highly enjoyable — 10 No enjoyment at all

7. Does the pain interfere with your sleep?

0 Not at all — 10 All the time

Fig. 2 **Pain assessment chart for chronic pelvic pain.**

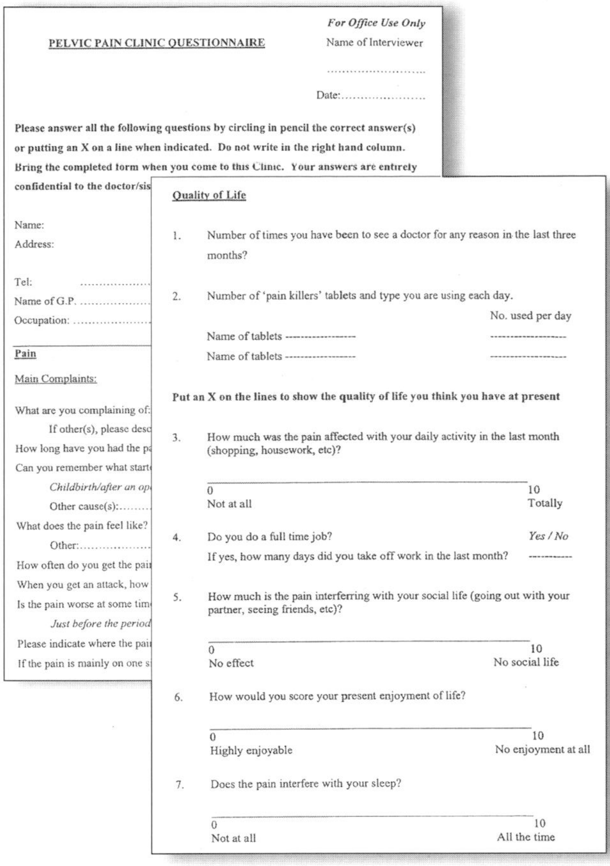

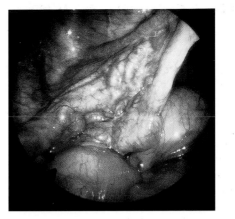

Fig. 3 **Laparoscopic view showing dilated pelvic veins.**

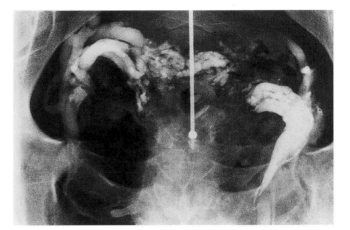

Fig. 4 **Venogram showing pelvic venous congestion.**

Management

The approach to this problem must be systematic to ensure early diagnosis of treatable pain and to allow a sympathetic approach to pain which may be persistent despite a diagnosis having been reached. Pain management may include suitable analgesia, nerve root injections, antibiotic therapy for pelvic infection (see p. 100), progestogens or gonadotrophin releasing hormone (GnRH) analogues for endometriosis (see p. 128), surgery for residual ovary syndrome or prolapse and a variety of therapies for bladder problems.

The pelvic pain syndrome has been characterized by the finding of dilated pelvic veins (Fig. 3) in these patients when examined with pelvic venography (Fig. 4). It is proposed that this is a response in some people to high oestrogen content in the blood and can be shown in the vessels draining the ovary with the developing follicle which thus have a higher oestrogen content. Treatment is directed to reducing the ovarian production of oestrogen – medroxyprogesterone acetate daily has been shown to be effective.

Ovarian suppression can be used as a diagnostic tool before proceeding with the more definitive management of removal of the pelvic organs. Total abdominal hysterectomy and bilateral salpingo-oophorectomy may give dramatic relief of pain but in premenopausal women loss of ovarian function may have long-term implications (osteoporosis, cardiovascular disease). Thus using ovarian suppression before surgery would allow a trial of whether ovarian removal would be likely to be associated with pain relief.

Psychotherapy will have an invaluable role in management of chronic pain and is probably the most reasonable approach in those with idiopathic pain. Helping the patient to understand the role that stress hormones play in exacerbating pain will encourage involvement in relaxation therapy. Better outcomes in pain management are achieved when incorporating this approach.

Acute and chronic pelvic pain

- Pelvic pain may be a sign of acute disease or of a more long-term nature.
- A good history may guide you to the source of the pain.
- Pelvic ultrasound may allow a diagnosis to be reached but also allows exclusion of some acute conditions.
- Pelvic pain syndrome is difficult to manage but may respond to progestogens, though best results are found in conjunction with counselling.

Endometriosis

Endometriosis is a common benign condition estimated to affect between 10 and 25% of women. It is commonest among European and nulliparous women and has its peak incidence between 30 and 45 years of age.

Pathology

Endometriosis may be defined as the presence of tissue outside the uterus that is histologically similar to that of the endometrium. This can be found within the pelvis or at more distant sites. The site will in turn determine the presenting symptoms and signs as the ectopic endometrial tissue will continue to bleed (Table 1) on a cyclical basis under hormonal control.

Endometriosis can be diagnosed accurately by visualization and inspection. Histological confirmation is not usually required. Endometriosis involving the ovaries may lead to endometriomas ('chocolate cysts'; Figs 1 and 2).

Aetiology

There is uncertainty surrounding the aetiology of this common condition (Table 2). An immunological

Table 2 **Possible aetiologies of endometriosis**
■ Retrograde menstruation and implantation
■ Lymphatic and haematogenous spread
■ Transformation of coelomic epithelium
■ Genetic and familial aspects
■ Implantation at operation

mechanism may account for why certain susceptible individuals go on to develop the disease. Antigens, produced by degrading endometrial proteins, have been identified which stimulate an immune response characterized by peritoneal irritation and fibrosis. There appears to be evidence of decreased cellular immunity to endometrial tissue in sufferers.

Another theory is that of transformation of coelomic epithelium which proposes that adult cells undergo de-differentiation by metaplasia back to their primitive origin and then transform to endometrial cells, influenced by prolonged oestrogen stimulation.

Vascular and lymphatic embolization to distant sites outside the peritoneum are probable and endometriotic tissue has been found within lymph channels, lymph nodes and pelvic veins.

There are racial differences and a higher incidence of endometriosis is encountered in the first-degree relatives of patients.

Presentation

The most common site for endometriosis is the ovary, followed by the pelvic peritoneal surface, the uterosacral ligaments and the posterior aspect of the uterus.

The classic symptom of endometriosis is pain – deep dyspareunia, secondary dysmenorrhoea or pelvic pain. 'Crescendo' dysmenorrhoea is typical, where the pain precedes the onset of menstruation by several days, reaches a climax, and is relieved when bleeding commences. There is a wide variation – some women are asymptomatic yet have a severe degree of endometriosis on laparoscopy, others have only one or two localized deposits and experience considerable pain.

Endometriosis is associated with infertility. Luteal phase defiency and luteinized unruptured follicles (LUf) syndrome occur with increased frequency. Dyspareunia may reduce the frequency of intercourse and inhibit penetration.

Diagnosis

There may be cervical excitation on bimanual assessment. The uterosacral ligaments may feel scarred, nodular and irregular, and there may be exquisite tenderness in the pouch of Douglas. Adnexal endometriomas may be palpable. Chronic pelvic infection (see p. 100) should be excluded as this can also present with dysmenorrhoea, pelvic pain, deep dyspareunia and infertility. Corroboration is by diagnostic laparoscopy – the appearance of endometrial peritoneal deposits varies (Fig. 2).

The typical lesion is the slate-grey powder burn. Other appearances include white opacification of the peritoneum, red flame-like lesions (Fig. 2a), glandular excrescences, subovarian adhesions in the fossa ovarica (Fig. 2d), yellow-brown peritoneal patches, and café-au-lait spots (Fig. 2c). Accumulation of scar tissue may deform the surrounding

Table 1 **Documented sites of endometriotic implants with associated symptoms**		
	Site	**Symptoms**
Intrapelvic (common)	Ovarian, uterosacral ligaments, pelvic peritoneal surfaces, e.g. broad ligament, tubes	Dysmenorrhoea, lower abdominal pain, pelvic pain dyspareunia, low back pain, ovarian accident – torsion or rupture of endometrioma, infertility
Extrapelvic (rare)	Small bowel	Obstruction
	Appendix	Pseudoappendicitis
	Rectum	Cyclical rectal bleed, tenesmus, cyclical pain with defecation/altered bowel habits
	Ureters	Ureteric obstruction
	Bladder	Cyclical haematuria/dysuria
	Lungs	Cyclical haemoptysis
	Surgical scars, e.g. caesarean or hysterectomy scar, vaginal vault	Cyclical pain and bleeding
	Umbilicus	Cyclical pain and bleeding
	Limbs/joints/skin	Cyclical pain and swelling

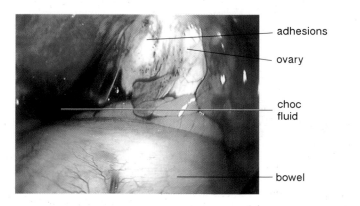

— adhesions
— ovary
— choc fluid
— bowel

Fig. 1 **Ovarian endometriosis.** A pseudo ('chocolate') cyst has been created (containing altered blood and breakdown products) surrounded by dense fibrosis.

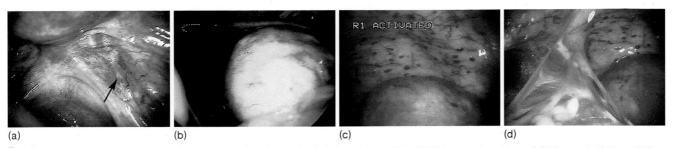

Fig. 2 **Laparoscopic appearance of endometriosis. (a)** Endometriotic deposits – red 'flares'. **(b)** Intact endometrioma. **(c)** Uterovesical fold – café-au-lait spots. **(d)** Filmy adhesions over ovarian cyst.

peritoneum resulting in the development of adhesions between adjacent pelvic structures leading to a 'frozen pelvis'.

Attempts to find a non-invasive test for endometriosis include serum markers, ultrasonography, computerized tomography, magnetic resonance imaging and immuno-scintigraphy. The latter is an attempt to combine tissue labelling and isotope-labelled marker with gamma camera imaging. Unfortunately the results still show great overlap with other conditions, particularly pelvic inflammatory disease.

Many centres have introduced the American system of charting the degree of endometrial deposits to stage the severity of the disease. This is particularly useful if subsequent laparoscopy is performed to evaluate response to treatment.

Treatment
Endometriosis is a particularly difficult disease to treat. Medical treatment relies on 'suppression therapy' for 6–9 months, creating either a pseudopregnancy or a pseudomenopause (Table 3). The endometrial deposits regress, but eventually recur in up to 60% of cases. Counselling and self-help groups may be beneficial.

Radical surgery should be reserved for patients with unsuccessful medical treatment who have severe intractable pain and who have completed their family or who have no desire to maintain their fertility but would rather improve their quality of life. In cases requiring total abdominal hysterectomy and bilateral salpingo-oophorectomy most clinicians would agree that progestogen should be prescribed with oestrogen replacement for 6 to 9 months following surgery to prevent reactivation.

Endometriosis can be reactivated in postmenopausal women by hormone replacement therapy.

Adenomyosis
This is a term used to describe ectopic endometrium which penetrates deep within the myometrium and produces a bulky, tender, smooth, globular uterus (Fig. 3). It usually presents with dysmenorrhoea and menorrhagia and affects a different population to that affected by endometriosis, e.g. multiparous patients. It is only diagnosed after hysterectomy.

Table 3 **Treatment modalities for endometriosis**	
Medical	
Pseudo pregnancy	
Combined oral contraceptive pill	Use continually with no pill-free intervals
	Use a monophasic pill with an androgenic progestogen
Didrogesterone (Duphaston)	10 mg b.d./c.d.s. continuously. Side effects: weight gain, acne, mastalgia, PMT symptoms, depression
Medroxyprogesterone acetate (Provera)	10 mg bd/tds continuously. Side effects: as above
Norethisterone (Primulut)	5 mg bd/qds continuously. Side effects: as above, probably more pronounced as more androgenic
Danazol (Danol)	200 mg od/bd (max. dose qds) Side effects: weight gain, acne, nausea, dizziness, virilization, receding hairline, deepening voice in a few cases
Gestrinore	2.5 mg twice weekly for 6–9 months. Side effects: as above
Pseudo menopause	
GnRH analogues	Implants: goserelin (Zoladex)
	Injections: leuprorelin (Prostap), goserelin (Zoladex)
	Nasal spray: buseralin (Suprecur), nafarelin (Synarell)
	Side effects: climacteric symptoms, prolonged therapy will cause osteopenia therefore will need 'add back' hormone replacement therapy
Surgical	
Conservative	
Laparoscopic diathermy or laser ablation therapy	Certain deposits near the ureters or rectum may not be amenable to treatment without risk of damage
Laparotomy, tubal reconstruction, adhesion lysis, enucleation of endometriomas with ovarian reconstruction	Surgery may be difficult with variable results
Radical	
Total abdominal hysterectomy and bilateral salpingo-oophorectomy with excision of all deposits	Difficult dissection, risk of bowel and bladder damage, loss of fertility

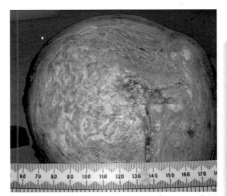

Fig. 3 **Adenomyosis.** The cut surface of the uterus showing the typical interdigitating whirled appearance.

Endometriosis

- This is a common condition affecting 10–25% of women.
- Peak incidence is 30–45 years of age.
- The main symptom is pain; there is an association with infertility.
- Diagnosis is by laparoscopy.
- Medical treatment relies on suppression therapy.
- Surgical treatment can be radical or conservative.
- Treatment can be difficult, relapses can occur, support groups are helpful.

Investigation of infertility

Infertility exists when a couple trying for pregnancy have not achieved this after 12 months. Eight in 10 healthy couples will become pregnant in the first 12 months of trying, so it is reasonable to commence investigations if pregnancy has not been achieved in this time.

Physiology

The sperm meets the egg in the tubal ampulla and an understanding of the complexity of the process leading to that moment and the subsequent fertilization (Fig. 1) and implantation is important to the understanding of infertility. The human female starts life with many eggs and 'wastes' most:

Fetus	2 000 000 ova at about 20 weeks
Birth	750 000 ova
Puberty	250 000
Reproductive life	200–300 ovulations
Menopause	a few residual ova but unresponsive to follicle stimulating hormone.

Eggs are held in prophase of first meiosis. Meiotic division resumes as the follicle matures and is complete by the time of ovulation. A regular 28-day menstrual cycle results in 13 ovulations per year. Couples should be encouraged to have regular intercourse throughout the menstrual cycle.

The early conceptus produces human chorionic gonadotrophin (hCG) which is necessary for the continuation of the pregnancy and is the basis of urine and blood tests to confirm pregnancy. The production of progesterone by the corpus luteum is also essential for at least the first 9 weeks of pregnancy, until placental production takes over this role.

Infertility affects 1 in 10 couples with varying causes predominating in different countries. The common causes of infertility in the UK (usually a combination of causes) are:

▪ unexplained	28%
▪ sperm problem	21%
▪ ovulatory failure	18%
▪ tubal damage	14%
▪ endometriosis	6%
▪ coital problems	5%
▪ cervical mucus hostility	3%
▪ other male problems	2%

In the USA the male factors can account for 40% of cases of infertility. Female factors (e.g. tubal blockage secondary to pelvic inflammatory disease) are high in the Caribbean and West Indies. The tendency for women in 'advanced' countries to delay childbearing whilst establishing a career may result in more cases of infertility as fecundity decreases with increasing maternal age. There are increasing numbers of anovulatory cycles and the oocytes are ageing whilst there is a lower frequency of sexual activity with increasing age.

Investigations

Investigation of an infertile couple (Fig. 2) needs to rapidly assess ovulation, patency of tubes and presence of sperm. A diagnosis allows formulation of a management plan to help allay anxiety and ensure that older couples do not miss the chance of assisted conception (see p. 132).

Check the rubella status and offer vaccination if negative – remember to advise avoiding pregnancy within 1 month of vaccination. Advice to take folic acid whilst trying to conceive is appropriate, along with advice to stop smoking and reduce alcohol intake to a minimum. A body mass index (BMI) over 30 necessitates a supervised weight loss

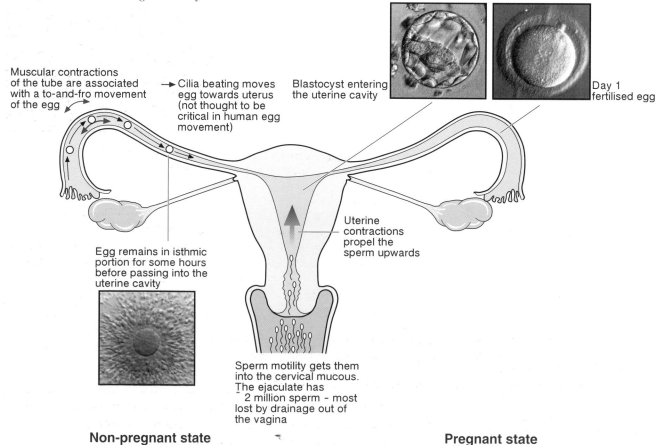

Muscular contractions of the tube are associated with a to-and-fro movement of the egg

→ Cilia beating moves egg towards uterus (not thought to be critical in human egg movement)

Blastocyst entering the uterine cavity

Day 1 fertilised egg

Egg remains in isthmic portion for some hours before passing into the uterine cavity

Uterine contractions propel the sperm upwards

Sperm motility gets them into the cervical mucous. The ejaculate has 2 million sperm - most lost by drainage out of the vagina

Non-pregnant state

Pregnant state

Fig. 1 **The physiology of fertilization.**

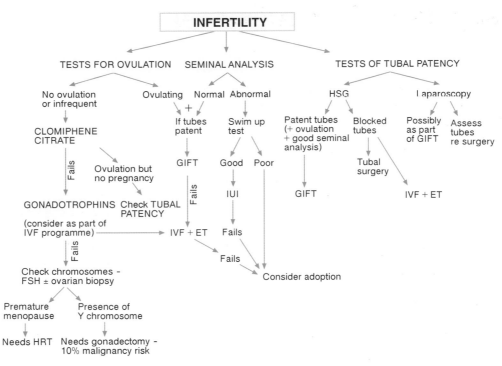

Fig. 2 **Investigation of the infertile couple.**

programme. The male partner should also be advised to stop smoking and limit alcohol to optimize his reproductive performance. Intercourse two to three times per week throughout the cycle should optimize the chance of conception.

Semen analysis
The World Health Organization normal values are:

- volume   2–5 ml
- sperm count   > 20 million sperm per ml
- motility   > 50% progressive motility
- morphology   > 30% normal forms
- white blood cells   < 1 million/ml
- liquefaction time   within 30 mins

Counts below 20 million sperm per ml are associated with lower pregnancy rates. Over recent years decreased sperm counts have been noted – possibly due to environmental pollutants such as agricultural chemicals, stress, intercurrent illness and jet lag. With azoospermia, luteinizing hormone (LH) and follicle stimulating hormone (FSH) should be checked – high FSH suggests failure of sperm production and needs further investigation with chromosome study. Normal FSH may imply a blockage to the outflow of sperm.

A sperm migration test will assess the number of viable sperm with good forward motility (normal value > 5 million/ml). Antibodies can be detected in semen (IgA and IgG) using immunofluorescent techniques.

Antibodies may be found on the head (affecting ability to fertilize the egg) or tail (affecting sperm motility).

Tests of ovulation
Measurement of serum progesterone in the mid-luteal phase confirms ovulation if > 30 nmol/l. Ultrasound 'tracking' of the ovaries can follow developing follicles during ovulation induction cycles (Fig. 3).

Tubal function
Hysterosalpingography (HSG) and diagnostic laparoscopy are complementary methods for assessment of tubal patency. Before instrumentation of the uterus, screen for *Chlamydia trachomatis* or give appropriate antibiotic prophylaxis. At HSG, radio-opaque dye is introduced through the cervix and outlines the uterine shape and fallopian tubes, determining their patency (Table 1).

Laparoscopy allows assessment of the pelvis for endometriosis (see p. 128) and peritubal adhesions due to infection (see p. 100). There may be an obvious corpus luteum (evidence of ovulation) and free fluid from the pouch of Douglas can be assessed bacteriologically to rule out pelvic infection. Dye injected through the cervix can be observed flowing from the fimbriae of the tubes in healthy cases.

A sensible investigation plan allows speedy diagnosis of the problem and the most appropriate management.

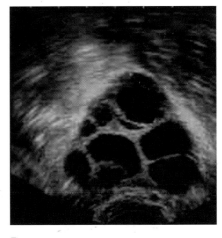

Fig. 3 **Ultrasound scan showing a follicle being measured.**

Table 1 **Assessing the results of hysterosalpingography**

Findings at HSG	Presumptive diagnosis
Uterine synechiae	Asherman's syndrome
Irregular uterine cavity	Uterine fibroids
Septum in cavity	Congenital abnormality of uterus
Cornual blockage	Spasm of tubes
Tubal distension	Blocked tubes
Peritoneal spread of dye	Normal tubal patency

Investigation of infertility

- Infertility investigations can commence after 12 months of intercourse not resulting in pregnancy.
- An investigation plan should enable couples to learn rapidly the cause of their infertility.
- Investigation should always be in parallel for male and female partners.

Management of infertility

Management of anovulation

Clomifene citrate

Clomifene citrate is used in cases of anovulation or infrequent ovulation found in the presence of normal seminal analysis before any further investigation is needed. The oestrogen-like structure of clomifene confers anti-oestrogenic properties and induces a rise in follicle stimulating hormone (FSH) and luteinizing hormone (LH) output possibly by affecting gonadotrophin releasing hormone (GnRH) release. Treatment is given on days 2–6 of the menstrual cycle in the UK (to avoid the anti-oestrogenic effect on the cervical mucus), though in the USA, where treatment is given on days 5–9, similar results are obtained. The starting dose is 50 mg daily with step-wise increase until ovulation is achieved – as evidenced by appropriate rise in the mid-luteal progesterone. Seventy-five percent of pregnancies occur in the first three ovulatory treatment cycles.

Conception rates, if no other causes of infertility are present, approach normal (80–90%). There is a cumulative rise in pregnancy rate up to 9 months of treatment so alternative therapies should be considered at this stage. If used in conjunction with intrauterine insemination (see below) timing of ovulation is important. Once ultrasound shows a follicular diameter of 18–20 mm or appropriate serum estradiol levels, a human chorionic gonadotrophin (hCG) injection can be given – usually around day 11. Ovulation occurs 36–40 hours later and sperm can be introduced at this stage.

Side effects of clomifene include a 15% incidence of poor cervical mucus, which may hamper sperm transport. A multiple pregnancy rate of 5% is reported. There may be a slight increase in risk of ovarian carcinoma with clomifene, but not if used for fewer than 12 cycles. Ovarian hyperstimulation (see below) is rare but can occur particularly in association with polycystic ovarian syndrome (PCOS). Headaches, dizziness and abdominal discomfort are also reported.

Gonadotrophins

The gonadotrophins are controlled by gonadotrophin releasing hormone (GnRH) from the hypothalamus and manipulation of their levels is used to affect egg production. FSH is used to achieve ovulation in women with clomifene-resistant PCOS. GnRH analogues can be used to suppress endogenous activity in the pituitary–ovarian axis but there is no increase in pregnancy rate in women with clomifene-resistant PCOS and there may be an increased risk of ovarian hyperstimulation (see below).

Down-regulation with a GnRH analogue allows exact timing of ovulation so that it coincides with theatre time if a gamete intrafallopian transfer (GIFT – see below) cycle is in progress or the presence of an embryologist if an in vitro fertilization (IVF) cycle is planned. The analogue is commenced during the middle of the cycle prior to the procedure (long cycle) or on day 1 of the treatment cycle (short cycle). Once low FSH, LH and estradiol are achieved, FSH is commenced at 150 IU per day until three or four 18–22 mm follicles are produced (follicle maturation) as followed by ultrasound tracking.

During IVF and GIFT procedures the gonadotrophins are used to produce more than one egg per cycle (superovulation). Purified FSH is given starting with a low dose and monitoring the response with serum estradiol and ultrasound scanning of the ovaries. When three or four follicles 18–22 mm diameter are noted, hCG is given to mature the eggs prior to harvesting. Spare eggs may be frozen for use in subsequent cycles.

Egg collection

The technique is by transvaginal scan using a needle guide to ensure correct placement of the needle (Fig. 1) and harvesting the eggs using suction. This allows the eggs to be fertilized in vitro and replacement of up to three embryos per cycle into the uterine cavity. The legal limit of three embryos per cycle (UK) maximizes the chance of a successful pregnancy whilst minimizing the risk of a high-order multiple pregnancy, though many units replace two routinely.

Gamete intrafallopian transfer (GIFT)

This procedure was introduced for the management of unexplained infertility and is now used also with mild oligospermia or mild endometriosis. As ovulation timing is difficult to predict in a natural cycle, and usually produces only one or two eggs, gonadotrophins are used (see above). Egg collection is carried out at laparoscopy, allowing replacement of eggs and 'washed' sperm into the fallopian tube at the same time. Two or three oocytes per tube are placed just proximal to the tubal ampulla. There has been an increased incidence of corpus luteal dysfunction in these cycles so progesterone 400 mg is given twice daily for 2 weeks after the GIFT procedure.

In vitro fertilization and embryo transfer (IVF and ET)

The classic indication for this is in the patient with tubal disease which is not appropriate for surgery. The tube is by-passed, and multiple oocytes are collected and made available – allowing in vitro fertilization with sperm (Figs 2, 3, 4). If more than three embryos develop, the extra ones can be cryopreserved, allowing two or three IVF cycles to be achieved from one ovulation induction cycle. There is at least a 25% loss of embryos at defrosting. The

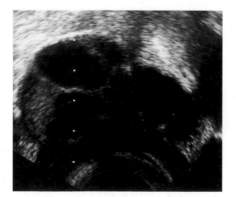

Fig. 1 **Ultrasound scan of egg collection.**

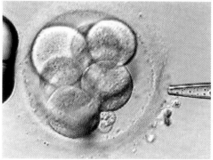

Fig. 2 **The zona pellucida is chemically eroded to assist access to the eggs.**

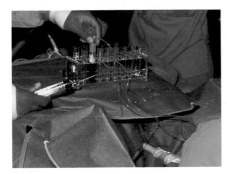

Fig. 3 **Ultrasonically guided egg retrieval via posterior fornix.**

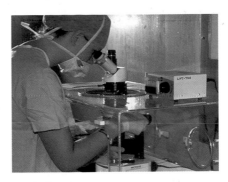

Fig. 4 **Incubation process for egg fertilization.**

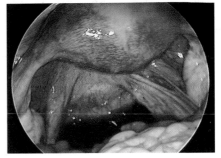

Fig. 6 **Laparoscopic view showing damaged tubes.**

pregnancy rate is often higher in the cycle where no ovulation induction is needed, but remains only ~ 20–25%.

Intracytoplasmic sperm injection (ICSI) and embryo transfer

This overcomes any problem with the sperm penetrating the zona pellucida. It also ensures that only one sperm fertilizes the egg (Fig. 5). It is indicated when IVF has failed to generate embryos, where sperm have been recovered from the epididymis or testis by aspiration, or when seminal analysis shows sperm with very poor motility. The technique enables men to father children themselves rather than resorting to AID (artificial insemination with donor sperm – see below).

Intrauterine insemination (IUI)

This technique is used in cases of unexplained infertility, male antisperm antibodies, post-vasectomy antibodies, if white blood cells are found in semen, or possibly if borderline oligospermia is detected. Coital difficulty may also be managed this way. The semen sample is washed, centrifuged and the sperm pellet suspended in medium. The healthy sperm swim into the medium and 0.1–0.2 ml is injected directly into the uterine cavity. This avoids the cervical mucus barrier and the washing removes the prostaglandin content of the seminal fluid which can cause intense uterine contractions. Artificial insemination with donor sperm may be indicated in cases of azoospermia or severe oligospermia.

Tubal surgery

The role of surgery on damaged tubes (Fig. 6) has advocates who usually feel it is essential that the surgeon is specifically trained and uses microscopic techniques but many feel that it wastes resources. If the fallopian

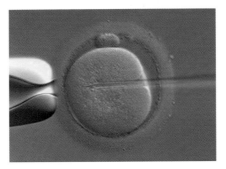

Fig. 5 **Intracytoplasmic sperm injection.**
The egg is held by a suction pipette (left) and the sperm injected into the cytoplasm.

tube is obviously enlarged and has been damaged for a number of years, the chance of restoring function is very small, so IVF may be more cost- and time-effective. However, if there is minimal fimbrial clubbing laparoscopic laser surgery may be able to achieve a good result. In patients wishing reversal of their sterilization, high success rates can be achieved using a microsurgical technique.

Unexplained infertility

After appropriate investigation there will be a group of patients whose tests are normal and who have unexplained infertility. The decision on when to treat will depend on the duration of infertility, the woman's age and the previous pregnancy history. It is reasonable to wait for up to 3 years with no treatment in younger women.

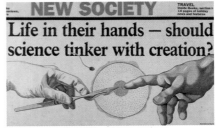

Fig. 7 **An area of controversy.**

IUI with ovarian stimulation, GIFT or IVF are all effective treatments in this group (Fig. 7).

Ovarian hyperstimulation

Ovarian hyperstimulation syndrome (OHSS) is a potentially serious side effect of ovulation induction and is associated with large ovarian cysts. There is increased vascular permeability leading to ascites, pleural effusions and intravascular hypovolaemia. Thrombosis may ensue. OHSS is found particularly in patients with polycystic ovarian syndrome and older women. The mild form, found in approximately 30% of patients, responds to conservative management and no further ovarian stimulation. The severe form (found in < 2%) requires fluid replacement, antithrombotic measures and bed rest.

Management of infertility

- Clomiphene citrate in women with PCOS may enable them to achieve near normal conception rates.
- Multiple pregnancy is increased with any ovulation induction and patients should be counselled accordingly; the possibility of fetal reduction may be discussed.
- Tubal surgery should only be performed by those with specific training using microsurgical techniques.
- Advances in freezing/defrosting techniques have improved the outlook for infertile couples, making the cost of each cycle of treatment more attainable.

Cervical intraepithelial neoplasia (CIN)

Definition
Cervical intraepithelial neoplasia (CIN) is a premalignant condition of the cervix. It is usually asymptomatic and is detected by routine cytological screening. The degree of severity is graded CIN 1 to CIN 3.

Aetiology
The causes of CIN are the same as those of cervical carcinoma, since one is a precursor of the other (Table 1).

At puberty, the squamo-columnar junction corresponds to the anatomical external os. Hormonal changes cause cervical oedema with exposure of the columnar epithelium – an ectropion; common misnomer, 'an erosion'. The exposure of the fragile columnar cells to vaginal acidity stimulates squamous metaplasia. Tongues of squamous cells grow inwards to cover the exposed columnar epithelium. It takes approximately 3 months for this metaplasia to mature into stable squamous epithelium. Early sexual intercourse will expose immature stable metaplasia to several potentially oncogenic agents. The area of previously exposed columnar epithelium that undergoes squamous metaplasia is known as the transformation zone (TZ) (Fig. 1).

Screening
Screening for CIN is based on a cervical smear – sampling surface cells from the cervix with a spatula. The success of any screening programme depends on the age screening commences and finishes, how frequently it is performed (1- to 3-yearly) and the reliability of the cytology laboratory (the number of false positive and false negative results).

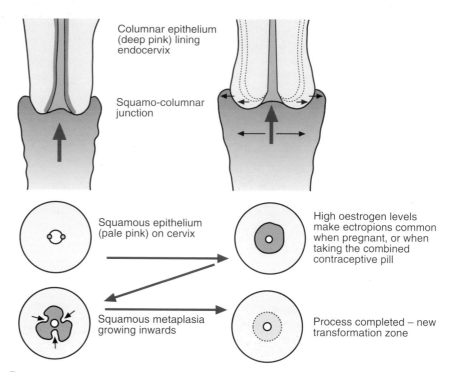

Fig. 1 **Ectropion and transformation of the transformation zone.**

Diagnosis
To obtain a complete diagnosis the triage of cytology, colposcopy and histological biopsy are needed, as smears are often under reported (Fig. 2).

Cytology
Dyskaryosis is a cytological term. It describes features of individual cells such as size and staining of nuclei and the amount of cytoplasm (Fig. 3).

Indirectly, it is commenting on the degree of cellular maturation, since parabasal cells should not be present at the surface of the epidermis and accessible to cellular sampling. Cytology reports *always highlight the most immature cells present.*

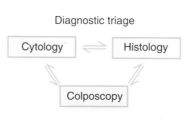

Fig. 2 **Diagnosis of CIN.**

Histology
Dysplasia is a histological term. It requires a full-thickness biopsy for diagnosis (Fig. 4). Carcinoma-in-situ and CIN 3 are more or less synonymous. The basement membrane remains intact. Precancerous lesions have also been identified for adenocarcinoma, termed mild or severe glandular atypia.

Colposcopy
The colposcope is a low-power binocular microscope which allows the cervix to be viewed stereoscopically (Fig. 5), at magnifications of ×6 to ×40. In dysplastic tissue the normal pattern of blood vessels becomes distorted and punctation (Fig. 6) and mosaicism (Fig. 7) are seen. Abnormal tissue stains white with acetic acid but will not take up the brown iodine stain. Studying the vessel patterns and staining reactions, a colposcopist gauges the degree of CIN present. Colposcopically directed biopsies are taken from suspicious areas to exclude the presence of invasive disease. The extent of the lesion must

Table 1 **The risk factors for CIN and cervical carcinoma**	
Young age at first intercourse	Exposure to tumour promoters has a greater influence on immature cells
Number of sexual partners	
Smoking	Increases the risk of cervical cancer four-fold; the risk remains elevated in ex-smokers
Poor uptake of screening programme	
Long-term use of the contraceptive pill	Pill takers do not necessarily use barrier methods – increasing exposure to seminal fluids
Male-related risk factors	The number of the partner's previous sexual relationships is relevant
	Cervical cancer risk increased if partner has penile cancer
	Cervical cancer risk increased if partner's previous sexual contact had cervical cancer
Immunosuppression	Risk increased with immunosuppressed renal transplant patients, and in HIV-positive women
HPV infection	Mainly subtype 16

Mild dyskaryosis
- Superficial cell
- Normal-sized nucleus
- Mild nuclear abnormalities
- Abundant cytoplasm
- Angular cell borders

Moderate dyskaryosis
- Intermediate cell
- Nucleus larger than normal, but < 50% of cell

Severe dyskaryosis
- Parabasal cell
- Nucleus > 50% of cell
- Cell border rounded
- Nucleus darker (hyperpicnotic)
- Nucleus irregular

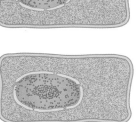
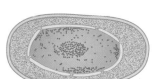
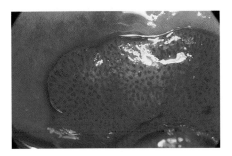

Fig. 3 **Cytology of CIN.**

CIN 1
- Upper $^2/_3$ of epithelium exhibits reasonable differentiation
- Mild nuclear abnormalities, most marked in basal layer
- Few mitotic figures, confined to basal $^1/_3$

CIN 2
- Upper $^1/_2$ of epithelium well differentiated
- Moderate nuclear cell abnormalities
- Mitotic figures (some abnormal) present in basal $^2/_3$

CIN 3
- Maturation confined to superficial $^1/_3$ (or absent)
- Nuclear abnormalities marked and throughout full thickness
- Mitotic figures numerous, bizarre and at all levels

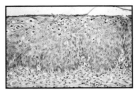
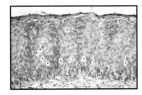

Fig. 4 **Histology of CIN.**

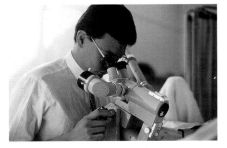

Fig. 5 **Colposcope.**

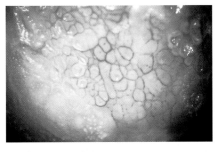

Fig. 7 **Mosaicism.**

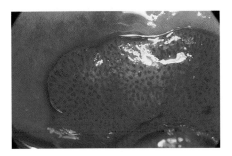

Fig. 6 **Punctation seen with carcinoma-in-situ and microinvasion.**

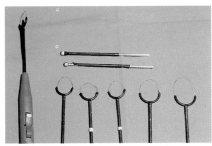

Fig. 8 **Loop diathermy apparatus.**

also be defined. If the lesion enters the endocervical canal the colposcopist must be sure that the upper limit is clearly visualized. This will determine whether the lesion is suitable for local destructive techniques or if a cone biopsy is required. Destruction is carried out by an expert. There must be adequate cytology and colposcopy follow-up.

Local treatment
There are several different treatment modalities including cryocautery, cold coagulation, electrodiathermy, carbon dioxide laser, loop diathermy. Small localized lesions of CIN 1 and possibly of CIN 2 may be treated by cryocautery. Lesions entering the canal and those that look more severe require either

laser ablation or loop wedge excision. Laser treatment destroys the tissue by evaporation and coagulation. It has been superseded by loop diathermy which involves running an electric current through a thin loop of varying size and shape (Fig. 8). The tissue is excised rather

than ablated and, therefore, pathology can be reviewed if questions arise later. It is an easier technique to learn.

Cone biopsy
Cone biopsy is reserved for when the upper limit of the lesion cannot be seen, when there is a suspicion of invasive disease and if cytology is persistently positive with negative colposcopy. Most cone biopsies are now performed by loop diathermy. Some situations require knife cones. Complications include haemorrhage (10%), cervical stenosis or incomplete excision. Stenosis is related to the depth of the cone excised. Hysterectomy should be considered for a patient with recurrent abnormal smears suffering from menorrhagia and, in the case of an incomplete cone biopsy, when the family is complete. In a woman with a uterine prolapse, a vaginal hysterectomy would be ideal.

If a hysterectomy is performed because of abnormal smears, annual vault smears should be performed.

There is growing evidence to suggest a psychosexual morbidity following investigation. Patients need to be approached with confidence and sensitivity.

Cervical intraepithelial neoplasia

- CIN is a premalignant condition of the cervix characterized by specific cytology (dyskaryosis) and histological (dysplasia) features.
- Aetiological factors are similar to those of cervical carcinoma.
- It is usually asymptomatic; diagnosis requires cytology, colposcopy and histology.
- Cone biopsies are taken if the upper limit of the lesion is not clearly visualized.
- Loop excision is currently the most common treatment modality; laser is useful if dysplastic areas extend into the vaginal fornices.

Cervical carcinoma

Epidemiology

Worldwide, cancer of the cervix is the second most common malignancy in women after breast cancer – 77% of cases occur in developing countries. Finland, which has an advanced population-based screening programme, has one of the lowest rates in the world. Israel has a low incidence as a result of conservative sexual practice.

Approximately 2000 deaths occur annually in the UK. A bimodal distribution with an initial peak of incidence for women in their 30s, and a larger peak for women in their 50s has emerged. The incidence of cervical cancer is higher in lower socio-economic groups.

Risk factors

The main aetiological agent is infection with certain subtypes of human papilloma virus (HPV). Several risk factors have also been identified (see p. 134).

HPV infection is far more common than the development of cancerous change, so other factors must influence the malignant potential between one individual and another (Fig. 1).

HPV subtype 16 appears to be the main oncological agent. It is present in:

- only 5% of cytologically normal women
- up to 50% of smears containing CIN 1
- over 90% of invasive cervical cancer.

HPV subtypes 18, 31 and 33 may also be implicated.

Pathology

Malignant tumours of the cervix may be squamous (85–90%) or glandular

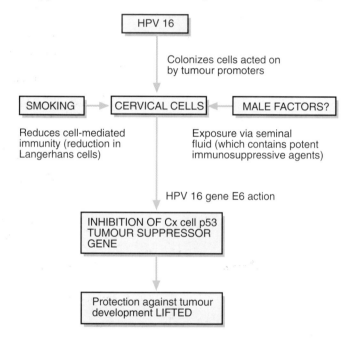

Fig. 1 **Possible aetiological pathway for CIN and carcinoma.**

Fig. 2 **Cervical carcinoma.** Exophytic lesion.

(10%) in type. Microinvasion (stage 1a) is defined as invasion that is less than 5 mm from the basement membrane.

Most squamous cell carcinomas involve the external os and are visible on speculum examination. The lesion may be either exophytic, growing outwards in a papillary or polypoidal excrescence, (Fig. 2), or endophytic, infiltrating the surrounding structures. Ulceration and excavation frequently occur. Invasive squamous cell carcinomas vary in their degree of cellular differentiation, but often attempt to form a keratin pearl.

Assessment

Presentation

Many women are asymptomatic. More advanced disease will present with symptoms (Table 1). Screening for cervical cancer has resulted in an increase in the number of women found to have asymptomatic disease (Table 1).

Staging

Accurate staging of the disease determines the treatment and prognosis (Table 2). Early detection is associated with significantly better survival rates. Clinical staging is based on an examination under anaesthesia (EUA). This should include:

- cervical biopsy
- cystoscopy
- a rectal examination including sigmoidoscopy
- dilatation and curettage.

The patient should undergo an intravenous pyelogram (IVP) and a chest X-ray. Magnetic resonance imaging (MRI) is useful in assessing

Table 1 **Symptoms and signs of cervical carcinoma**	
Symptoms	**Signs**
Confined to cervix	At routine examination
■ Postcoital bleeding	■ Cervix looks suspicious at time of smear
■ Postmenopausal bleeding	■ Abnormal cells, indicative of invasive carcinoma on
■ Intermenstrual bleeding	cytology
■ Offensive, blood-stained vaginal discharge	
	At colposcopy
Spread to adjacent structures	■ Heavy, contact bleeding
■ Fistulae – passage of urine, faeces or flatus vaginally	■ Irregular surface contour
(if bowel/ bladder involved)	■ Atypical vessels – capillaries of irregular calibre and
■ Renal failure – bilateral ureteric obstruction	branching pattern
■ Deep visceral or nerve root pain (if sacral nerve root	
involved)	
■ Lower limb oedema – extensive pelvic side wall	
infiltration	

Table 2 Staging and survival rates of cervical carcinoma

	5-year survival rate
Stage 1: Tumour confined to the cervix	
a Microinvasive carcinoma	
a1 Stromal invasion ≤ 3 mm depth and ≤ 7 mm horizontal spread	95.1%
a2 Lesions with a depth > 3 mm, but ≤ 5 mm, and a horizontal spread ≤ 7 mm	94.9%
b Clinical lesions confined to the cervix	
b1 Tumour diameter < 4 cm	80.1%
b2 Tumour diameter ≥ 4 cm	
Stage 2: Spread beyond the cervix, but not to the pelvic side wall, with involvement of upper two-thirds of the vagina	
a Vaginal spread, but no obvious parametrial spread	66.3%
b Parametrial spread, but not as far as pelvic side wall	63.5%
Stage 3: Spread in the pelvis	
a Involvement of lower one-third of the vagina	33.3%
b Extension to the pelvic side wall or hydronephrosis	38.7%
Stage 4: Distant spread	
a Spread to involve adjacent organs (bladder, rectum)	17.1%
b Distant spread	9.4%

FIGO classification, Montreal 1994. FIGO Data for survival 1990–1992 (n = 11 945).

early-stage disease and tumour extension into the bladder, rectum, vagina and pelvic floor. Computed tomography (CT) scanning or MRI can be used in later-stage disease. CT scanning is now routinely used for radiotherapy treatment planning. MRI is the imaging modality of choice when salvage surgery is indicated for an isolated central pelvic recurrence.

Treatment options

Microinvasive disease
In the woman who has not yet completed her family, it is possible to adopt a conservative approach. A knife cone biopsy will provide both diagnosis and treatment and preserve the uterus. Ablative techniques are inappropriate.

Stage 1a superficial invasion only occurs with squamous cancers of the cervix because the lesion spreads contiguously. Adenocarcinomas are known to have skip lesions in separate crypts and cannot be treated in a similar conservative fashion.

Follow-up is indicated with cytology and colposcopy. Once the family is complete a hysterectomy may be appropriate. The vaginal approach is preferred as it is easy to remove a small cuff of vagina with the specimen.

Invasive disease
Radical treatment is indicated for stages 1b, 2a and some cases of 2b. Either surgery or radiotherapy can be first-line treatment. Both modalities produce equivalent cure rates for patients with stage 1b cervical cancer. Surgery offers several advantages:

- it allows preservation of the ovaries (radiotherapy will destroy them)

- there is better chance of preserving sexual function (vaginal stenosis occurs in up to 85% of irradiated patients, although use of topical oestrogens vaginally has reduced this)
- a more accurate prognosis can be obtained as surgery allows nodal sampling. (Total staging is not possible from an EUA.)

The classical surgical procedure is the Wertheim's radical hysterectomy including pelvic lymphadenectomy and 3 cm vaginal cuff. The original operation conserved the ovaries, since squamous carcinoma does not spread directly to these tissues. Oophorectomy should be performed in cases of adenocarcinoma of the cervix as there is a 5–10% incidence of ovarian metastases. Some surgeons remove the ovaries if the lesion is large (stage 1b2) or if there is a poorly differentiated tumour on biopsy.

Postoperative radiotherapy is given in all cases where there is proven lymph node involvement.

Radiotherapy is recommended as first-line treatment in the following circumstances:

- when surgical expertise is not available
- in women with a tumour greater than 4 cm in diameter

- in women who are not medically fit for surgery.

Obesity makes surgery more difficult, but may also compromise the delivery of radiotherapy.

Some centres now perform laparoscopic lymphadenectomy, in conjunction with the radical vaginal hysterectomy – this may represent less morbidity than a radical abdominal operation. These new combinations await full evaluation.

Advanced disease (stage 4)
Combinations of chemo- and radiotherapy are used but the overall survival rate is very poor.

Follow-up
Follow-up is for 5 years with more frequent clinic visits initially as 90% of relapses present within the first 3 years. Recurrent disease may present with weight loss, leg oedema, pelvic, leg or back pain, supraclavicular lymphadenopathy, vaginal discharge, renal failure, bone pain or haemoptysis. The most frequent sites of recurrence are in the pelvis, lung, para-aortic nodes, liver, bone, vulva, inguinal nodes and supraclavicular nodes. There are four possible therapeutic options for recurrent disease:

- radiotherapy
- chemotherapy, e.g. platinum, bleomycin or ifosfamide
- surgery, generally exenterative
- palliation.

The role of surgery for recurrent disease is confined to specific subgroups of patients, where there is evidence of central pelvic recurrence without metastatic disease and where the patient accepts such radical intervention. As 40% of patients with cervical carcinoma will eventually die, palliative care for the terminally ill is very important. The objective is to relieve or control any symptoms affecting the patients' quality of life whilst maintaining dignity.

Cervical carcinoma

- Cancer of the cervix is still quite common – reduction in incidence depends on the quality of the screening programme.
- The aetiology appears to be multifactorial; the prime oncogenic agent is probably HPV-16.
- Microinvasive squamous tumours carry a good prognosis, allowing conservative treatment initially if required.
- Early invasive squamous disease, stages 1b, 2a (and some cases of 2b) may be treated by either a Wertheim's hysterectomy or radiotherapy as first-line treatment.
- Glandular tumours (adenocarcinomas) are not detectable by screening, are associated with skip lesions and require radical surgery.

Carcinoma of the uterus

Carcinoma of the endometrium forms the most common type of uterine cancer. These are mainly adenocarcinomas derived from endometrial glandular cells. There are some rare variations, e.g. adenoacanthoma. Sarcomas which are derived from stromal cells may be endometrial or myometrial in origin. Prognosis and treatment are different for these two categories of uterine cancer.

Endometrial carcinoma

This is a disease which predominantly presents in the postmenopausal years (over 75% of cases). Around 3–5% of cases will present under the age of 40 years. Over one-third of the premenopausal patients present with heavy, but regular periods. The incidence of endometrial cancer is highest in white North Americans, who have a rate approximately seven times higher than the Chinese.

Risk factors for endometrial carcinoma

Most of the known risk factors for carcinoma of the corpus uteri share a common basis – that of excessive, unopposed oestrogen stimulation of the endometrium (Table 1). A doubling in body weight results in a doubling of peripheral conversion of androgens to oestrone in the fat cells. In polycystic ovarian syndrome there is an increase in the free, unbound oestrogen fraction available to stimulate the endometrium (see p. 114).

There appears to be an association between endometrial cancer and non-insulin-dependent diabetes mellitus (NIDDM). Although rare, the granulosa–theca cell ovarian tumours secrete excess oestrogen – 10% of cases are associated with endometrial cancer and 50% are associated with endometrial hyperplasia. Mucinous carcinomas, endometrioid carcinomas and Krukenberg tumours (squamous ovarian tumours) have also been associated with an increase in oestrogen secretion.

Care must be taken when prescribing hormone replacement therapy (see p. 150). The administration of unopposed oestrogens leads to a risk of developing endometrial carcinoma 7–10 times higher than that of the general population. Tamoxifen used in the treatment of breast cancer has also been associated with endometrial hyperplasia and cancer as it has both oestrogenic and anti-oestrogenic properties. Smoking appears to be protective.

Presentation and investigation

The commonest presentation of endometrial carcinoma is postmenopausal bleeding. Pain may indicate metastatic disease. Discharge is often associated with the presence of a pyometra. Although postmenopausal bleeding is the commonest presentation for endometrial cancer, and occurs in 80% of cases, endometrial cancer is not the commonest cause of postmenopausal bleeding (Table 2).

All cases of abnormal bleeding must be thoroughly investigated including irregular and/or heavy regular bleeding in the premenopausal group.

Ultrasonography provides a useful screening tool. Atrophic endometrium has a thickness of 3 mm or less – thickened endometrium in a postmenopausal woman is therefore suspicious. Some centres use 5 mm as a cut-off point but 6% of cancers will be missed. With a cut-off point of 4 mm most cancers are detected. Demonstration of fluid in the endometrial cavity is associated with uterine and extrauterine malignancy in 25% of cases and warrants a careful inspection of the adnexa.

Outpatient endometrial sampling techniques have been introduced together with visualization of endometrial tissue via the 3-mm hysterosope (Table 3 and p. 124). There is always a small risk of uterine perforation in the presence of friable cancerous tissue.

Introduction of the sonohysterogram (SHG), seems to improve the detection of endometrial polyps, submucous fibroids and focal thickening of the endometrium. Further techniques under evaluation include 3-D scanning and colour Doppler blood-flow imaging.

Pathology

Endometrial carcinoma appears as a raised, rough or even papillary area and often arises in the fundus. The internal os is rarely involved early in the disease (Fig. 1). Endometrial carcinoma has several distinct sub-types; the commonest is the endometrioid adenocarcinoma, when the glandular pattern generally resembles a normal proliferative phase endometrium (Fig. 1).

Prognosis

A number of prognostic factors have been identified. Clearly, the stage and

Table 3	Investigation of postmenopausal bleeding
History	Look for relevant risk factors
Examination	To exclude pelvic masses, assess uterine size and mobility
Ultrasound	Transabdominally or transvaginally (TVS) to assess endometrial thickness and presence of intracavity fluid
Endometrial biopsy	Pipelle, 'Z' sampler, Vabra aspirator
Hysteroscopy	Under general anaesthetic or as outpatient procedure
Dilatation and curettage	Endometrial sampling under general anaesthesia
Sonohysterography	The instillation of fluid into the uterine cavity during scanning
3-D scanning (still in semi-experimental stage)	Facilitates accurate volume measurements
Doppler and colour flow imaging (still in semi-experimental stage)	Used to detect changes in uterine and endometrial blood flow with malignancy

Table 1	Risk factors for carcinoma of the uterus
■ Obesity
■ Impaired glucose tolerance
■ Nulliparity
■ Late menopause
■ Unopposed oestrogen therapy
■ Functioning ovarian tumours (granulosa–theca cell tumour)
■ Family history of carcinoma of breast, ovary or colon

Table 2 Causes of postmenopausal bleeding	
Benign causes – 88% of cases	Malignant causes – 12% of cases
Atrophic vaginitis	Endometrial carcinoma (8%)
Endometrial polyps	Cervical carcinoma
Endometrial hyperplasia	Ovarian tumours
	Rare uterine tumours
	Extragenital tumours, bladder, colonic and rectal cancers

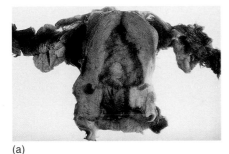 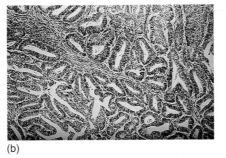

(a)   (b)

Fig. 1 **Endometrial carcinoma. (a)** View of cut surface of the uterus. **(b)** High-power view of Grade 1 cancer.

Table 4 **Prognostic factors**	
Age	Older women have a worse prognosis
Body shape	Obese, diabetic, hypercholesterolaemic (better differentiated tumours/better prognosis)
Stage of the disease	Myometrial invasion Peritoneal cytology Lymph node involvement
Histological subtype	
Degree of differentiation	
Steroid receptor status	
Lymphatic/vascular involvement	

grade of the disease are of paramount importance. Lymph node involvement and evidence of vascular spread reduce the survival rate (Tables 4 and 5).

Patients with tumours involving the cervix have a higher risk of metastases to other pelvic organs and lymph nodes. The survival rate is approximately 20% less than those with tumour confined to the corpus. Cancer of the corpus uteri is staged surgically (Table 5).

Treatment

Treatment will depend on both the stage of the disease and the fitness of the patient. The patient must be accurately assessed preoperatively to exclude suspicious lymphadenopathy, ascites or organomegaly. Renal and hepatic function tests, tumour markers, chest X-ray and possibly an intravenous urogram will need to be undertaken. The CA125 level increases with increasing spread of the disease.

The operation of choice is a total abdominal hysterectomy and bilateral salpingo-oophorectomy. Removal of a vaginal cuff does not reduce the recurrence rate or improve survival. The pelvic and the para-aortic nodes should be removed if the cervix or adnexa are involved, or if the myometrium is obviously deeply infiltrated.

Radiotherapy is indicated if the histology shows a poorly differentiated or high-grade tumour, if the nodes are involved, or if staging at the time of surgery scores more than a Ib.

The stage 3 patient should have further imaging to determine whether the disease is confined to the pelvis. If possible, radical surgery with radiotherapy should be offered. Stage 4 disease most commonly spreads to the lungs followed by peripheral lymph nodes and the bladder.

Approximately 70% of recurrences following primary treatment occur within the first 2–3 years. Early recurrences carry a grave prognosis as

Table 5 **Grading and staging of carcinoma of the uterus**					
Grading		**Staging**			**5-year survival**
Gx	Grade cannot be assessed	Stage 0		Atypical hyperplasia/carcinoma-in-situ	
G1	Well differentiated				
G2	Moderately differentiated	Stage 1a		Tumour limited to endometrium	90.9%
G3	Poorly or undifferentiated		1b	Invasion < 50% myometrium	88.2%
			1c	Invasion > 50% myometrium	81.0%
Differentiation refers to the degree to		Stage 2a		Endocervical glandular involvement only	76.9%
which the tumour resembles			2b	Cervical stromal invasion	67.1%
adenocarcinoma. The more squamous		Stage 3a		Tumour invades the serosa of the corpus and/or adnexa, ± positive cytology	60.3%
or solid growth, the less differentiated			3b	Vaginal metastases	41.2%
			3c	Metastasis to pelvic or para-aortic nodes	31.7%
		Stage 4a		Invasion of bladder and/or bowel mucosa	20.1%
			4b	Spread outside pelvis, including intra-abdominal spread/distant organs and/or inguinal nodes	5.3%

As per FIGO classification, 1988. FIGO Data for Survival 1990–1992.

they indicate an aggresive tumour. Radiotherapy is of great value for palliation. Medroxyprogesterone acetate has been widely used for distant recurrence – the response rate is 15–20%.

Tamoxifen and aminoglutethimide (an aromatase inhibitor) have also been assessed for stage 4 disease, i.e. to shrink distant spread.

Uterine sarcoma

Endometrial stromal sarcomas and mixed Müllerian tumours rarely occur.

Myometrial tumours

Leiomyosarcoma

This is the malignant counterpart of the benign leiomyoma (fibroids) and is the most common pure sarcoma of the uterus. The gross appearance is similar to that of a leiomyoma, although the cut surface may be paler and more yellow, with areas of haemorrhage and necrosis.

The majority present with irregular or postmenopausal bleeding, vaginal discharge, pelvic pain or pressure symptoms. In some situations the sarcoma is detected when fibroids enlarge rapidly. Only 5–10% of leiomyosarcomata arise from pre-existing fibroids and these have a better prognosis. Surgery is the treatment of choice.

Carcinoma of the uterus

- Endometrial carcinoma commonly presents with postmenopausal bleeding, but endometrial carcinoma *is not* the commonest cause of postmenopausal bleeding.

- Most of the known risk factors for endometrial cancer involve excessive unopposed oestrogen stimulation of the endometrium.

- The differentiation (grading) and staging of the disease are the most important factors influencing survival.

- Total abdominal hysterectomy and bilateral salpingo-oophorectomy is the treatment of choice (for stage 1 disease).

- Sarcomas carry a much worse prognosis than endometrial cancer, but are a much rarer tumour.

Benign ovarian conditions

Figure 1 shows the stages of ovarian development from the primordial ridge. Cells in the ovary may develop from all three types, hence the diversity of problems that may be found within the ovary. The mesodermal ridge is covered in epithelium for development of gonads and invagination of the coelomic epithelium forms the Müllerian duct. Primordial germ cells migrate from the yolk sac.

Physiological cysts

The physiological cysts are a persistence of structures found during normal ovarian function. They are largely asymptomatic and frequently undergo spontaneous resolution. They may present with pain and need investigation. Rupture or torsion may both present with an acute abdomen needing surgical intervention (see below). Haemorrhage into the cyst, although painful, may be managed conservatively and laparoscopy is only performed if the symptoms fail to settle.

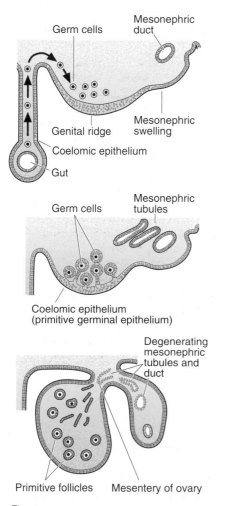

Fig. 1 **Development of the ovary.**

Table 1 **Pathological ovarian cysts**	
Derivation	**Pathology**
Coelomic epithelium	Serous cystadenoma
	Mucinous cystadenoma
	Brenner cell tumour
	Endometrioid cystadenoma
Germ cells	Cystic teratoma (dermoid cyst)
	Solid teratoma
Sex cord cells	Granulosa/theca cell tumours
	Fibroma
	Sertoli–Leydig cell
	(arrhenoblastoma) tumour

Follicular. These cysts are small (but may reach 10 cm diameter), unilocular, common, lined by oestrogen-producing granulosa cells and contain clear fluid rich in hormones. They are particularly likely in patients undergoing ovulation stimulation.

Luteal. These may present with intraperitoneal haemorrhage. Luteal cysts are formed when the corpus luteum does not regress.

Pathological cysts

The pathological cysts and their derivation are shown in Table 1.

Serous cystadenoma. The most common presenting cyst (Fig. 2) is unilocular with papilliferous growths on the inner surface (may also be on the outer surface making distinction from a malignant tumour very difficult). The fluid content is thin and serous, epithelial lining is cuboidal or columnar

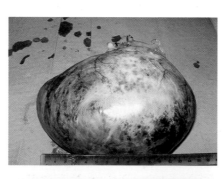

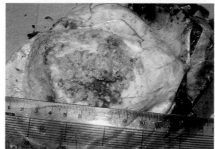

Fig. 2 **Serous cystadenoma.**

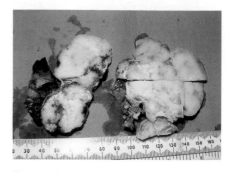

Fig. 3 **Mucinous cystadenoma.**

epithelium and they occasionally contain calcified granules known as psammoma bodies.

Mucinous cystadenoma. These are unilateral, multilocular, full of thick mucin, lined by columnar mucin-secreting epithelium and may reach great size (recorded up to 100 kg) (Fig. 3). Rarely they rupture, releasing mucin-producing cells which may implant and continue to secrete mucin which compromises bowel function and gives rise to significant mortality (pseudomyxoma peritonei).

Brenner cell tumour. A rare presentation with islands of transitional epithelium in dense fibrotic stroma. They are usually small and may secrete oestrogen, so they can present with abnormal vaginal bleeding.

Endometrioid cystadenoma. This is seldom distinguishable from a cystic patch of endometriosis.

Dermoid cyst (cystic teratoma). This is the commonest cyst presenting in young women (Fig. 4). Their derivation from the pluripotential germ cells means that all tissue types may be found with hair, sebaceous cells, fat cells and teeth being most common. One cell-line may predominate (e.g. struma ovarii with hormonally-active thyroid tissue). They are mostly asymptomatic but may tort or rupture.

Solid teratoma. Another rare presentation which will be benign if it contains mature tissues. Immature tissues are malignant.

Granulosa cell tumour. The commonest hormone-secreting tumour – 25% of which are malignant.

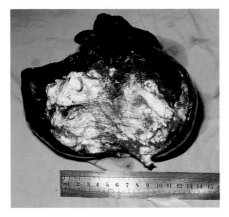

Fig. 4 **Opened dermoid cyst.** Showing hair, fat tissue and peripheral infarction due to ovarian torsion.

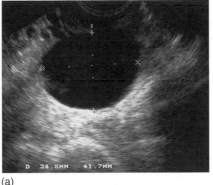
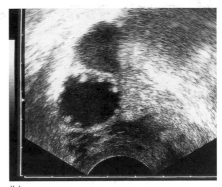

(a)   (b)

Fig. 6 **Ultrasound examination of ovarian cyst. (a)** Smooth outline in a non-malignant cyst. **(b)** Projections into a malignant cyst.

Symptoms found with ovarian cysts include:

- pain – due to torsion or haemorrhage
- asymptomatic – especially physiological cysts
- abdominal swelling – large cyst or associated ascites (fibroma)
- pressure symptoms – affecting bladder and bowel function
- menstrual upset due to hormone secretion.

Investigations

Bimanual examination (Fig. 5). This may allow distinction between an enlarged fibroid uterus and an ovarian cyst but ultrasound may also be necessary.

Ultrasound scan. The cyst fluid will show as dark on the picture (see follicular cyst) with a white-flecked appearance if blood is present. Dermoid cysts appear more complex. It is important to look for features which may suggest malignancy (Fig. 6) (protrusions inside the cyst, multilocular, neovascularization, ascitic fluid in pouch of Douglas).

Hormone assays. If the main symptoms suggest hormone-producing cysts (such as menstrual upset, hirsutism or virilization) check oestrogen and androgen levels.

CA125. This tumour marker will be modestly raised in the face of endometriosis but a high value is suggestive of malignancy. Unfortunately a low value does not completely exclude malignancy.

Diagnostic laparoscopy. This allows visualization of the cyst, peritoneal washings for cytology if concerned about possible malignancy and treatment by laparoscopic removal if appropriate (see below).

Treatment

Asymptomatic cysts less than 5 cm in diameter in a young woman require no action as these will usually undergo spontaneous resolution.

Asymptomatic cysts greater than 5 cm in diameter in a young woman should be rescanned in 6 weeks. The cyst will be either smaller (or the same size) and need no action, or enlarged in size, possibly with blood in the fluid, and would be best removed to avoid the risk of torsion and loss of the ovary.

A cyst that is symptomatic or rapidly enlarging requires removal. The traditional approach is by laparotomy. An ovarian cystectomy conserving all normal ovarian tissue and restoring the ovarian surface to normal with

minimal chance for adhesion formation is the aim. This ensures that future fertility is not compromised. A fine, inert suture is used on the ovary to excite less tissue reaction and peritoneal lavage used to remove all blood, which would promote development of adhesions. The need to limit adhesion formation has encouraged the development of laparoscopic techniques to allow removal of the cyst with minimal tissue handling. The contents of a dermoid cyst, if spilled into the peritoneal cavity, may cause a chemical peritonitis so this may be best managed through a mini-laparotomy incision.

Laparoscopic management of simple cysts can be performed by drainage of the cyst contents then peeling off the cyst capsule, which is sent for histological examination. In the case where the cyst may be malignant it is sometimes appropriate to offer laparoscopic oophorectomy. This will be considerably less invasive for the patient than the previous practice of total abdominal hysterectomy with bilateral salpingo-oophorectomy and omentectomy in any woman over 45 years old found to have an ovarian cyst. The ovary is captured in a bag and removed intact from the abdomen so there is no risk of peritoneal seeding if any tumour exists. The patient may not require to proceed with more major surgery if histology confirms benign disease.

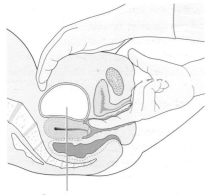

Ovarian cyst

Fig. 5 **Bimanual examination for ovarian cyst.**

Benign ovarian conditions

- Asymptomatic, simple cysts in young women may be managed conservatively.
- Torsion of an ovarian cyst is an emergency – the ovarian blood supply must be restored to prevent necrosis.
- Ultrasound examination allows distinction between ovarian cysts and fibroids.
- Laparoscopic management allows minimal tissue handling which should help to limit adhesion formation within the pelvis.

Ovarian carcinoma

The peak incidence is between 50 and 70 years and carcinoma is more likely with nulliparity and in those with a positive family history. The use of the combined oral contraceptive protects, probably because it reduces the number of ovulations, which is thought to be an aetiological factor. Presentation is usually with abdominal pain and swelling, but may be with urinary frequency, weight loss, dyspeptic symptoms or abnormal menses. Three-quarters of cases have spread outside the pelvis at presentation (to the peritoneum, diaphragm, para-aortic lymph nodes, liver and lung); hence the overall 5-year survival of only 29%. Epithelial tumours account for 80% of all ovarian neoplasms and 90% of all primary malignant ovarian tumours.

Management
Malignancy in an ovarian cyst is more likely in those > 45 years, or in whom cysts are bilateral, or where there is ascites, or solid areas within the cyst, or an irregular growth on the capsule or where the cyst is fixed.

Staging (see Table 1)

Investigations and treatment
Initial investigations should be with ultrasound scanning (USS) (± computed tomography (CT) or magnetic resonance imaging (MRI)), measurement of urea and electrolytes (U & Es), liver function tests (LFTs), a cancer antigen 125 test (CA125) and chest X-ray α-fetoprotein (AFP), human chorionic gonadotrophin (hCG) and estradiol should also be measured if a sex-cord/stromal or germ cell tumour is suspected). Peritoneal fluid cytology

may demonstrate malignant cells. Pleural fluid, if present, may also demonstrate malignant cells and this should be aspirated prior to surgery. CA125 is not a specific marker and may be elevated with many intra-abdominal problems including pelvic inflammatory disease, endometriosis and after surgery itself. Preoperative bowel preparation should be given if bowel surgery is anticipated. On opening the peritoneum, peritoneal fluid should be aspirated or washings taken with saline. Conservative surgery (with removal of one ovary) may be warranted if the patient is young, plans further family, has unilateral disease and has no ascites. A peroperative frozen section may be used, but is often difficult to interpret. Otherwise, total abdominal hysterectomy, bilateral salpingo-oophorectomy and infracolic omentectomy should be performed. Peroperative rupture of intact cysts probably has no adverse prognostic effect providing careful peritoneal toilet is performed. If there is extensive disease, cytoreductive surgery (debulking) is appropriate to improve quality of life, improve response to chemotherapy, prolong remission and increase median survival. Some surgeons would consider pelvic and para-aortic node sampling to ensure accurate staging in apparent 1a and 1b cases.

Postoperative chemotherapy is usually given for epithelial tumours if the staging is > 1a (or for 1a if poorly differentiated), ideally with a platinum-based agent in combination with Taxol. Germ cell tumours are very sensitive to chemotherapy, so fertility-conserving surgery in the young patient is appropriate and the majority

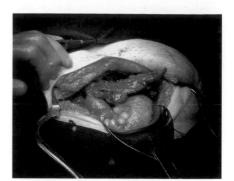

Fig. 1 **Omental 'cake' in a stage 3c ovarian adenocarcinoma.**

of these are cured even if metastatic disease is present. Sex-cord/stromal tumours may occur at either end of the age spectrum. Most are stage 1 at presentation and can be effectively treated with conservative surgery if the patient is young.

Recurrent disease
Most women with advanced epithelial ovarian cancer relapse after primary management. There is considerable potential for palliative therapy in such instances. New chemotherapaeutic agents have traditionally been first evaluated in such patients, but if a patient is offered palliative experimental chemotherapy in this way, it is vitally important to consider the side effects, as these can considerably impair a patient's quality of life. If relapse occurs more than a year after platinum-based chemotherapy, the disease will often respond again and patiens may gain useful palliation in this way.

Screening for ovarian cancer
The poor survival rates associated with advanced ovarian cancer have contributed to the concern that effective screening tests be developed. Presently there is no evidence that screening the general population is useful or cost effective. Women with a family history who are deemed to be at high risk should be considered for the national familial ovarian cancer screening study run through clinical genetics centres.

Familial ovarian cancer
Although overall there is an increased risk of ovarian cancer in those with a family history (relative risk 1.1 for mother, 3.8 for sister and 6.0 for

Table 1	**FIGO staging of ovarian cancer**	
Stage	**Definition**	**5-year survival**
1a	One ovary	60–70% but can be 95% for 1a
1b	Both ovaries	
1c	1a or 1b with ruptured capsule, tumour on the surface of the capsule, positive peritoneal washings or malignant ascites	
2a	Extension to uterus and tubes	30%
2b	Extension to other pelvic tissue, e.g. pelvic nodes, pouch of Douglas	
2c	2a or 2b with ruptured capsule, positive peritoneal washings or malignant ascites	
3a	Pelvic tumour with microscopic peritoneal spread	10%
3b	Pelvic tumour with peritoneal spread < 2 cm	
3c	Abdominal implants > 2 cm ± positive retroperitoneal or inguinal nodes (Fig. 1)	
4	Liver parenchymal disease. Distant metastases. If pleural effusion, must have malignant cells	10%

daughter), the risk is small for most categories except those with more than one affected relative. If one affected primary relative has ovarian cancer and it was diagnosed when she was < 50 years old, the risk increases to 1 : 20 (5%). If there are two affected primary relatives and both developed disease under the age of 50 years there is a > 50% chance of the disease being hereditary. The lifelong risk of a family member with this family history developing ovarian carcinoma is 25%.

5–10% of cases of ovarian carcinoma are attributable to hereditary factors, particularly the breast–ovarian cancer tumour suppressor BRCA1 and BRCA2 genes, which are associated with a 10–50% lifetime risk of developing ovarian carcinoma. Mismatch repair genes, associated with cancer of the colorectum, endometrium, stomach, urinary tract and small bowel, are also responsible for a small proportion of this group. BRCA1 mutations are found in ~ 80% of families with histories of both ovarian and breast cancer, but overall this mutation accounts for only 2% of cases of breast cancer and 3% of cases of ovarian cancer. Those with these genes may warrant screening every 6–12 months with CA125 and USS. Bilateral oophorectomy after completion of the family may also be advocated, but this does not offer complete protection, probably because of 'ovarian carcinoma' arising de novo from the peritoneum.

Pathology of ovarian tumours
(see Table 2)

Neoplasms can arise from any of the elements that comprise a mature ovary, including its surface serosal or mesothelial elements. A number of simpler themes can be drawn from a diversity of tumour types, namely: epithelial tumours, which are by far the most common (70% of primary ovarian tumours), sex-cord–stromal tumours, germ-cell tumours and metastatic tumours. Most of the epithelial tumour types can be further broadly classified as benign, borderline or malignant.

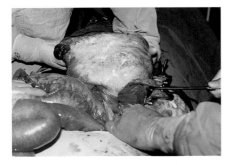

Fig. 2 **Huge stage 1a borderline ovarian tumour.**

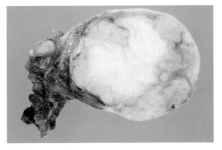

Fig. 3 **Fibrothecoma.**

Table 2 **Pathology of ovarian tumours**			
Origin	Class	Type	Details
Epithelial	Serous, mucinous, endometrioid	Benign or malignant	Commonest malignant ovarian tumour. Rupture of mucinous tumours may lead to pseudomyxoma peritonei (may lead to death from small bowel obstruction and cachexia)
	Borderline tumours (Fig. 2)		These are a separate entity and are defined as carcinoma of low malignant potential lacking stromal invasion, but they may have apparent extra-ovarian spread. They carry a better prognosis (e.g. 5-year survival stage 1 97%, stage 3 85%). Nonetheless, ≈50% will eventually die from the disease
Sex cord/stromal tumours	Granulosa cell tumours	Adult	Rare. Usually occur at extremes of age, and many secrete sex hormones, particularly oestrogen
		Juvenile	Rare. Rarely malignant
	Thecoma (Fig. 3)		Rare. These are solid, yellow, usually postmenopausal and almost always benign
	Androblastoma	Sertoli	Usually benign, but most secrete sex hormones
		Leydig cell	Very rare
		Mixed Sertoli/Leydig	Very rare
Germ cell tumours			These are the commonest tumours in the < 30-year-old age group but overall are more common > 40. Only 2–3% are malignant (although ≈30% are malignant in those < 20 years old)
	No differentiation	Dysgerminoma	Very radio- and chemosensitive
	Extra-embryonic differentiation	Malignant ovarian choriocarcinoma	Very rare. Secrete hCG and may present with precocious pseudopuberty. They have a poor prognosis
		Yolk sac tumours	Very rare. These occur in the 14–20 age group and secrete AFP
	Embryonic	Mature cyst (dermoid)	90% occur in women of reproductive age. 10% are bilateral. They are usually unilocular, often with squamous epithelium and skin appendages. Usually benign
		Immature solid tumour	These are rare, malignant and secrete hCG and AFP
Metastases			From gastric, breast and colonic tumours. A Krukenberg tumour is a metastasis from any mucus-secreting adenocarcinoma

Ovarian carcinoma

- Presentation is insidious, and disease may be advanced at presentation.
- Management is with optimal debulking ± chemotherapy, ideally with a platinum-based agent in combination with Taxol.
- 5–10% of cases of ovarian carcinoma are attributable to hereditary factors and there may be a role for screening in this group.

Benign vulval conditions

Anatomy

The vulva consists of the mons pubis, labia majora, labia minora, clitoris and the vestibule. It is covered with keratinizing squamous epithelium, unlike the vaginal mucosa which is covered with non-keratinizing squamous epithelium. The labia majora are hair-bearing and contain sweat and sebaceous glands: from an embryological viewpoint, they are analogous to the scrotum. Bartholin's glands are situated in the posterior part of the labia, one on each side of the vestibule. Its lymphatics drain to the inguinal nodes and then to the external iliac nodes, and the area is richly supplied with blood vessels.

Bartholin's cyst

The greater vestibular, or Bartholin's, glands lie in the subcutaneous tissue below the lower third of the labium majorum and open via ducts to the vestibule between the hymenal orifice and the labia minora. They secrete mucus, particularly at the time of intercourse. If the duct becomes blocked a tense retention cyst forms, and if there is superadded infection the patient develops a painful abscess (Fig. 1). The abscess can be incised and drained, usually under general anaesthesia. Antibiotics are usually only necessary if there is additional cellulitis.

Pruritus vulvae

This is commoner in the > 40 age group and has numerous aetiologies:

- infection (*Candida*, pediculosis, threadworms)
- eczema
- dermatitis
- irritation from a vaginal discharge
- lichen sclerosus
- lichen planus
- vulval intraepithelial neoplasia (VIN)
- vulval carcinoma
- medical problems, e.g. diabetes mellitus, uraemia or liver failure.

A biopsy may be necessary to establish the diagnosis. If no cause is found, irritants and bath water additives should be avoided, soap substitutes used, the area dried gently (e.g. with a hairdryer), loose cotton clothing worn and nylon tights avoided. A strong cream b.i.d. for 3 weeks followed by milder hydrocortisone cream 1% daily as maintenance is useful, as is the use of soap substitutes (e.g. Oilatum). Antihistamines may also be of help. Primary or secondary depression may also warrant treatment.

Vulvodynia

This is chronic vulvar discomfort, especially that characterized by the complaint of pruritus, burning, stinging, irritation or rawness. No one factor can be identified as the specific cause and indeed there appear to be no clinically definable differences between groups of patients. It may occasionally be associated with previous sexual abuse. Vulvar vestibulitis is a chronic clinical syndrome with erythema, severe pain on entry or to vestibular touch, and tenderness to pressure localized within the vestibule. If symptoms are of less than 3 months' duration, there is often response to topical corticosteroids. If they are chronic, treatment is empirical and symptomatic, with vestibular resection being considered only as a last resort. Essential vulvodynia refers to the description of constant, unremitting burning localized to the vulva which may respond to low-dose tricyclic antidepressants (e.g. amitriptyline).

Urethral caruncle

A urethral caruncle is a polypoidal outgrowth from the edge of the urethra which is most commonly seen after the menopause. The tissue is soft, red, smooth and appears as an eversion of the urethral mucosa. Most women are asymptomatic but others experience dysuria, frequency, urgency and focal tenderness. If there are any suspicious features, an excision and biopsy may be required to exclude the rare possibility of a urethral carcinoma.

Ulcers

Ulcers of the vulva may be:

- aphthous (yellow base)
- herpetic (exquisitely painful multiple ulceration, see p. 104)
- syphilitic (indurated and painless, see p. 104)
- associated with Crohn's disease ('like knife cuts in skin')
- a feature of Behçet's syndrome (a chronic painful condition with aphthous genital and ocular ulceration. Treatment is difficult; the combined oral contraceptive or topical steroids may be tried)
- malignant
- associated with lichen planus or Stevens–Johnson syndrome
- tropical (lymphogranuloma venereum, chancroid, granuloma inguinale).

Simple atrophy

Elderly women develop vaginal, vulval and clitoral atrophy as part of the normal ageing process of skin. In severe cases the thin vulval skin, terminal urethra and fourchette cause dysuria and superficial dyspareunia. The labia minora fuse and bury the clitoris. Introital stenoses can make coitus impossible. Treatment is with oestrogen replacement, and may need to be for a few months. There is a small amount of systemic absorption with topical therapy and, if this route is chosen, treatment should be for no more than 2 or 3 months without either a break or a short course of progesterone to prevent endometrial stimulation. If the oestrogen is given orally, progesterone should be added as for any HRT.

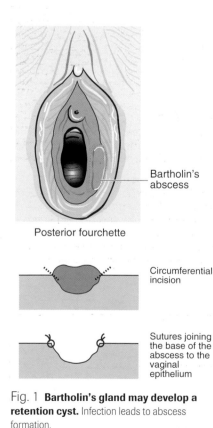

Bartholin's abscess

Posterior fourchette

Circumferential incision

Sutures joining the base of the abscess to the vaginal epithelium

Fig. 1 **Bartholin's gland may develop a retention cyst.** Infection leads to abscess formation.

Benign vulval diseases

These are classified as:

Lichen sclerosus. This can present at any age, but is more common in the older patient and usually presents with pruritus, and less commonly with dyspareunia or pain. The skin appears white, thin and crinkly but may be thickened and keratotic if there is coexistent squamous cell hyperplasia. There may also be clitoral or labial adhesions. Diagnosis is by biopsy and there is an association with autoimmune disorders in < 10% (pernicious anaemia, thyroid disease, diabetes mellitus, systemic lupus erythematosus, primary biliary cirrhosis or bullous pemphygoid). It is non-neoplastic but may coexist with VIN and there is an association with subsequent development of squamous cell carcinoma of the vulva (probably between 2–9%) (Fig. 2). Long-term follow-up is probably warranted. Treatment is required only if symptomatic, e.g. Dermovate twice daily initially, reducing gradually to hydrocortisone twice daily, once daily, or less as symptoms require. Eosin paint may also be of help. Vulvectomy has no role, the recurrence being ≈ 50%.

Squamous cell hyperplasia. This frequently presents in premenopausal women with severe pruritus. Diagnosis is again by biopsy and treatment is with hydrocortisone as for 'lichen sclerosus'.

Other dermatoses. These include:

- *Allergic/irritant dermatosis.* This may be caused by detergents, perfume, condom lubricants, chlorine in swimming pools or podophyllin paint. There may be secondary infection. Irritants should be removed and the area treated with emollients ± topical corticosteroids.

- *Psoriasis.* The vulva is an unusual site for this, but if present, moderately potent steroids are better than coal tar.
- *Intertrigo with candida.* This responds to antifungal preparations.
- *Lichen planus.* This appears as purple-white papules with a shiny surface and keratinized area and may respond to strong steroids ± azathioprine or PUVA. It is usually idiopathic, but can be drug related, and tends to resolve within 2 years. Surgery should be avoided.

Varieties of intraepithelial neoplasia (i.e. the presence of neoplastic cells within the confines of the epithelium).

Squamous VIN. This is classified as 1, 2 or 3 depending on the severity ('Bowen's disease' and 'Bowenoid papulosis' have been used to describe atypical squamous lesions, but are part of the same process of VIN). It is considered that human papilloma virus (HPV) may be important in aetiology. Many are asymptomatic although pruritus is present in between one-third and two-thirds, and pain is an occasional feature. Lesions may be papular and rough surfaced resembling warts, or macular with indistinct borders. White lesions represent hyperkeratosis, and pigmentation is common. The lesions tend to be multifocal in women under 40 and unifocal in the postmenopausal age group. Diagnosis is by biopsy, which may be taken at vulvoscopy, using 5% acetic acid as at colposcopy, under either local or general anaesthesia. The opportunity should be taken to look at the cervix as well, as there is an association between cervical intraepithelial neoplasia (CIN) and VIN. As the natural history is so uncertain, treatment is controversial. Regression has been observed (particularly in low-grade VIN) but progression of high-grade VIN to invasion may occur in approximately 6% of cases and up to 15% of those with VIN 3 may have superficial

invading vulval cancer. Treatment of VIN may be indicated in those > 45, those who are immunosuppressed and those with multifocal lower genital tract neoplasia. The main treatment is wide local excision (the exception is VIN 3 on the clitoris in young women – use an Nd-YAG laser). A colposcope should be used to inspect the vulva (keratinization may make visualization of abnormal cells difficult) and then take a biopsy with a 4-mm trephine under local or general anaesthesia (Fig. 3). It is also necessary to check the perianal area as there may also be anal intraepithelial neoplasia.

Melanoma in situ. This is uncommon.

Non-squamous VIN (Paget's disease). This is also uncommon. There is a poorly demarcated often multifocal eczematoid lesion associated in 25% with adenocarcinoma either in the pelvis or at a distant site. Treatment is by wide local excision.

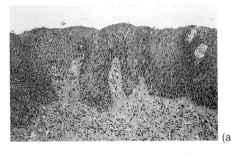
(a)

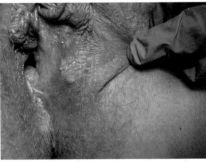
(b)

Fig. 3 **Squamous VIN. (a)** There is a superficial hyperkeratosis. Hyperchromatic nuclei are seen within all cells from the basement membrane to the epithelial surface. **(b)** There is a raised wart-like area of leukoplakia on the medial aspect of the left labia majora. A biopsy is required to differentiate this from other conditions with a similar appearance.

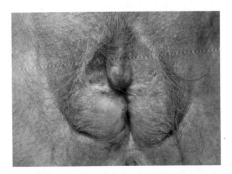

Fig. 2 **Lichen sclerosus has a small association with carcinoma of the vulva.**

> ### Benign vulval conditions
>
> - Pruritus vulvae has numerous aetiologies.
> - Appearances are often not diagnostic and biopsies are often required.
> - Lichen sclerosus is common, associated with autoimmune disorders, and only rarely with VIN are vulval carcinoma.
> - The natural history and optimal treatment of VIN are uncertain.
> - There is an association between VIN and CIN.

Vulval carcinoma

Vulval cancer is not a common disease – approximately 800 new cases are registered annually in the UK. It is an unpleasant but potentially curable disease – even in elderly, unfit ladies if they are diagnosed and referred early.

Vulval cancer should be referred to specialist centres where adequate numbers are seen to maintain a level of expertise.

Treatment requires a multidisciplinary approach with adequate supportive care and counselling facilities. The patients are usually elderly and often have coexisting disease.

Aetiology

The majority of vulval carcinomas are squamous in origin with a number of much rarer cancers contributing to the remaining 10%. Basal cell carcinoma and verrucous carcinoma represent uncommon squamous subtypes. Malignant melanomas and Bartholin gland tumours can occur. Several risk factors have been identified for vulval carcinoma:

- other genital cancers
- smoking
- prior history of genital warts
- vulval carcinomas in situ (VIN)
- chronic vulval inflammatory disorders.

Several conditions are thought to have malignant potential (Table 1) although progression to carcinoma has not yet been proven. Vulval intraepithelial neoplasia is graded in order of severity in a similar fashion to cervical intraepithelial neoplasia (CIN) (see p. 135). Patients with precursor lesions should undergo continued surveillance. Early biopsy is recommended if there is any change in

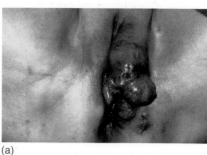
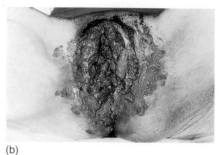

(a) (b)

Fig. 1 **Vulval carcinoma. (a)** Polypoidal lesion. **(b)** Ulcer.

symptoms or appearance of the lesion. Multifocal or multicentric disease can be very difficult to manage.

Diagnosis

Most patients with invasive disease complain of irritation or pruritus (71%) and 57% notice a vulval lesion, which may be a polypoidal mass or an ulcer (Fig. 1). The presentation of symptoms and the appearance of the epithelium may be quite varied. Vulval symptoms in a postmenopausal woman should be promptly examined and atypical areas biopsied. One of the most worrying features of this disease is the delay between the onset of the first symptoms and the diagnosis of the condition – delays of over 12 months have been reported.

Warts are not common in postmenopausal women and should be treated with suspicion.

Lesions that fail to respond to simple first-line treatment in premenopausal women should be investigated.

Assessment

Diagnosis should be confirmed by appropriate biopsy so that definitive management can be planned. It may be appropriate to remove a large ulcerated or fungating mass completely at the first sitting, so that excision both provides a biopsy specimen and achieves symptomatic relief in the very frail. Small lesions (less than 2 cm in diameter) may be removed by a wide local excision as both biopsy and curative procedure.

Once a diagnosis has been confirmed the patient requires a full explanation of the situation. Preoperative assessment must be thorough as the majority of patients affected are elderly and may have other medical conditions. In a younger patient who remains sexually active there are both psychological and psychosexual connotations involved.

Female lower genital tract cancer is often multicentric and the investigation of a patient with vulval cancer must include inspection of the cervix and up-to-date cervical cytology. Nodal involvement, if present, must be identified before surgery. Full blood count, biochemical profile and chest X-ray are necessary. An electrocardiogram (in the elderly patient), intravenous urogram or lymphangiogram may be required. A magnetic resonance imaging (MRI) scan may be helpful if there is nodal involvement in defining the extent of the spread.

Management

The management of vulval carcinoma depends entirely on the stage of the disease at presentation. Early invasion of the vulva is termed 'superficially invasive vulval cancer' and is analogous to stage 1a cervical cancer. This is rarely associated with lymph node metastasis. The risk of metastasis increases with the depth of invasion of the tumour – tumours showing less than 1 mm depth of invasion appear to have a negligible risk of lymph node spread (Table 2).

Table 1 **Precursor lesions**	
Lesion	**Lifetime risk of vulval carcinoma**

Vulval intraepithelial neoplasia (VIN)
 Histologically recognizable atypia present
     VIN 1 – mild
     VIN 2 – moderate
     VIN 3 – severe
 (Full thickness abnormalities, disordered maturation, excess mitotic figures)
	5–10% (range quoted at 2–80%)

Paget's disease A disorder of skin adnexal structures (apocrine sweat glands)	Rare. In 20% of cases, there is evidence of malignancy elsewhere
Lichen sclerosus Cause unknown, associated with autoimmune disorders	3–5%

Table 2	**Staging of vulval carcinoma**
Stage	
0	Carcinoma-in-situ, intraepithelial neoplasia grade 3
1a	Lesion confined to the vulva, diameter < 2 cm with < 1 mm invasion, superficially invasive vulval carcinoma
1b	Lesion confined to the vulva, diameter < 2 cm, depth > 1 mm no nodal metastasis
2	Lesion confined to the vulva, and/or perineum, diameter > 2 cm – no nodal metastasis
3	Lesion of any size extending beyond the vulva with adjacent spread to lower urethra and/or vagina, or anus, without grossly positive groin nodes Lesion of any size confined to the vulva and having nodal metastasis (unilateral or regional)
4a	Tumour invades any of the following: upper urethra, bladder mucosa, rectal mucosa, pelvic bone and/or bilateral nodes
4b	Any distant metastasis, including pelvic lymph nodes

As per FIGO classification, including 1994 modifications.
*The depth of the invasion is defined as the measurement of the tumour from the epithelial stromal junction of the adjacent, most superficial dermal papilla, to the deepest point of invasion.

Table 3	**Complications of radical surgery**
Short-term	
■ Wound infection and breakdown	
■ Deep vein thrombosis, pulmonary embolism	
■ Pressure sores	
Long-term	
■ Introital stenosis, dyspareunia	
■ Urinary and faecal incontinence	
■ Rectocele	
■ Lymphoedema/lymphocyst	
■ Hernias	
■ Psychological and psychosexual problems	
■ Recurrence	

Spread can either be direct (to adjacent organs), lymphatic, or, in very late cases, haematogenous. The femoral and inguinal nodes are the sites of regional spread. Involvement of pelvic lymph nodes, (external iliac, hypogastric, obturator and common iliac nodes) is considered distant spread. Lymphatic drainage from the vulva and perineum is complex. Tumours that are close to midline structures, e.g. the clitoris, can spread quickly bilaterally.

Management of early stage disease

The high morbidity associated with radical surgical treatment of vulval cancer has prompted the development of more conservative, but effective, alternatives. Early stage disease is best treated by wide radical local excision, which should remove all areas of atypical epithelium – although this may be difficult to achieve in multifocal disease. In these situations, multiple diagnostic biopsies must be considered as it is important to try to exclude areas of occult invasion. The decision to perform groin node dissection would depend on the depth of the lesion (if > 1 mm).

The site of the lesion will determine whether unilateral or bilateral groin dissection is required. For stage 1b and stage 2 tumours the triple incision technique is employed – excision of the vulval tumour and then excision of the groin nodes via separate incisions (Fig. 2). This avoids the prolonged

healing associated with the classical butterfly incision of radical vulvectomy.

Advanced vulval disease

The management of stage 3 disease will require radical dissection. There are no data available to support the use of the triple incision technique for stage 3 tumours when the nodes are obviously involved. In these situations radical vulvectomy via the butterfly incision with complete node dissection en bloc is the standard technique. Healing is by granulation (Fig. 3), unless skin flaps or skin grafting is employed. Wound breakdown still affects 30 to 50% of cases (Table 3). Consider reconstructive surgery at the time of radical excision.

Preoperative radiotherapy with or without concurrent chemotherapy can cause tumour shrinkage – this may allow for urinary and anal sphincter conservation.

Postoperative radiotherapy is considered valuable if two or more nodes are found positive, and if the primary tumour has not been adequately excised.

Recurrent disease

Local recurrence is associated with inadequate excision margins and is more likely with verrucous and basal cell carcinomas. Radiation may be useful and further excision may be possible in previously irradiated cases. Erosion into the femoral artery is the usual long-term outcome.

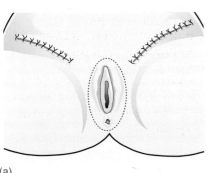
(a)

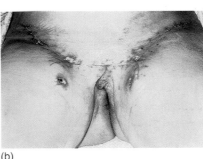
(b)

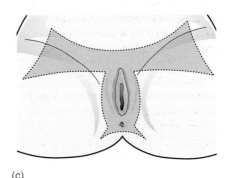
(c)

Fig. 2 **Surgery for early stage vulval carcinoma. (a and b)** Triple incision technique. **(c)** Butterfly incision.

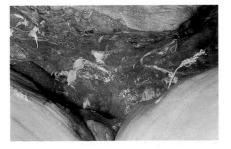

Fig. 3 **Healing by secondary intention**.

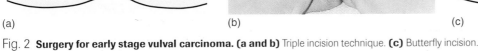

Vulval carcinoma

■ Vulval carcinoma is an uncommon gynaecological cancer affecting mainly the elderly age group.

■ 90% of vulval cell carcinomas are squamous.

■ Lesions less than 1 mm in depth have a negligible risk of lymph node metastasis.

■ Early stage disease can be treated with wide radical local excision.

■ Advanced disease is still treated by radical vulvectomy with en bloc node dissection.

Menopause: physiological changes

Definitions

The menopause is the final act of menstruation. The climacteric is the phase in the ageing process when a woman passes from the reproductive to the non-reproductive stage. Thus the menopause is a single event and the climacteric is a period of time during which a woman may experience a considerable number of symptoms and signs (Table 1).

The menopause may be physiological or artificial, induced by radiation, surgery (e.g. oophorectomy), or hormonal therapy (e.g. gonadotrophin releasing hormone analogues). This chapter deals with the physiological menopause, although the changes are common to both. Spontaneous cessation of menses before the age of 40 years is termed premature ovarian failure.

Pathogenesis

There are 7 million oogonia in the fetal ovary at 20 weeks' gestation. After the seventh month of gestation no new oocytes are formed. At the time of birth, the number has already dropped to 2 million and by puberty there are only 30 000 oocytes. Continued reduction follows. These large numbers are lost mainly due to the process of atresia, although some are lost through ovulation.

At the menopause the sensitivity of oocytes to respond to gonadotrophin stimulation disappears. Estradiol levels are therefore low, removing negative feedback to the hypothalamus and pituitary, leading to very high levels of gonadotrophins, luteinizing hormone (LH) and follicle stimulating hormone (FSH) (see p. 120).

Hormonal changes

Changes occur in four different hormonal groups after the menopause: androgens; oestrogens; progesterone; gonadotrophins.

There is a 50% reduction in circulating androstenedione. Adrenal androgens fall by 60–80% with age.

The fall in testosterone is minimal. There is 14% conversion from androstenedione, but the majority is produced by hilar and luteinized stromal cells within the ovary that do respond to the increased gonadotrophin outpouring. The relative increase in testosterone compared to the other androgens may be manifest in a receding hairline, hoarse voice and the facial hair sometimes seen in elderly ladies.

Estrone is the oestrogen of the menopause, mainly produced by the adrenals – although peripheral conversion from androstenedione doubles. Some estrone and testosterone peripherally convert to estradiol, accounting for the small percentage of estradiol still available. Cessation of ovulation heralds a 70% reduction in progesterone as there is no further corpus luteal production. Adrenal production continues. Pituitary LH and FSH levels rise considerably as estradiol levels fall, but are still released in a pulsatile fashion.

Signs and symptoms

Reproductive tract

Although abrupt cessation of menses can occur, it is more usual to have oligomenorrhoea with increasing cycle irregularity. Polymenorrhagia with heavier and more frequent menses is uncommon and warrants endometrial assessment (see p. 138). The vaginal and cervical skin become thinner, drier and more fragile. The vaginal cytology confirms surface cells that are less mature and less keratinized. This results in vaginal soreness and dryness with superficial dyspareunia, postcoital bleeding and intercurrent infections.

The uterus also undergoes changes. The normal endometrium becomes thin and inactive (see p. 138). The myometrium shrinks. The ovaries also atrophy. Easily palpable ovaries are suspicious and warrant further investigation. Ligaments and connective tissue lose tone and elasticity which predisposes to uterovaginal prolapse.

Urinary tract

As the bladder and vagina both share the same embryological derivation from the urogenital sinus, the urethra and trigone are predisposed to similar atrophic changes. This can give rise to symptoms of frequency and urgency, often mistaken for cystitis.

External changes

Breast tissue regresses in size and tends to sag. There is generalized thinning and loss of elasticity in the skin leading to wrinkling. The hair changes in pattern with sparser axillary and pubic hair and increased, coarse terminal hair.

Psychological and emotional changes

Psychiatrists report a premenopausal peak incidence of affective disorders relating to negative feelings regarding the onset of ageing and loss of fertility, especially in western cultures. Gynaecologists ascribe the increased incidence of tearfulness and depression to falling levels of estradiol and progesterone. Oestrogen receptors have been identified in the limbic system of the brain. The situation is complex – life crises can occur in this age group and genuine endogenous depression may also be present.

Vasomotor symptoms

Flushes normally start on the face and spread downwards across the neck and chest. They may last a few seconds or

---

Table 1 **Signs and symptoms of the menopause**

General problems	Sexual problems
Daytime sweats and flushes	Vaginal dryness/soreness
Night time sweats and flushes	Vaginal itching
Poor sleep pattern	Dyspareunia
Tiredness	Postcoital bleeding
Loss of energy	Loss of libido
General aches and pains	Difficulty achieving orgasm
Generalized pruritus	
Formication (sensation of something crawling over the skin)	**Urinary problems**
	Frequency
	Urgency
Emotional problems	Urge incontinence
Tearfulness	Stress incontinence
Depression	Nocturia
Feelings of unworthiness	Enuresis
Irritability	
Anger	**Period problems**
Bitterness	Erratic cycles
Panic attacks	Lighter menstrual loss/heavier loss
Palpitations	Intermenstrual bleeding
	Postmenopausal bleeding (bleeding after 1 year's amenorrhoea)
Personality problems	
Loss of memory	
Loss of concentration	
Feelings of personality disintegration	

10 minutes and can occur from once to 20 times a day. Night sweats may lead to chronic sleep depletion. Seventy percent of women exhibit vasomotor symptoms for 1 year, 30% for 5 years and 10% for 10 years. There appears to be a temporal relationship between flushes and pulsatile release of LH.

Osteoporosis

Osteoporosis represents reduction in bone mass and micro-architectural disruption leading to enhanced bone fragility and increased fracture risk. The World Health Organization (WHO) definitions are as follows:

- osteopenia (1–2.5 SDs below adult reference peak bone mass)
- osteoporosis (> 2.5 SDs below adult reference peak bone mass).

The bone remodelling process involves four processes (Fig. 1). Formation takes longer than resorption – the two are linked, or coupled. At the menopause the remodelling cycle becomes imbalanced, or uncoupled. The osteoclasts produce larger cavities which the osteoblasts do not completely fill with osteoid, resulting in a net decrease of bone mass. Oestrogen has an anti-resorptive effect.

In women, peak bone mass is achieved in the early 30s. It is influenced by diet (including calcium intake), exercise, genetics and environment. Subsequently bone mass is lost gradually until the menopause, when falling oestrogen levels accelerate the process. When bone density falls below a critical level (the fracture threshold) the risk of fracture is increased. There is a 50% loss of trebecular bone and a 5% loss of cortical bone (Fig. 2). The commonest fracture sites are vertebral body, upper femur, distal forearm, humerus, ribs. The incidence of these fractures varies with age (Fig. 3). One in four women in the 60s suffer vertebral crush fractures, causing pain, shortened stature and spinal curvature – the classical 'dowager's hump' (Fig. 4).

Cardiovascular changes

Ischaemic heart disease (IHD) represents the biggest cause of death in women. Men suffer from IHD more commonly than women until women reach the menopause – subsequently catching up rapidly. Comparing age-matched groups of premenopausal and postmenopausal women, the incidence of IHD is found to rise with increasing age, but is consistently less in the premenopausal groups at all ages. This would suggest that oestrogen has a protective effect.

Total cholesterol is made up of low density lipoprotein (LDL) and high density lipoprotein (HDL) fractions. The former is easily deposited on damaged endothelium and predisposes to atherogenic change. At the menopause, total cholesterol, LDL-cholesterol and triglyceride levels rise. HDL-cholesterol and in particular the HDL 2 subfraction falls. Oestrogen reverses these trends and appears also to act at the cellular level.

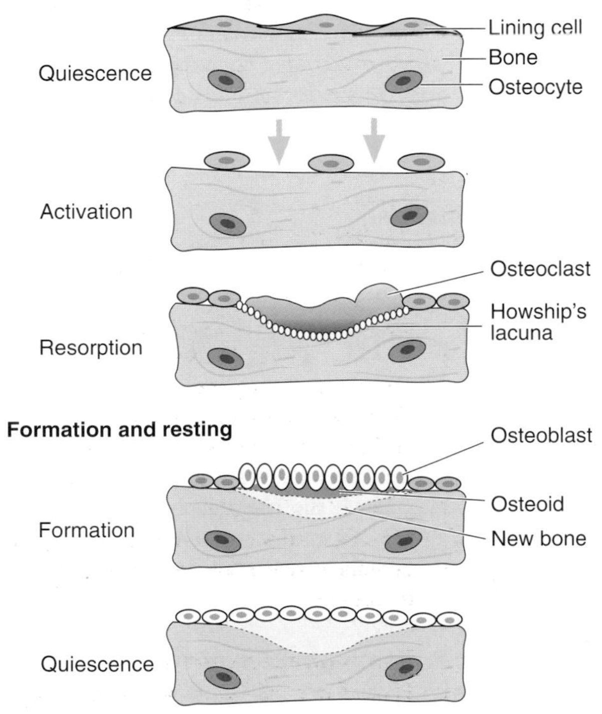

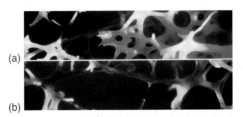

(a)

(b)

Fig. 2 **(a) Normal and (b) osteoporotic bone.**

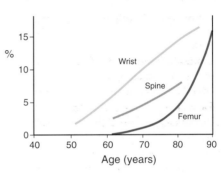

Fig. 3 **Incidence of different types of fractures with age.**

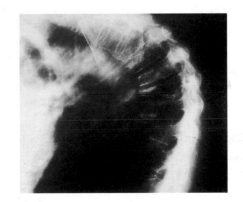

Fig. 4 **X-ray showing wedge fracture of the spine.**

Resting and resorption

Quiescence — Lining cell / Bone / Osteocyte

Activation

Resorption — Osteoclast / Howship's lacuna

Formation and resting

Formation — Osteoblast / Osteoid / New bone

Quiescence

Fig. 1 **The bone remodelling process.**

Menopause: physiological changes

- Loss of oestrogen production has a profound effect on several systems.
- Periods usually become lighter and less frequent.
- Estrone replaces estradiol as the chief oestrogen produced.
- Testosterone is relatively the most important androgen.
- Symptoms may be severe and prolonged.
- Bone loss is accelerated at the menopause, predisposing to fractures.
- The lipid profile alters to become more atherogenic.
- Oestrogen possesses anti-resorptive properties in bone and reverses the trends in the HDL/LDL ratio.

Menopause: management

Hormone replacement therapy (HRT) is widely accepted as a treatment for symptoms of the menopause and osteoporosis. Epidemiological data suggest a role against ischaemic heart disease (IHD) and, from more recent evidence, Alzheimer's disease.

Hormone replacement therapy

HRT combines natural oestrogen with progestogens, synthetic derivatives of progesterone (Table 1). 19-nortestosterone derivatives are androgenic and produce more side effects (e.g. bloating, mood swings and mastalgia). C21-progesterone derivatives are more progesterone-receptor specific and produce fewer side effects. Micronized progesterone is available in Europe and America. There are several oestrogens available.

Progestogen is administered either cyclically for 12 to 14 days a month (a sequential combined therapy, SCT), or continuously (a continuous combined therapy, CCT) (Fig. 1). The former will promote a monthly withdrawal bleed. The continuous combined preparations are reserved for women who have been amenorrhoeic for 12 months and do not wish to bleed. One preparation offers the chance of 3-monthly withdrawal bleeds (seasonal bleeds).

Unopposed oestrogen may only be prescribed to hysterectomized women, as oestrogen induces endometrial hyperplasia and long-term use may promote endometrial cancer. The incidence of cystic hyperplasia varies between 7 and 20%. Even after cessation of unopposed oestrogens, the increased risk of endometrial cancer persists for up to 14 years. The added progestogen effects protection by secretory transformation.

Several routes of administration are available (Table 2). No one preparation is better than another, but there is a wide variation in patients' needs, requiring a flexible approach to treatment. Oral HRT enters the enterohepatic circulation, activating hepatic enzymes that accelerate metabolism. Systemic HRT achieves 'liver bypass' entering the circulation directly. Patches or gels may therefore be better for epileptics, tablets for those with hypercholesterolaemia or skin conditions. Estradiol implants are useful for long-term therapy

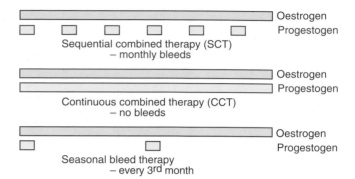

Fig. 1 **Sequential combined therapy, continuous combined therapy and seasonal bleeds.**

Table 1 **Components of hormone replacement therapy and related preparations**

Oestrogens
- Conjugated equine oestrogens (CEEs)
- 17 beta estradiol (plant extract oestrogens)
- Estradiol valorate (plant extract oestrogens)
- Estrone

Progestogens
- Progesterone (the natural hormone)
- Progesterone analogues, C21 derivatives
  - didrogesterone
  - medroxyprogesterone acetate
- 19-nortestosterone derivatives
  - norethisterone/norethisterone acetate
  - levonorgestrel

Gonadomimetics
- Tibolone (containing oestrogenic, progestogenic and androgenic components)

Selective oestrogen receptor modulators (SERMs)
- Raloxifene (modified oestrogen molecule stimulating bone receptors, but not endometrial and breast receptors; also reduces cholesterol levels)

Phyto-oestrogens
- Natural dietary fibre oestrogens, obtained from a health food shop

Table 2 **Routes of administration of HRT available**

Oestrogen
- Oral
- Transdermal, patches or gel
- Nasal spray
- Implants
- Vaginal preparations, cream, pessary and ring

Progesterone
- Oral
- Vaginal, gel or pessary

Progestogens
- Progesterone analogues, C21 derivatives
  - oral
- Testosterone analogues 19-nortestosterone derivatives
  - oral
  - transdermal (as sequential combined and continuous combined preparations)

Gonadomimetics
- Oral

SERMs
- Oral

and can be given in conjunction with testosterone. Careful monitoring of the serum estradiol level is required to prevent tachyphylaxis. The body adapts to supraphysiological levels of oestrogen resulting in severe symptoms, even though levels are well above the accepted therapeutic range.

Tablets, gels and nasal spray are administered daily, patches either once or twice a week and implants 6-monthly. Vaginal preparations may be useful for relief of vaginal dryness.

Approach to treatment

Many women show great interest in HRT, but some express reservations. Main concerns focus on side effects, weight gain, risk of cancer and withdrawal bleeds. A structured approach to treatment includes information, counselling and HRT.

Every woman should be fully counselled as to the risks and benefits of treatment (Table 3) and should be included in the decision-making process. Information should include what routes of administration and types of HRT are available, how long therapy should continue (for adequate bone protection a minimum of 5 years' therapy is advised), and what side effects may be encountered. Bleeding usually lessens over four to six successive cycles to a light, regular 3- to 5-day loss. Minor transient side effects may occur and the patient should be encouraged to persevere. Changing brands every 1–2 months promotes problems.

Table 3 **Risks and benefits of HRT**	
Benefits	**Risks**

■ Protection against osteoporosis and reduced fracture rates (may 'buy back' some lost bone)
■ Reduction in incidence of colonic cancer
■ Protection against IHD (controversial):
  – increases HDL/LDL ratio
  – reduction in insulin resistance
  – reduction in android fat distribution
  – enhanced coronary artery blood flow
  – beneficial effects on renin–angiotensin system
■ Delay in onset of Alzheimer's disease (controversial) (improvement in mild to moderate disease)
	■ Increased incidence of breast cancer – duration of use effect:
	  – background population risk increased by 2 per 1000 if used from 50–55 years
	  – background population risk increased by 6 per 1000 if used from 50–60 years (*but* 5-year survival rates are better in women developing breast cancer on HRT compared to non-users)
	■ Increased incidence of thromboembolism
	■ Increased risk of endometrial cancer (very small if progestogens are used correctly)
	■ Urogenital atrophy/vaginal soreness

Table 4 **Absolute contraindications to HRT**
■ Severe hepatic impairment ■ Recurrent idiopathic thrombosis ■ History of recent breast cancer ■ Irregular vaginal bleeding of unknown origin ■ Myocardial infarction and stroke

Table 5 **Factors that indicate risk of osteoporosis**
■ Family history of osteoporosis ■ History of spontaneous fractures ■ Premature ovarian failure ■ Oophorectomy or ovarian ablation ■ Long-term steroid therapy ■ Chronic immobilization ■ Hyperthyroidism
Weaker and less accurate predictors:
■ Thin individual with slight frame ■ Caucasian or Asian ■ Low calcium intake ■ Caffeine or alcohol excess ■ Smoking

Assessment and screening

Diagnosis is normally made on clinical grounds. A follicle stimulating hormone (FSH) level may be performed if there is doubt, e.g. severe premenstrual syndrome. Independent medical conditions may coexist; both hypothyroidism and endogenous depression can mimic climacteric symptoms. Thyroid function tests and a fasting lipid profile are useful baseline tests. Pre-existing diabetes and hypertension should be adequately controlled prior to commencing HRT, but are not contraindications to treatment (Table 4). A personal or family history of thrombosis should prompt a full thrombophilia screen including anti-thrombin III, protein C, protein S, activated protein C resistance

HRT increases breast tissue density – which makes interpretation more difficult. A decision to perform mammography more frequently may also be taken.

Bone densitometry is expensive and not routinely available. It is performed in high-risk groups (Table 5). If symptoms are present that require treatment, HRT is prescribed in a bone-sparing dose. Bone density measurements, including single or dual X-ray absorptiometry, are made over the lower lumbar spine and left hip (Fig. 2). The results are plotted against accepted norms for the age and sex of the patient (Fig. 3).

The follow-up appointment

The follow-up visit is normally at 4 months, then 6- to 12-monthly

thereafter if the patient is stable. A review is made at each visit of symptom control, side effects and the bleeding pattern achieved if on a sequential combined therapy. Weight and blood pressure are checked at each visit. If there is irregular bleeding, an initial response would be to adjust the HRT regimen. If this fails to achieve control, the bleeding should be investigated.

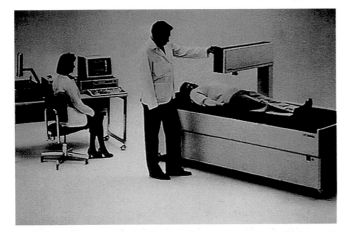

Fig. 2 **Bone densitometry equipment.**

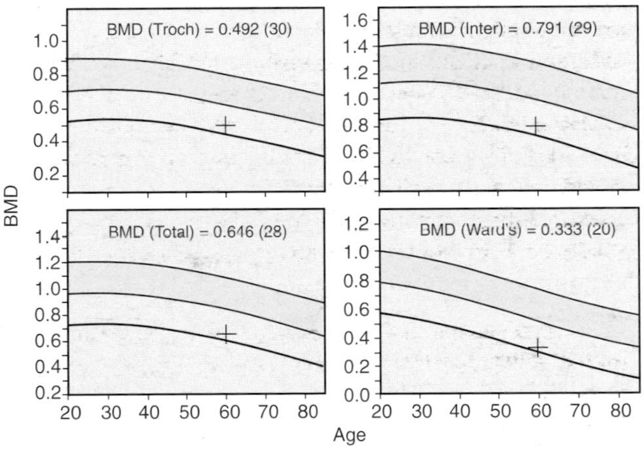

Fig. 3 **Bone densitometry plot for hip.**

BMD (Troch) = 0.492 (30)
BMD (Inter) = 0.791 (29)
BMD (Total) = 0.646 (28)
BMD (Ward's) = 0.333 (20)
BMD
Age

(APCR), anti-nuclear factor, lupus anticoagulant and anti-cardiolipin antibodies. A cervical smear need only be performed at the initial assessment if it is overdue.

Mammography is routinely offered in many countries. In the UK screening is 3-yearly between the ages of 50 and 65 years. If HRT is commenced before the age of 50 years, mammography is not routinely performed. If there is a family history of breast cancer, or a past medical history of benign breast disease, baseline imaging prior to treatment is useful, as

Menopause: management

■ There is a wide variety of HRT regimens available and treatment should be tailored to the individual's needs.

■ Clear explanations and adequate counselling improve compliance.

■ Medical conditions mimicking climacteric symptoms should be excluded.

■ Unopposed oestrogen increases the risk of uterine cancer and must be given in conjunction with progestogens, either cyclically or continuously.

■ The risk of breast cancer with HRT is duration-dependent, but remains small for 5 years of use after the age of 50.

■ Regular follow-up should assess symptom control, side effects and bleeding pattern.

■ Abnormal bleeding should be investigated.

■ HRT should not be prescribed in the presence of undiagnosed abnormal bleeding.

Uterovaginal prolapse

Uterovaginal prolapse is rare in quadripeds, but evolution to an upright posture has added additional strain to the biped pelvic floor.

Aetiology

The pathogenesis of prolapse is thought to be multifactorial, with congenital weakness of supporting structures, damage to pelvic floor musculature during childbirth, menopausal atrophy of the tissues and raised intra-abdominal pressure. Potential aetiological factors include the following.

Congenital weakness

A deficiency of the supporting tissues may be important. There are families where prolapse is noted through the generations. Nulliparae may also develop prolapse. This may be a less extreme form of cases where herniae formation are well recognized.

Childbirth

It is well recognized that childbirth damages the pelvic floor innervation and the secondary muscle atrophy predisposes to uterovaginal prolapse. Caesarean section appears to afford some degree of protection over vaginal delivery. It has been assumed that the length of the second stage of labour and heavy birth weight would be factors associated with prolapse, but surprisingly studies have not confirmed this. Tearing of tissue, as might occur with a precipitous labour, may be a factor.

Menopause

After the menopause there is marked atrophy of the vaginal tissues. While this may be associated with stenosis of the vagina, it is more common to find some form of prolapse.

Raised intra-abdominal pressure

Chronic cough or the presence of an intra-abdominal mass is associated with raised intra-abdominal pressure and may be a factor in the development of prolapse. Work has shown that obesity is not a factor in transmission of raised pressures to the urinary tract, thus it is of questionable importance in the genesis of prolapse.

Other factors

Chronic straining at stool with perineal descent may damage pelvic floor innervation, thus putting the connective tissue supporting structures under additional strain. The type of connective tissue found in those with prolapse may predispose them to tissue failure contributing to the genesis of prolapse.

Presentation (Table 1, Fig. 1)

History

Commonly the patient complains of a lump or fullness within the vagina which may have been first noticed during a lifting episode or be of gradual occurrence. It is commonly worse in the evening, after standing. There is often associated back pain (possibly due to tension on the utero-sacral ligaments), and bleeding and discharge may be present if the prolapse has ulcerated. Care should be taken not to miss a coincidental endometrial carcinoma. Associated symptoms may be urinary incontinence and frequency (see p. 154) or problems with defecation – or, less commonly, faecal incontinence. Patients may mention the need to reduce a posterior prolapse in order to complete defecation or a cystocele to aid voiding.

Examination

On examination there may be signs of vaginal wall laxity at rest – asking the patient to bear down or cough should demonstrate the problem. Urinary incontinence may also be demonstrable. The patient is then placed in the Sims' position and examined using the Sims' speculum

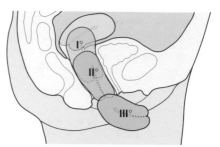
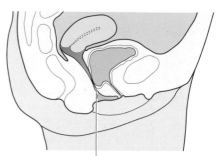

Cystourethrocele

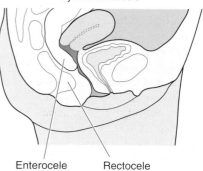
Enterocele   Rectocele

Fig. 1 **Types of uterovaginal prolapse.**

(see p. 86), examining first the anterior vaginal wall with cough to demonstrate urinary incontinence and then the posterior vaginal wall by reversing the speculum. The patient is then returned to the dorsal position and a bimanual examination performed to assess the size of the pelvic organs. Neurological examination as in cases of urinary incontinence (see p. 154) may be appropriate. Urinary symptomatology may necessitate urodynamic investigation (see p. 154).

Management

The management may be conservative or surgical, the conservative approach being appropriate in patients who prefer this, who wish to avoid surgery or who may be unfit for surgery. Surgical treatment includes anterior colporrhaphy, Manchester repair (anterior repair and cervical amputation – rarely performed), vaginal hysterectomy, posterior repair, repair of enterocele and vault fixation.

Table 1	**Types of prolapse**
Name	**Condition**
Cystocele	Prolapse of the anterior vaginal wall and bladder
Urethrocele	Prolapse of the anterior vaginal wall and urethra – often found with cystocele
Rectocele	Prolapse of the posterior vaginal wall and rectum
Enterocele	Prolapse of the upper posterior vaginal wall (posterior fornix) and pouch of Douglas
Uterine prolapse 1st degree	The cervix uteri descends within the vagina but does not pass outside the introitus during straining
Uterine prolapse 2nd degree	The cervix uteri protrudes beyond the introitus during straining
Uterine prolapse 3rd degree (procidentia)	Total prolapse of the uterus and cervix outside the vaginal introitus, dragging the vaginal walls and associated structures with it

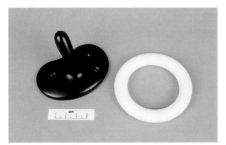

Fig. 2 **The shelf pessary (black) may be needed if the perineum is deficient or the prolapse pushes out the ring pessary (white).**

Conservative (Fig. 2)

A ring pessary made of a circle of pliable plastic is inserted by compressing it into an oval shape. When it regains its circular shape in the vaginal fornices it is then larger than the vaginal outlet and keeps the vaginal walls elevated. Patients should be unaware of it once it is correctly positioned and should be able to lead a normal life including sexual intercourse. It is changed every 6–12 months and oestrogen cream may improve tissue quality, preventing ulceration of the ring site. A shelf pessary may be used in very unfit patients not suitable for surgical correction where the ring pessary will not stay in place. Vaginal cones may be used to strengthen the pelvic floor in more mild degrees of uterovaginal prolapse (see p. 155).

Surgical

Numerous operations exist for correction of prolapse. The principle behind them all remains the same – that of correction of the protrusion with placement of supporting sutures and tissues to prevent recurrence. The problem with this approach is that the tissues have failed in their supporting role already and thus may fail again, so the patient should be warned of this before surgery is undertaken.

Anterior colporrhaphy (or anterior repair). The anterior vaginal wall is opened, the bladder and urethra dissected free, and sutures placed from the pubocervical fascia under the bladder neck to the pubocervical fascia on the other side, giving support and continent function. The operation is completed with supporting sutures to the bladder base, if possible, repairing the fascia under the bladder (Fig. 3).

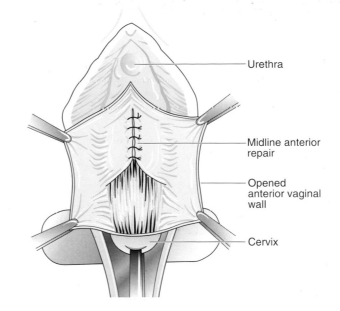

Fig. 3 **Anterior repair.**

Urethra

Midline anterior repair

Opened anterior vaginal wall

Cervix

Posterior colporrhaphy or colpoperineorrhaphy (or posterior repair). The posterior vaginal wall is opened in the midline and tissues dissected free from the vagina until the fascial plane is clear. An overlapping fascial repair is performed above the rectum. The tissue has already failed, so its strength is questionable. If there is also an enterocele, the hernial sac should be located, a purse-string suture applied round this and the uterosacral ligaments brought together in the midline to supply support underneath this. There is usually an associated deficiency of the perineum, corrected by sutures to the superficial perineal muscles.

Vaginal hysterectomy. This procedure is seldom carried out alone for prolapse but often in combination with anterior and/or posterior repair as the descent of the uterus usually drags other structures with it (Fig. 4). Operating from the vagina, the uterus is removed and the uterosacral ligaments used to provide support to the vaginal vault.

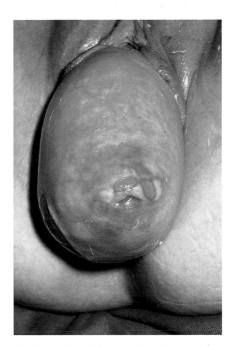

Fig. 4 **A procidentia (whole uterus outside the body) may be best treated with a vaginal hysterectomy.**

Clinical note

Bleeding from an ulcerated prolapse may mask endometrial carcinoma – assessment with ultrasound and endometrial sampling is important to exclude this.

Uterovaginal prolapse

- Prolapse is caused by childbirth, menopause and/or congenital weakness.
- It is important to establish any history of associated urinary and bowel problems.
- Examination should include use of Sims' speculum and neurological examination.
- Conservative management with pelvic floor exercises may supplement surgery to correct the prolapse.

Urinary incontinence

The main conditions affecting women are urodynamic stress incontinence (USI) and detrusor overactivity (DO). Between them these comprise over 90% of female incontinence with 45–50% being USI. The remaining 5–10% are a mixture of congenital abnormality, neurological problems resulting in overflow incontinence, and postsurgical or postdelivery problems. Urinary symptomatology may trouble a woman at any stage in her life but onset is particularly prevalent any time after childbirth and through into the postmenopausal phase.

Genitourinary fistulae have an unknown incidence as many affected women throughout the world do not seek medical help. In developing countries, fistulae are mainly of obstetric origin due to obstructed labour leading to pressure necrosis or due to a traumatic delivery with injury to the urinary tract. In developed countries, most genitourinary fistulae are due to pelvic surgery, malignancy or radiation therapy and if of obstetric origin are likely to be the result of forceps delivery, caesarean section or peripartum hysterectomy.

Symptoms

The symptoms show wide variation and include stress incontinence, urgency, urge incontinence, frequency and nocturia (Table 1). Enquiry for voiding disorder includes completeness of bladder emptying, straining to initiate micturition, and whether the urinary stream has a good volume and is constant. However, the history is a surprisingly poor discriminator of the different diagnostic groups. This makes investigation important.

Examination

Examination of the patient should include general examination, including the chest for signs of chronic obstructive airways disease resulting in chronically raised intra-abdominal pressure, and general neurological examination – especially testing S2,3,4 perianal sensation, informing on the innervation of the bladder. Abdominal palpation should rule out the presence of a full bladder or pelvic mass (see p. 86).

Pelvic examination is performed first in the dorsal position. The health of the vaginal tissues is determined and whether there is any redness due to incontinence. Parting the labia to reveal the external urethral meatus allows demonstration of stress incontinence with coughing. If the jet of urine is not simultaneous with the cough it may point to cough-induced detrusor overactivity.

An assessment of the degree of prolapse is performed in Sims' position. Examination is completed by a bimanual examination, during which assessment is made of the strength of pelvic floor muscle contraction.

Investigations

Mid-stream urine examination for infection is always the first investigation as many of the patient's symptoms may be caused by urinary tract infection. Uroflowmetry will allow assessment of the voiding time and also the peak flow rate achieved. In females this is commonly 50 ml/sec as the short, wide urethra allows rapid voiding (Fig. 1). The lower normal limit is 15 ml/sec, although voiding disorder is quite uncommon in the female patient.

Subtracted cystometry is performed to assess the detrusor pressure during filling of the bladder and voiding. Intravesical pressure is a mix of intra-abdominal pressure and intravesical pressure. By measuring intrarectal pressure and subtracting this from intravesical pressure, detrusor pressure or pure bladder pressure is measured (Fig. 2a).

The standard approach is to use fast-fill cystometry (50–100 ml per minute),

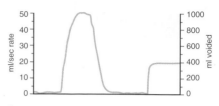
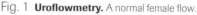

Fig. 1 **Uroflowmetry.** A normal female flow.

which is a provocative manoeuvre for detrusor contraction whilst the patient attempts to inhibit this. The usual bladder capacity is ~ 500 ml and during filling there should be no appreciable rise in detrusor pressure. Other provocations used during filling include coughing, listening to the sound of running water, and change of position. The patient coughs when standing. Should coughing produce incontinence with a flat detrusor pressure the diagnosis is USI. Various patterns of raised detrusor pressure are noted which make the diagnosis of DO (Fig. 2b).

The patient then voids on a commode while the pressures are still being measured, allowing an assessment of whether voiding is by abdominal straining, detrusor contraction, or purely by pelvic floor relaxation. These basic investigations may not result in a diagnosis in all patients and improved sensitivity may be obtained by using ambulatory cystometry or filling using contrast medium to allow visualization of the urinary tract (videocystometry). Pelvic ultrasound can assess whether the patient voids to completion and investigation of the kidneys with intravenous urography may be appropriate if haematuria is noted. Cystoscopy may also be indicated.

Management

Once the diagnosis is made a decision about the type of management is necessary. For both USI and DO there are conservative and surgical options.

Conservative management of USI

Conservative management of USI centres around controlling and improving pelvic floor function. There are many ways to do this. The physiotherapist teaches pelvic floor exercises, either using digital examination and teaching the patient to do this herself whilst contracting the pelvic floor, or aided by the use of a perineometer which grades the strength of contraction achieved.

Table 1 **Symptoms of urinary incontinence**	
Symptom	**Meaning**
Stress incontinence	Leakage of urine during raised intra-abdominal pressure, e.g. coughing, laughing
Urgency	Uncontrollable desire to micturate, necessitating rushing to toilet
Urge incontinence	Urinary leakage associated with uncontrollable need to micturate
Frequency	Voiding more than seven times during day
Nocturia	Woken to void twice or more at night
Continuous leakage	Possible genitourinary fistula
Enuresis – childhood or adult onset	Bed-wetting – not woken with the desire to void

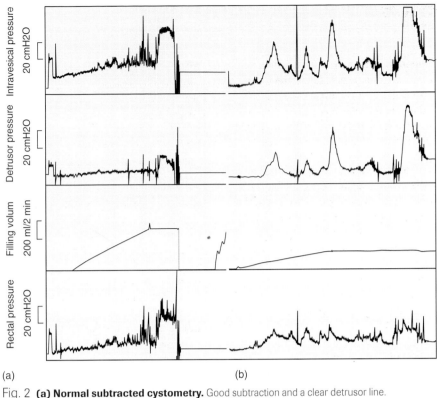

Fig. 2 **(a) Normal subtracted cystometry.** Good subtraction and a clear detrusor line.
(b) Systolic detrusor overactivity with detrusor contractions provoked by bladder filling.

The long-acting formulation is associated with fewer side effects and tolterodine also has a better side effect profile. Imipramine or antidiuretic hormone may be helpful with adult enuresis.

Surgical management of USI

Various surgical procedures may be appropriate with the colposuspension often being first-line in a case where there is adequate vaginal mobility to allow the elevation of the vaginal mucosa towards the ileopectineal ligaments. This raises the level of the bladder outlet and as a first time procedure would result in ~ 90% of patients being dry.

The TVT (tension-free vaginal tape) procedure, which aims to reproduce the action of the pubourethral ligaments, has similar results to the colposuspension but is performed under local or regional anaesthesia. Long-term follow-up for TVT is awaited.

Surgical management of DO

Surgical management of DO is used only if bladder drill and medical treatment have failed to control the symptoms. The surgical approach attempts to denervate the bladder, with varying success. The 'Clam' ileocystoplasty inserts an ileal patch and allows the raised pressure during a contraction to be dissipated.

Surgical management of fistula

Unless the fistula is detected within a few days of its formation, conservative management with continuous catheter drainage in the hope of spontaneous closure has little to offer. The principles of surgical management include antibiotics to ensure no infection in the field, wide mobilization of the tissues around the fistula, a layered tension-free closure, augmentation of the repair by use of surrounding healthy tissue or omental graft, and adequate urine drainage postoperatively.

Vaginal cones are a set of graduated weights (Fig. 4) used to improve the pelvic floor muscle strength and can demonstrate the improvement the patient is making, thereby aiding compliance.

Interferential therapy stimulates pelvic floor muscles and improves their strength by application of two currents set to form an interference pattern at the level of the pelvic floor. This allows greater stimulation of the muscle than a direct application of current which has to overcome skin resistance.

Having been objectively assessed all these methods are now in more common use than in the 1970s when surgery was the first-line treatment for many women.

Conservative management of DO

Bladder drill is the main conservative method of managing DO. This involves teaching the patient to retrain her bladder by regular, timed voiding and step-wise increasing of the time between voids. This may be useful in 80% of patients, is non-invasive, and if a relapse occurs they may try the same treatment again. Combining this with drug therapy may improve results though admission of patients for inpatient retraining has not been shown to be superior.

As the cause for detrusor overactivity is unknown, treatment has to be symptomatic. Anticholinergic medication will damp down smooth muscle contractions but side effects include dry mouth, constipation, and trouble with visual acuity. A commonly used drug is oxybutinin hydrochloride with the dose titrated against the patient's symptoms and side effects.

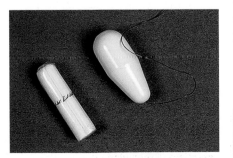

Fig. 4 **Vaginal cone.** Tampon pictured for size comparison.

Urinary incontinence

- Urodynamic stress incontinence (USI) and detrusor overactivity (DO) are the two main causes of female incontinence.

- The incidence of genitourinary fistulae is unclear due to the large numbers of women who do not seek medical help.

- Investigation of urinary symptoms is needed as there is large overlap in symptoms between DO and USI.

- Surgery or conservative therapies are appropriate for USI and DO but the balance favours surgery for USI and conservative treatment for DO.

Emotional disturbances in gynaecology

It is important to think holistically when assessing a woman presenting with emotional lability. A number of different possibilities must be considered:

- endogenous depression
- reactive depression
- thyroid imbalance
- severe premenstrual tension
- pregnancy
- perimenopausal or menopausal status.

It is easy to distinguish between some of these possibilities, but in other cases diagnosis is more difficult. Women in their late 40s often have increasingly severe premenstrual tension. It is quite easy to confuse severe premenstrual with perimenopausal women who have mood swings, but the latter may have an elevated basal follicle stimulating hormone (FSH).

Women entering the menopause are not immune from other problems. There is often a change in the psychodynamics of the family unit at this time. Children grow up and leave home; the woman who until now has worked part-time to be available for the family may feel isolated and under-valued. The desire to go back to work full-time may be hindered by loss of self-esteem and self-confidence. Marital relationships may deteriorate and a long-standing partner leaving for a younger woman further reinforces feelings of low self-esteem and unworthiness.

Financial considerations represent an added burden. Redundancy, early retirement due to ill health, or sudden bereavement may leave the woman in financial difficulties. These women often present as withdrawn and tearful and need careful assessment to establish what proportion of their symptoms are hormonally-related and what are due to reactive depression.

Endogenous depression may arise without any precipitating extrinsic factors. A family history of depression, a previous history of postnatal depression, or severe premenstrual tension may act as warning signs. The patient usually presents with classic symptoms of early morning waking, inability to cope and a withdrawn and blunt affect. She may need assessment by a psychiatrist, or counselling and therapy from a clinical psychologist. If the general practitioner has known the patient for a long time and has a good

rapport, he/she is in an excellent position to supervise and maintain treatment.

Premenstrual syndrome

Premenstrual syndrome (PMS) is a disorder of unknown aetiology. It may represent an exaggerated response to the physiological levels of ovarian hormones through the cycle. There is a wide range of proposed theories.

Symptoms

Classically, the symptoms occur in the luteal phase. In primary PMS, the symptoms resolve completely by the end of menstruation, whereas in secondary PMS the symptoms improve by the end of menstruation but do not disappear. The improvement should be sustained for at least 1 week. The range of symptoms reported are numerous but fall mainly into four categories:

- mood, including irritability, tearfulness, depression and hostility
- cognitive function, including poor concentration, forgetfulness and confusion
- somatic manifestations, including bloating, mastalgia, headaches,

tiredness and both appetite and sleep disturbance
- behavioural change, including social withdrawal and inability to cope.

It is often helpful to have the patient score the severity of her symptoms (Fig. 1). It is also important to assess the

Please mark ALL symptoms with a tick √. Score 0 if you have never experienced that symptom, 1 if mild, 2 if moderate and 3 if severe

	0	1	2	3
Muscle stiffness				
Headache				
Cramps				
Backache				
Fatigue				
General aches and pains				
Lowered work performance				
Stay at home				
Avoid social activities				
Decreased efficiency				
Dizziness				
Cold sweats				
Nausea, vomiting				
Hot flushes				
Affectionate				
Orderliness				
Excitement				
Feelings of well being				
Bursts of energy				
Insomnia				
Forgetfulness				
Confusion				
Lowered judgement				
Difficulty				

Fig. 1 **Premenstrual symptom questionnaire.**

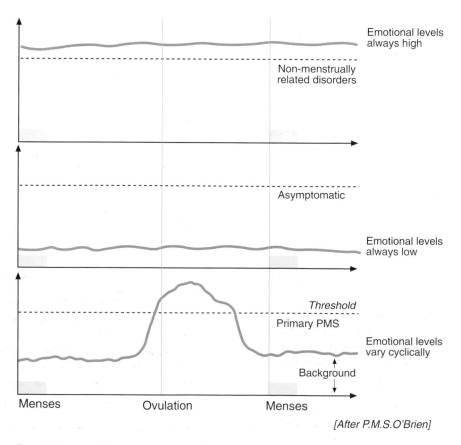

Fig. 2 **Menstrual diary evaluation of PMS.**

[After P.M.S.O'Brien]

degree of underlying psychological dysfunction using established psychiatric questionnaires. Quality-of-life questionnaires will assess the degree to which the woman's life is disrupted.

Diagnosis

This is based on the history and supported by cycle charting (Fig. 2). Symptom charting is required to obtain a sound diagnosis and to monitor therapeutic interventions. Cycle charting increases patient insight into the condition and empowers her to take control of her own experiences. Charting will clearly differentiate cyclical symptoms with a symptom-free week from those where the symptoms are continuous, e.g. endogenous depression, hypothyroidism, lethargy due to anaemia.

It is important to differentiate cyclical from non-cyclical breast pain which may require mammography or ultrasonography. Breast cancer must be excluded.

Few women exhibit significant fluid retention with PMS – daily weighing may differentiate.

In ambiguous cases a therapeutic 3-month trial of a gonadotrophin releasing hormone (GnRH) analogue to suppress ovarian function is very helpful. If symptoms persist, despite amenorrhoea, the diagnosis cannot be PMS.

Management

The list of therapies employed in PMS is extensive, partly because the theories of aetiology are numerous. It is reasonable to start with simple, non-hormonal approaches (Fig. 3) and ask the woman to complete a stress management diary. There may be certain situations which trigger stress or inability to cope. These are best avoided in the premenstrual phase. Exercise may reduce stress by enhancing endorphin metabolism in the luteal phase.

Some women report benefit from caffeine withdrawal. An evening meal which is carbohydrate-rich and protein-poor has been recommended – this could have an effect via serotonin metabolism.

Circadian modification has been shown to reduce the severity of PMS symptoms. The manoeuvre involves sleep deprivation for 1 night early in the luteal phase. Postulated mechanisms involve melatonin secretion. PMS appears to be a seasonal variation disorder, as it is less troublesome in the summer.

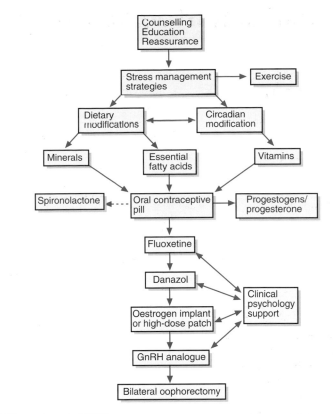

Fig. 3 **Management of PMS.**

If non-medical treatments are unsuccessful, a combination of oil of evening primrose, vitamin B6 or calcium and magnesium supplements may be considered. Some also make claims for zinc and copper supplements. Oil of primrose contains the polyunsaturated essential fatty acids linoleic and gamma linolenic acids, which are the dietary precursors of several prostaglandins, mainly E1 and E2. Efficacy and treatment has probably been over-stated, but some studies do demonstrate benefits over placebo. Many patients will have self-prescribed before seeking medical treatment; one problem with this approach is cost.

Ovulation suppression with the pill or depot progestogens is successful. Danazol is helpful, but because of its side-effect potential is not first-line therapy. Natural progesterone

suppositories have been used extensively, but no study has demonstrated a benefit superior to that of placebo.

Diuretics, e.g. aldosterone antagonists, should be reserved for those who demonstrate true fluid retention.

Antidepressants have been used with some benefit. The selective serotonin re-uptake inhibitors appear to be especially beneficial, e.g. fluoxetine (Prozac). Oestrogens in the form of implants or transdermally as patches have produced measurable benefits. For the intractable, severe cases of PMS it may be necessary to refer to a clinical psychologist to offer group and individual therapy. No woman should be subjected to bilateral oophorectomy as a treatment until a proven benefit from ovarian suppression has been confirmed.

Emotional disturbances

- In the perimenopausal age group, severe premenstrual tension, endogenous or reactive depression may present with emotional lability.
- The patient must be treated with care and sensitivity, or background social and emotional problems may be missed.
- The diagnosis of PMS depends on proven, cyclical variation with 1 week clear of symptoms, or at least a reduction in severity of symptoms.
- Ovulation suppression will eradicate symptoms; failure to do so puts the diagnosis in question.
- Treatment options are varied, but should involve the woman and ideally start with non-hormonal therapies.

Psychosexual disorders

Psychosexual disorders are very prevalent. They may be secondary to a physical problem or the primary aetiology may be psychogenic or psychosocial. Often women are reluctant to admit to problems and find it easier to consult their doctor about 'discharge' or 'general malaise', hoping their real concern will eventually be addressed. Sometimes the problem is more obvious, e.g. non-consummation, and the partner or the family, concerned about lack of offspring, may demand referral.

Physiology of sexual arousal

Human sexual response is a specialized autonomic reflex, which is extensively modulated by the higher centres of the central nervous system. There are several discrete, yet inter-related physiological and psychosensorial components (Fig. 1). Sexual response can be triggered and developed psychogenically by stimuli arising within the central nervous system, or reflexogenically in response to tactile stimulation of the genitalia or other erogenous zones. When arousal reaches a threshold level, orgasm is triggered (Fig. 2). Following orgasm, loss of arousal to prestimulation levels occurs, so-called resolution, if the stimulus is withdrawn. In women, continued stimulation may result in a series of orgasms known as a multi-orgasmic response. Three factors are involved in this model of arousal:

- effective stimulation
- sexual drive and sexual desire
- sexual arousal and sexual excitement.

Many women increase psychogenic stimulation during sexual activity by sexual fantasies to enhance their arousal. Reflexogenic sexual stimulation is a partly learned phenomenon. Negative stimuli include anxiety, guilt, feelings of inadequacy, low self-esteem and pre-occupation with other issues.

Sexual arousal in women induces local vasocongestion, which makes the organs turgid and spongy, providing a cushioning effect against possible trauma caused by penile penetration. Simultaneously, vaginal transudation provides increased lubrication. The upper two-thirds of the vagina balloon and the uterus and cervix move away from the penetrating object. Some women have an inability to associate these physiological changes with erotic feelings.

Taking a sexual history

There is a wide range of sexual problems. Sexual dysfunctions, e.g. lack of libido, aversion to penetration, difficulty in obtaining orgasm or superficial and deep dyspareunia, are the most common problems seen in gynaecology. A full history should be taken (Table 1). A sex therapist or psychosexual counsellor will interview both partners and may spend 3 or 4 hours with the couple. A gynaecologist or general practitioner is less able to afford this time, but often each appointment will last 1 hour. It is important to modify the history to assess the main points, e.g. was sexual function always difficult or has there been a recent deterioration? Can triggering factors be identified? Is there interest in or desire for sexual activity, or does the act cause revulsion? During sexual activity does adequate excitement and lubrication occur? If there is adequate stimulation is orgasm unreasonably delayed?

Care must be taken in eliciting whether there is genuine loss of libido

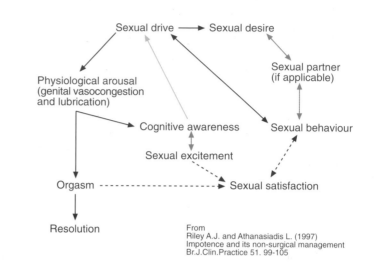

From
Riley A.J. and Athanasiadis L. (1997)
Impotence and its non-surgical management
Br.J.Clin.Practice 51. 99–105

Fig. 1 **Physiological model of female sexual function.**

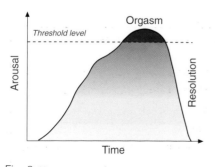

Fig. 2 **Human sexual response.**

Table 1 **Areas to cover in a sexual history**	
Details of the problem	**Nature, duration and development**
Relationship history	With current and previous partners – quality of general relationship, separation, infidelities, areas of conflict, hopes
Sexual development	Puberty, menarche, menopause (and attitude to these changes), sexual experiences (both positive and negative), masturbation
Past medical and surgical history	Including past and current medication and contraceptive history
Past psychiatric history	Any current psychiatric illnesses, any previous sexual/relationship difficulties
Family history	Parental relationships, family and religious influences, relationship with in-laws and children
Social history	Education, leisure activities, work history, occupational factors – e.g. shift work, time away from home, periods of unemployment
Alcohol intake/drug usage	
Sex education	Level of sexual knowledge, patient's beliefs and expectations of sexual function, aims and goals of seeking therapy

Courtesy of Dr Lynne Webster, Consultant Psychiatrist with a special interest in Psychosexual Medicine, Manchester Royal Infirmary.

or sexual drive. A woman who presents with loss of urge to have sex with her partner, but who masturbates regularly and who can generate sexual fantasies, has an intact sexual drive but an absent sexual desire directed to her partner. A women who experiences no desire to masturbate and is unable to generate any sexual fantasies appears to have a sexual drive disorder which may be organic in origin.

It is important to exclude organic or psychiatric conditions. Hyper-thyroidism reduces sexual drive; testosterone deficiency, hyperprolactinaemia and hypothyroidism affect arousal. Brain trauma (e.g. head injury, tumour or stroke) may impact on sexual drive and arousal. Conditions affecting the spinal cord (e.g. multiple sclerosis, syringomyelia and tabes) and those affecting peripheral nerves (e.g. diabetes, alcohol abuse, vitamin deficiency, prolapsed intervertebral disc, lumbar canal stenosis and multiple sclerosis) also have an effect. Epilepsy can be implicated.

Dopamine agonists (e.g. neuroleptics and metoclopramide) and depressants (e.g. sedatives, hypnotics and alcohol) will reduce both sexual drive and arousal. Alpha adrenoserotonin antagonists, antidepressants, pelvic inflammatory disease (by causing pain), sympathectomy and pelvic surgery may affect the ability to achieve orgasm.

Counselling skills

The physician must build a rapport with the patient, as intimate and sensitive areas are being discussed. Some factors will prevent this happening:

- embarrassment
- powerlessness
- poor communication skills.

If either the patient or the doctor is embarrassed, this can effectively put an end to any further useful communication. The doctor may feel out of his/her depth, that a consultation will get out of control, that issues will be raised that the doctor is unable to answer. If revulsion is shown at any stage this reinforces the patient's feeling of guilt and inadequacy. Taking a useful sexual history requires a great degree of trust and openness in the consultation – particularly if both partners are present. Any doctor should be able to at least identify that there is a problem

and to offer the patient hope that therapy or treatment is possible, referring her to someone who can provide it.

Painful penetration

The causes of painful penetration are numerous (Table 2). It is important to exclude anatomical or pathological causes by examination. Vaginismus and painful penetration are closely linked. Vaginismus or involuntary tightening of the vaginal musculature can be a cause of superficial pain, but may have originally occurred secondary to infection and become a conditioned reflex as the woman continues to anticipate pain.

Vaginismus may be secondary to a psychogenic cause, e.g in situations of non-consummation where the woman, for whatever reason, is scared of penetrative intercourse. Due to her fear there is inadequate arousal leading to poor lubrication, pain and resulting vaginismus. Ultimately the vaginismus becomes a primary event, further enhancing the negative feedback. Pain on palpating the pelvic floor muscles indicates vaginismus.

The treatment of painful penetration will depend on the cause. Management may involve advice on how to cope with the pain. Practical measures include artificial lubricants, relaxation techniques, pelvic floor exercises and experimenting with different coital positions. Often an explanation of the physiology of arousal and the effects of stress and fear on the arousal mechanism is all that is required. If there is no organic cause for the problem, then exploration of possible psychogenic causes will be necessary.

Pelvic floor exercises help with involuntary spasm of the vaginal muscles. Graded tasks might start with the woman self-exploring initially with one digit, then two, or possibly with graded dilators, leading eventually to penetration. The sensate focus technique requires the couple

to learn to explore each other physically without penetration, focusing on personal experience rather than pleasing the partner. Contact is then gradually increased.

Specific situations

Loss of interest in sex may persist after delivery; fatigue, especially in breast-feeding women, and physical discomfort are common reasons given. Poor libido at the menopause may be due to poor sleep, sweats and vaginal dryness, responding to oestrogen, or lack of testosterone, especially after a surgical menopause.

Table 2	Causes of painful penetration	
Anatomical		Intact hymen/hymenal remnants
		Vaginal stenosis
		'Ridged' symphysis
Pathological		
Superficial		Vulval and vaginal
		allergica
		atrophic changes
		bartholinitis
		Candida
		eczema
		herpes
		psoriasis
		vestibulitis
		genital warts
		Trichomonas
		bacterial vaginosis
	Urethral	
		cystocele
		urethral caruncle
Deep	Uterus	
		endometritis/myometritis
		fibroids
	Adnexa	
		endometriosis
		pelvic inflammatory disease
		ovarian cysts
	Bladder	
		cystitis
	Bowel	
		constipation
		irritable bowel syndrome (and inflammatory bowel)
Iatrogenic		
Medical		Beta-blockers
		High-dose anxiolytics
Surgical		Episiotomy
		Anterior and posterior vaginal repair, vaginal hysterectomy

Psychosexual disorders

- Women are reluctant to admit to sexual difficulties and often repeatedly present with trivial problems.
- Tact and diplomacy are needed in taking an accurate and full psychosexual history.
- Genuine loss of sexual desire must be distinguished from difficulties with the current relationship.
- Vaginismus is a common cause of painful penetration.
- Sexual difficulties following delivery are not uncommon.
- Loss of libido at the time of the menopause may be primary, requiring testosterone, or secondary, responding to hormone replacement therapy.

Postoperative care

Postoperative gynaecological care has been radically changed, aiming to manage most patients as day cases (approximately 70%). Outpatient procedures frequently replace the need for admission (see p. 116). Surgical procedures that require hospital admission are discharged earlier. The aim is to increase patient throughput and reduce bed occupancy. An abdominal hysterectomy may stay for 2–4 days (previously 7) and vaginal hysterectomies may be discharged within 1–3 days. Endometrial ablative techniques and laparoscopically-assisted vaginal hysterectomy (LAVH) are being performed in some centres – the former as day cases, the latter with overnight stay.

Work has been done with community teams of multi-skilled nurse practitioners who will visit the patients at home once they have fulfilled guideline criteria to be discharged from hospital. Others have looked at the American model of discharging the low-risk patient from the hospital ward to a hotel-style setting where the patients are more ambulant and nursing care is less labour intensive.

The postoperative patient is entitled to high-quality care and the traditional approach to postoperative management continues – common to all surgical specialties. The management of fluid balance, drains and catheters, and the ability to detect the signs of postoperative complications and act upon them remain essential. Within each specialty however, particular skills and specialized requirements may be necessary.

Fluid balance

A patient's fluid requirement will vary depending on:

- the body mass index of the individual
- the ambient temperature which affects insensible loss
- the potential for fluid loss from various sites.

The input/output chart allows ongoing monitoring of the fluid received and lost by the patient, avoiding negative balance. This chart should be assessed daily and the infusion regimen adjusted accordingly, allowing for potential loss of electrolytes. When electrolyte derangement is likely, serum urea and electrolyte estimation should be performed daily until the patient is stable as the clinical consequences can be profound.

The use of catheters and drains

Prophylactic catheterization of patients aseptically in theatre for the first 24 or 48 hours reduces the incidence of postoperative urinary tract infection. Uncatheterized patients who do not void spontaneously require catheterization on the ward where the environment is less aseptic.

Spontaneous retention is more likely after large pelvic masses and posterior vaginal repairs where neurogenic retention can occur. For routine vaginal and abdominal surgery a urethral catheter is adequate. For surgery on the bladder neck a suprapubic catheter is usually inserted (see p. 155) and, after allowing periurethral oedema to settle, is clamped (Fig. 1). If the patient is unable to void, the clamp is released and the catheter left on free drainage for a longer period. Further instrumentation of the patient is thus avoided.

It is usual to leave a drain for difficult surgery, e.g. major oncological procedures, and where oozing is likely to occur, e.g. myomectomy or colposuspension. A closed-system drain allows blood loss to be assessed accurately and is left until the loss is less than 30–40 ml in a 24-hour period (Fig. 2). Surgery on a patient with established disseminated intravascular coagulation (DIC) will require a wide-bore rather than suction drainage, and clotting factors must be corrected.

Perioperative prophylactic management

Prophylactic antibiotic cover is widespread for vaginal surgery where vaginal flora may precipitate opportunistic infection if the patient's resistance is reduced. The antibiotic should be effective against anaerobes. The final decision as to which broad-spectrum antibiotics are used will depend on local bacterial factors and the patient's history of drug sensitivity.

The prophylactic use of anti-thrombogenic agents is now well recognized. Many will use them routinely for all gynaecological procedures, but specifically targeted

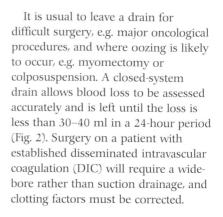

Fig. 1 **Suprapubic catheter.**

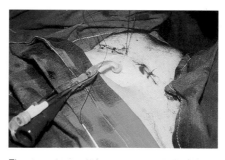

Fig. 2 **Closed-system drainage unit.**

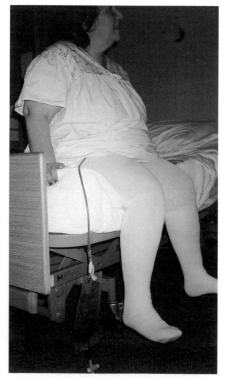

Fig. 3 **Postoperative measures to avoid thrombosis.** Patient wearing TED elastic stockings.

patients include the overweight, those with a previous history of thromboembolism, and surgery for pelvic carcinoma involving node dissection or a pelvic mass. Elastic stockings (Fig. 3) are routinely applied to reduce the risk of deep vein thrombosis, but extensive pelvic surgery carries the risk of pelvic venous thrombosis.

The new low molecular weight heparins appear to be safe and effective. These are administered subcutaneously until the patient is fully mobile. The dose prescribed will depend on the body mass index of the patient. Frail old ladies will require a lower dose than an obese patient. Full heparinization would only be indicated if deep vein thrombosis or pulmonary embolism developed.

Postoperative complicatons

Postoperative complications can be divided into immediate, intermediate and late. Some are common to all surgical procedures, e.g. wound infection or thromboembolism, some are confined to specific operations. The latter are dealt with in the relevant chapters. Prophylaxis has greatly reduced the incidence of complications, but an understanding of when they are likely to occur and the presenting symptoms is essential (Table 1). The early detection of complications is the main reason for daily postoperative ward rounds. It is also important that the patient feels that she has regular access to the medical team conducting her care, who should work in conjunction with the nurse practitioners.

Medicolegal aspects of care

The concept of risk management is now widespread and is based on the theory that if problems arise they should be recognized promptly, dealt with efficiently, and the patient kept fully informed at all times. Notes should contain a full and comprehensive account of all investigations, actions and discussions with the patient – particularly if the latter have been contentious. It is often advisable to conduct discussions with a third party present. It is always important to obtain senior help early if complications arise. Problems should be relayed to the consultant in charge of the case. Some hospitals have a specific risk management officer who acts as the liaison between clinical staff and the hospital's solicitors.

Table 1 Timescale of postoperative complications

Site	Timescale	Presentation	Predisposing factors
Chest			
Atelectasis	In first 24 hours	Poor basal air entry, spike of temperature 37.3	Poor lung expansion, poor drainage, lying flat on back
Pneumonia	2–3 days	Febrile, productive cough, inspiratory wheezes	Smoker, infection secondary to atelectasis
Urinary tract			
Cystitis	3–4 days	Moderate temperature 37.5 dysuria, frequency	Urogenital tract instrumentation, catheterization
Pyelonephritis	4–7 days	Rigors, nausea, vomiting, lower abdominal pains, loin pain	Poorly-treated UTI
Wound infection	4–5 days	Tense, tender erythematous wound ± fluctuation	Secondary to wound haematomas, poor aseptic technique
Thromboembolism	Day 4 onwards	Swollen, tense, tender calf, chest pain, dyspnoea, haemoptosis, cyanosis ± collapse (if PE)	Poor mobilization, inadequate prophylaxis, previous varicosities, pelvic mass at surgery, oncology case

The multidisciplinary approach to care

The standard of care for patients is greatly enhanced if all health-care professionals can work together in a constructive and integrated fashion. The physiotherapist has an important role teaching pelvic floor exercises, particularly relevant to vaginal and bladder neck surgery – in addition to the routine chest expansion, breathing and calf exercises that should be taught to all postoperative patients. Nursing staff mobilize patients early postoperatively to limit the risk of thromboembolism.

The nurse practitioner is emerging as a professional with added responsibilities and roles in the discharge process. Integrated care pathways (ICPs) set objectives and goals for routine postoperative management. It may be necessary to involve community nurses, carers or the local surgery practice nurse in postoperative management if the patient is unlikely to cope unaided and has little family support. Advanced oncology patients will require the involvement of the Macmillan nurses; urogynaecological patients may need the continence advisors. Both these specialized nurse practitioners will assess the patient on the ward and liaise with the medical team. Extensive ovarian cancer debulking requiring covering colostomy may need the involvement of stoma care sisters.

Throughout all of this it is important to remember the patient. Staff must be perceived to be friendly and approachable. Great emphasis must be placed on communication skills. Many units now run hysterectomy support groups allowing discussion of indications for surgery and giving the patient the chance to air her views and concerns. Leaflets are essential to reinforce any message. Research has shown that probably only 30% of verbally-given information is retained.

Ongoing postoperative management will vary and include hormone replacement therapy following oophorectomy, ongoing contraceptive issues following miscarriage or ectopic pregnancy and possibly suppression therapy following surgery for endometriosis. All of this must be explained with care to enhance subsequent compliance.

Postoperative care

- Patients are now discharged much earlier following gynaecological major surgery.
- Integrated care pathways establish goals and objectives for patient discharge.
- The routine use of prophylactic antibiotics and antithrombogenic agents has reduced postoperative complications.
- Routine catheterization for 24 to 48 hours reduces the risk of postoperative infection.
- Detailed notes and adequate communication with the patient reduce litigation.

Index